TREATING SUBSTANCE ABUSE

Treating Substance Abuse

Theory and Technique

Third Edition

Edited by

Scott T. Walters
Frederick Rotgers

THE GUILFORD PRESS
New York   London

The authors have checked with sources believed to be reliable in their efforts to provide information that is complete and generally in accord with the standards of practice that are accepted at the time of publication. However, in view of the possibility of human error or changes in behavioral, mental health, or medical sciences, neither the authors, nor the editors and publisher, nor any other party who has been involved in the preparation or publication of this work warrants that the information contained herein is in every respect accurate or complete, and they are not responsible for any errors or omissions or the results obtained from the use of such information. Readers are encouraged to confirm the information contained in this book with other sources.

Library of Congress Cataloging-in-Publication Data

Treating substance abuse: theory and technique / edited by Scott T. Walters, Frederick Rotgers.—3rd ed.
        p. cm.
    Includes bibliographical references and index.
    ISBN 978-1-4625-0257-8 (hardback)
    1. Substance abuse—Treatment.   I. Walters, Scott T.   II. Rotgers, Frederick.
    RC564.T734 2012
    362.29—dc23

                                                        2011040025

About the Editors

Scott T. Walters, PhD, is Professor of Behavioral and Community Health in the School of Public Health at the University of North Texas Health Science Center. His research focuses on the use of motivational interviewing and other brief interventions to help people make changes in substance abuse and other problem behaviors. Widely published, Dr. Walters has acted as a consultant for several agencies; is a frequent speaker to university, community, and medical groups; and has received national and international awards for his work integrating research and practice.

Frederick Rotgers, PsyD, ABPP, is Director of the Program for Motivation and Change at the Graduate School of Applied and Professional Psychology, Rutgers, The State University of New Jersey, and a psychologist in independent practice. He is a Fellow of the American Psychological Association (APA), is a past president of the Society of Addiction Psychology (APA Division 50), and is certified in clinical and cognitive and behavioral psychology by the American Board of Professional Psychology. The author or editor of numerous books on the assessment and treatment of substance use disorders, Dr. Rotgers is American Editor-in-Chief of the journal *Addiction Research and Theory*.

Contributors

Bryon Adinoff, MD, VA North Texas Health Care System and Department of Psychiatry, University of Texas Southwestern Medical Center, Dallas, Texas

Kristen L. Barry, PhD, Department of Psychiatry, University of Michigan Medical School, and Department of Veterans Affairs National Serious Mental Illness Treatment Research and Evaluation Center, Ann Arbor, Michigan

Gary R. Birchler, PhD, retired, Prescott, Arizona

Frederic C. Blow, PhD, Department of Psychiatry, University of Michigan Medical School, Ann Arbor, Michigan

Alan J. Budney, PhD, Department of Psychiatry and Behavioral Sciences, College of Medicine, University of Arkansas for Medical Sciences, Little Rock, Arkansas

Kathleen M. Carroll, PhD, Department of Psychiatry, Yale University School of Medicine, West Haven, Connecticut

Philip H. Chung, MD, Department of Psychiatry, University of Texas Southwestern Medical Center, Dallas, Texas

Jesse Dallery, PhD, Department of Psychology, University of Florida, Gainesville, Florida

Kevin A. Hallgren, MS, Department of Psychology, Center on Alcoholism, Substance Abuse, and Addictions, University of New Mexico, Albuquerque, New Mexico

Brian D. Kiluk, PhD, Department of Psychiatry, Yale University School of Medicine, West Haven, Connecticut

Benjamin O. Ladd, MS, Department of Psychology, Center on Alcoholism, Substance Abuse, and Addictions, University of New Mexico, Albuquerque, New Mexico

Wendy K. K. Lam, PhD, Duke Translational Medicine Institute, Duke School of Medicine, Chapel Hill, North Carolina

James MacKillop, PhD, Department of Psychology, University of Georgia, Athens, Georgia

James S. Marinchak, PsyM, Graduate School of Applied and Professional Psychology, Rutgers, The State University of New Jersey, Piscataway, New Jersey

Barbara S. McCrady, PhD, Department of Psychology, Center on Alcoholism, Substance Abuse, and Addictions, University of New Mexico, Albuquerque, New Mexico

Steven E. Meredith, MS, Department of Psychology, University of Florida, Gainesville, Florida

Thomas J. Morgan, PhD, Center for Applied Psychology, Rutgers, The State University of New Jersey, Piscataway, New Jersey

Theresa B. Moyers, PhD, Department of Psychology, Center on Alcoholism, Substance Abuse, and Addictions, University of New Mexico, Albuquerque, New Mexico

James G. Murphy, PhD, Department of Psychology, University of Memphis, Memphis, Tennessee

Joseph Nowinski, PhD, Correctional Managed Health Care Division, University of Connecticut Health Center, Tolland, Connecticut

Timothy J. O'Farrell, PhD, ABPP, Families and Addiction Program, Veterans Affairs Boston Healthcare System, Brockton, Massachusetts, and Harvard Medical School, Department of Psychiatry, Boston, Massachusetts

Gary S. Rose, PhD, Department of Clinical Psychology, Massachusetts School of Professional Psychology, Bedford, Massachusetts

Julie D. Ross, MD, PhD, Department of Psychiatry, University of Texas Southwestern Medical Center, Dallas, Texas

Frederick Rotgers, PsyD, ABPP, Graduate School of Applied and Professional Psychology, Rutgers, The State University of New Jersey, Piscataway, New Jersey

Edward M. Rubin, PsyD, Aurora Behavioral Health Services, Aurora Sinai Medical Center, Milwaukee, Wisconsin

Erin M. Tooley, MS, Department of Psychology, University of New Mexico, Albuquerque, New Mexico

Jalie A. Tucker, PhD, MPH, School of Public Health, University of Alabama at Birmingham, Birmingham, Alabama

Rudy E. Vuchinich, PhD, Department of Veterans Affairs, Residential Rehabilitation Treatment Program, Tuscaloosa, Alabama

Sidarth Wakhlu, MD, VA North Texas Health Care System and Department of Psychiatry, University of Texas Southwestern Medical Center, Dallas, Texas

John Wallace, PhD, private practice, Rochester, Massachusetts

Scott T. Walters, PhD, School of Public Health, University of North Texas Health Science Center, Fort Worth, Texas

Allen Zweben, PhD, School of Social Work, Columbia University, New York, New York

Contents

Introduction

Scott T. Walters
Frederick Rotgers

An old *Saturday Night Live* sketch depicts the medieval doctor "Theodoric of York: English Barber." Patients with a range of maladies are brought in for treatment, which consists of "state-of-the-art" medieval cures: bloodletting, leeches, and boar's vomit. At one point, the doctor expounds on recent advances in medical science: "Isabel is suffering from an imbalance of bodily humors perhaps caused by a toad or small dwarf living in her stomach. . . . You'll feel a lot better after a good bleeding." After a series of mishaps, a woman accuses the doctor of practicing shoddy medical science. In a moment of insight, he muses, "Perhaps I've been wrong to blindly follow the medical traditions and superstitions of the past centuries . . . maybe we should test those assumptions analytically through experimentation and the scientific method." He pauses in thought, before delivering the punch line, "Nah!"

The sketch is funny because it juxtaposes traditional medical quackery with a more effective, but more complicated, approach. We are left wondering how medieval societies could have been so stupid.

Fast forward to modern times. There is typically a lag between the development of an innovation and its adoption into everyday practice (Rogers, 2003); however, in substance abuse treatment the gap between research and practice has been, until recently, particularly wide. In 2003, Miller and colleagues reviewed nearly 400 alcoholism treatment trials (Miller, Wilbourne, & Hettema, 2003). They found strong evidence for approaches like brief interventions, motivational interviewing, community reinforcement, and behavioral approaches. Two pharmacotherapies—acamprosate and naltrexone—were also well supported in the alcohol treatment literature. However, they also noted a sad trend that still exists today. Although they identified a number of effective intervention approaches, the most *ineffective* treatments were most commonly used in practice. For instance, educational, confrontational, and general psychotherapy approaches, though widely used to address alcohol and drug use, have almost no evidence to suggest they change behavior.

This gap can be partly explained by the history of addiction treatment in the United States, which evolved relatively independently from mainstream medical and mental health care (Miller, Sorensen, Selzer, & Brigham, 2006). In fact, for many years, treatment was delivered almost exclusively by people who were themselves in recovery. The folk wisdom of this early approach led to a polarization of research versus practice and produced a veritable island of isolated addiction treatment services.

Things are changing. There are now hundreds of studies, and several dozen meta-analyses demonstrating effectiveness among "evidence-based" programs. These programs include many of those described in this book: motivational, contingency management, cognitive-behavioral, and family approaches are among those with a strong track record of success. We are at a tipping point in the delivery of services too. Many states now mandate that mental health providers document their use of evidence-based treatments, in much the same way as do medical providers. The American College of Surgeons mandates that all Level I trauma centers must provide an intervention for patients identified as problem drinkers. The U.S. Substance Abuse and Mental Health Services Administration (SAHMSA) has established a national registry of evidence-based programs (*www.nrepp.samhsa. gov*) and offers a searchable database of alcohol and drug treatment programs (*findtreatment.samhsa.gov*). The National Institute on Drug Abuse (NIDA) has established the Clinical Trials Network (*www.nida.nih.gov/ ctn*) and the Blending Initiative (*www.nida.nih.gov/blending*) to encourage community-based research and to translate research into practice. These efforts have created places where researchers, policymakers, and clinicians can work together to develop and disseminate the best treatment services.

This book fits in the mainstream of this effort. Like the previous two editions, this edition is organized into pairs of chapters around six treatment approaches. Each section is composed of a chapter on theory and a chapter on translation of theory into practice. The various approaches were selected on the basis of their strength of evidence and usefulness in practice. The final section shows how clinicians integrate the different treatment approaches in their clinical settings. Chapter authors include a mix of researchers and clinicians who are well recognized as experts in their field. In this way, the book is intended to bridge research, theory, and practical strategy.

What's New in the Third Edition?

Readers familiar with the first two editions will notice several changes. First, we eliminated the section on psychoanalytic approaches since they are not widely used clinically to treat substance use disorders. Second, we asked authors from the second edition to update their chapters to include the most current advances within their perspective, including research on effectiveness and likely mechanisms of change. In many cases there have been substantial advances in theory and technique since the last edition was published. Also, since addiction counseling is increasingly conducted within integrated settings, we also asked practice authors to address how their approach is typically implemented and integrated with other approaches. Finally, we reorganized the chapters to better reflect the sequence of how the approaches are most often used in practice. For instance, this edition presents motivational and contingency management approaches early, because they are more often used at the front of a treatment sequence to engage users in treatment.

In this edition, we have also added three new chapters. The second edition contained a single chapter on pharmacological approaches to treating substance use disorders. Because of the large amount of work that has recently been conducted in the area, this edition adds a parallel chapter to provide an overview of the biology of substance use disorders. This biology chapter rounds out the pharmacology section to make it consistent with the other approaches. Also, in the second edition, we included a single integrative chapter giving a clinician's perspective of how treatment is delivered in psychological practice. Because substance use treatment is increasingly delivered in nonspecialist settings, we asked two other author groups to write chapters describing how they address substance use disorders in brief medical settings and extended case management interactions. Thus, the final section of the book shows how experienced clinicians deliver substance abuse counseling in short, medium, and extended interactions.

As with the first two editions, authors in each section were asked to be advocates for their approaches. Theory chapter authors were asked to state the assumptions of their approach and to address a number of theory-relevant questions about etiology, maintenance, and mechanisms of change. Practice chapter authors were asked to translate their theoretical position into practical strategies. Among other things, practice chapter authors were asked to address sequencing of treatment activities, how "denial" and "resistance" are addressed, the role of self-help groups, how treatment termination is decided upon, how treatment modality (e.g., individual, group, family, marital) is selected, and how relapse is addressed. Finally, practice authors were asked to provide practical case examples of their work in action.

How Is the Book Organized?

The book begins with a pair of chapters focused on motivational interviewing (MI). Motivational approaches focus on increasing a person's perceived desire, ability, or reasons to change through modifying the kind of language that is exhibited during a counseling session. Since the time of the second edition, there has been a tremendous amount of research conducted on motivational approaches, and they now likely have the best evidence base of any therapy approach described in this book. For instance, a review of 119 studies concluded that MI was more effective than no treatment and generally equal to other longer treatments for a wide variety of problems (Lundahl & Burke, 2009). There has also been a substantial amount of work done on mechanisms of change in motivational approaches (Apodaca & Longabaugh, 2009), most focusing on the structure of language during MI sessions. This work has, in turn, substantially influenced the way that motivational approaches are delivered. Because of the strength of evidence and relative cost-effectiveness, motivational approaches have become a treatment of choice both as a stand-alone brief intervention and as a prelude to a more extensive treatment sequence.

The second set of chapters discusses behavioral economic theory and contingency management. Behavioral approaches modify drug use through changing environmental contingencies. The goal is to weaken the influence of reinforcement derived from drug use and to increase the reinforcement derived from healthier alternative activities, especially those that are incompatible with drug use. Like motivational approaches, there has been a substantial amount of research on behavioral approaches since the second edition. A review of 27 studies concluded that contingency management increased retention and lowered cocaine use when added to a treatment sequence (Knapp, Soares, Farrel, & Lima, 2007). Because of their strength of evidence and compatibility with other treatments, behavioral approaches are often used as preludes to more extensive interventions, to reinforce abstinence, and to maintain users early on in treatment.

The third pair of chapters covers cognitive-behavioral approaches. Cognitive-behavioral approaches combine behavioral theory with a focus on internal cognitions, such as automatic thoughts, cravings, and urges. A review of 53 controlled studies found that cognitive-behavioral therapy (CBT) was significantly more effective than comparison conditions, with the largest effect being found in marijuana studies (Magill & Ray, 2009). Since the second edition, cognitive behavioral approaches seem to have reached a period of "normal science" (Kuhn, 1970) in which efforts have focused on consolidating specific techniques, and integrating CBT with other approaches such as motivational interviewing and 12-step facilitation (e.g., COMBINE Study Research Group et al., 2006).

The fourth set of chapters discusses 12-step-oriented therapy. Approaches based on the Alcoholics Anonymous 12-step model still dominate the field of substance abuse treatment in the United States because of their low cost, structured approach, and wide availability (Ferri, Amato, & Davoli, 2006). This influence has no doubt been reinforced by research projects such as Project MATCH (Project MATCH Research Group, 1998) and COMBINE (Anton et al., 2006), which have provided evidence for the efficacy of 12-step facilitation, an individual 12-step counseling approach. There is evidence that individual and group 12-step approaches can reduce drinking and drug use, although the evidence base is admittedly not as strong as some other treatments (Ferri, Amato, & Davoli, 2006). Like cognitive-behavioral approaches, the basic 12-step theory is unchanged since the second edition. Recent work has focused on ways to better integrate 12-step principles with other approaches.

The fifth set of chapters presents couple- and family-oriented treatment. These approaches fulfill a unique role and have garnered substantial research evidence for their efficacy. For instance, community reinforcement and family therapy (CRAFT) is one innovative family approach that seeks to engage unmotivated clients into treatment. A recent review of studies found that CRAFT produced twice the engagement rates of the Johnson Institute intervention and three times the rates of Al-Anon/Nar-Anon (Roozen, de Waart, & van der Kroft, 2010). In addition to strong research support, these approaches provide a way to integrate aspects of a client's life into a more coherent support network that can help produce and maintain changes in substance use.

The last chapter pairing addresses pharmacological treatments for substance use disorders. Although some progress has been made in the last decade, pharmacological approaches are still vastly underused given their strong evidence of efficacy. There have been many treatment advances since the second edition, particularly with regard to medications for alcohol and opiate dependence. Recent reviews of acamprosate (Rosner, Hackl-Herrwerth, Leucht, Lehert, et al., 2010), naltrexone (Rosner, Hackl-Herrwerth, Leucht, Vecchi, et al., 2010), and buprenorphine (Veilleux, Colvin, Anderson, York, & Heinz, 2010) have concluded that they significantly improve treatment outcomes, compared with placebo medications. Particularly when used in combination with psychosocial treatments, psychopharmacological approaches are becoming an important treatment component for many people.

The final section of the book discusses treatment in three different clinical environments where substance use treatment is most often delivered: brief medical interactions, general counseling settings, and extended case management. Each of these chapters shows how clinicians have integrated different theoretical approaches to balance the clinical setting and the needs of the patient.

This volume is written for a broad audience. It is suitable for advanced undergraduates, beginning graduate students, and candidates who are undergoing certification as substance abuse counselors. Experienced substance abuse clinicians may find this book useful in broadening their knowledge of current treatment approaches. Finally, general psychotherapists and medical practitioners will find this book useful in learning how to approach substance abuse with clients who may be in treatment for other conditions. We recognize that this book is not comprehensive, nor do we intend it to be. Rather, it is a focused introduction to what we believe are the most prominent treatment theories and their derivative techniques. We believe the approaches covered here will form the core of effective substance abuse treatment for the coming decade and beyond.

References

Anton, R. F., O'Malley, S. S., Ciraulo, D. A., Cisler, R. A., Couper, D., Donovan, D. M., et al. (2006). Combined pharmacotherapies and behavioral interventions for alcohol dependence: The COMBINE study: A randomized controlled trial. *Journal of the American Medical Association, 295*(17), 2003–2017.

Apodaca, T. R., & Longabaugh, R. (2009). Mechanisms of change in motivational interviewing: A review and preliminary evaluation of the evidence. *Addiction, 104*(5), 705–715.

Ferri, M., Amato, L., & Davoli, M. (2006). Alcoholics Anonymous and other 12–step programmes for alcohol dependence. *Cochrane Database of Systematic Reviews, 3*, CD005032.

Knapp, W. P., Soares, B. G., Farrel, M., & Lima, M. S. (2007). Psychosocial interventions for cocaine and psychostimulant amphetamines related disorders. *Cochrane Database of Systematic Reviews, 3*, CD003023.

Kuhn, T. S. (1970). *The structure of scientific revolutions* (2nd ed.). Chicago: University of Chicago Press,

Lundahl, B., & Burke, B. L. (2009). The effectiveness and applicability of motivational interviewing: a practice-friendly review of four meta-analyses. *Journal of Clinical Psychology, 65*(11), 1232–1245.

Magill, M., & Ray, L. A. (2009). Cognitive-behavioral treatment with adult alcohol and illicit drug users: A meta-analysis of randomized controlled trials. *Journal of Studies on Alcohol and Drugs, 70*(4), 516–527.

Miller, W. R., Sorensen, J. L., Selzer, J. A., & Brigham, G. S. (2006). Disseminating evidence-based practices in substance abuse treatment: A review with suggestions. *Journal of Substance Abuse Treatment, 31*(1), 25–39.

Miller, W. R., Wilbourne, P. L., & Hettema, J. E. (2003). What works?: A summary of alcohol treatment outcome research. In R. K. Hester & W. R. Miller (Eds.), *Handbook of alcoholism treatment approaches: Effective alternatives* (3rd ed., pp. 13–63). Boston: Allyn & Bacon.

Project MATCH Research Group. (1998). Matching alcoholism treatments to client heterogeneity: Project MATCH three-year drinking outcomes. *Alcoholism, Clinical and Experimental Research, 22*(6), 1300–1311.

Rogers, E. M. (2003). *Diffusion of innovations* (5th ed.). New York: Free Press.

Roozen, H. G., de Waart, R., & van der Kroft, P. (2010). Community reinforcement and family training: An effective option to engage treatment-resistant substance-abusing individuals in treatment. *Addiction, 105*(10), 1729–1738.

Rosner, S., Hackl-Herrwerth, A., Leucht, S., Lehert, P., Vecchi, S., & Soyka, M. (2010). Acamprosate for alcohol dependence. *Cochrane Database of Systematic Reviews, 9*, CD004332.

Rosner, S., Hackl-Herrwerth, A., Leucht, S., Vecchi, S., Srisurapanont, M., & Soyka, M. (2010). Opioid antagonists for alcohol dependence. *Cochrane Database of Systematic Reviews, 12*, CD001867.

Veilleux, J. C., Colvin, P. J., Anderson, J., York, C., & Heinz, A. J. (2010). A review of opioid dependence treatment: Pharmacological and psychosocial interventions to treat opioid addiction. *Clinical Psychology Review, 30*(2), 155–166.

Chapter 1

Theories of Motivation and Addictive Behavior

Gary S. Rose
Scott T. Walters

A word after a word after a word is power.
—MARGARET ATWOOD, "Spelling"

For a detective, the easiest crimes to solve are those with an apparent motive: *He wanted her money, and so he killed her for it.* The crime makes sense. Crimes with no apparent motive are more difficult, such as when a person is attacked by someone unknown to him or her. But perhaps there are clues—a hair follicle, a scrap of clothing, or an eyewitness. The most difficult crimes of all are those that occur despite apparent countermotives: *He had spent his life savings to protect her, so why would he have killed her?* In this case, even the best detective is at a loss to explain why it happened.

Treatment providers can encounter similar puzzles when trying to explain the motivation behind substance abuse. Some people, particularly those in the early stages of addiction, seem to have clear motives for use. Perhaps they enjoy the pleasurable effects or use to minimize negative effects. However, people in later stages of addiction are more puzzling since they seem to use despite the effects. In fact, it's not uncommon for persons in later-stage addiction to say that they use drugs *despite* the effects rather than *because* of them. At the same time, people may feel that they *like* the drug less but *need* it more.

This chapter discusses motivational theories of addiction. Our goal is to explain why people use substances (sometimes despite their best interests) and the conditions under which people are more likely to make changes. The chapter begins with a review of motivational theories of addiction, in particular those that help explain the paradox of drug use despite an array of problems. We then discuss theories of motivational change, in particular focusing on factors that may make change more likely to "stick." Finally, we discuss the way that motivation connects to language, and how counselor and client words can shift the balance toward change.

Motivation and Addiction

There are many different ways to explain the acquisition and maintenance of addictive disorders. Berridge, Robinson, and colleagues (Berridge, 2009; Berridge, Robinson, & Aldridge, 2009; Robinson & Berridge, 2001, 2008) draw a distinction between two motivational factors: "liking" and "wanting." "Liking" refers to the immediate pleasure one gets from contact with a stimuli, such as with a pleasant taste or smell. "Wanting" refers to the "magnet quality" of something that makes it desirable. Wanting goes beyond our mere sensory experience and causes us to pay attention to something and seek it out. Furthermore, Robinson and Berridge (2001) argue that there are explicit and implicit factors that influence both liking and wanting. For instance, when people learn to expect a certain effect from a drug, this results in explicit learning about the effect one might reliably expect from use. However, there may also be implicit factors that are outside a person's immediate awareness, such as habit strength or environmental cues. Once started, drug use may play out automatically in much the same way as driving a car or tying a shoe. The distinction between liking and wanting, and explicit and implicit factors, can help us see why people might feel compelled to engage in behavior despite their best interests, or even outside their awareness.

Theories of liking are more straightforward, in part because they seem more rational. "Explicit liking" refers to the affective valence of an activity. Our bodies come programmed to seek reinforcement and avoid punishment. As such, theories of liking have focused both on the role that pleasure (positive reinforcement) and the avoidance of displeasure (negative reinforcement) play in acquiring and maintaining addictions.

Negative Reinforcement

People make choices, in part, to minimize undesirable effects. "Negative reinforcement" refers to the removal of an unpleasant state. For instance, aspirin is negatively reinforcing because it removes headache pain. The opponent process model, which combines Berridge's (2009) explicit affect dimension with classical conditioning, provides one explanation for opiate and alcohol dependence. In short, the model suggests that emotions are paired. When one emotion is experienced, another is suppressed. For instance, in a study of skydivers, Solomon and Corbit (1974) found that early skydivers had greater levels of fear upon jumping and less pleasure upon landing when compared to more experienced skydivers. In this instance, the opponent process was a shift from fear to pleasure after repeated jumps. Alcohol and opiates seem to function similarly. After a period of use, most individuals develop pharmacodynamic tolerance to the positive effects of the drug; their bodies adjust to the presence of the drug in order to maintain a homeostatic state. When the drug blood level drops, the person experiences unpleasant withdrawal symptoms, making him or her want to use again. The opponent process model of motivation suggests that drug use is rewarding because it decreases these noxious withdrawal symptoms. In other words, it is negatively reinforcing. This is the classic explanation for why people continue to use opiates. Although this commonsense explanation fits with the folklore that experienced drug users continue to use to feel "normal," observations of actual drug use patterns do not support the tenets of this model (Lyvers, 1998, 2000). Barring the existence of other medical disorders, opiate withdrawal is neither life-threatening nor markedly discomforting for most people. Moreover, many relapses seem to occur "out of the blue" long after any withdrawal symptoms have ceased. Because of this, there are likely to be other factors that motivate addictive behavior in addition to withdrawal relief (Lyvers, 1998).

Another negative reinforcement model suggests that people are motivated to use alcohol and other drugs to reduce stress. With particular application to alcohol abuse, the theory proposes that alcohol is negatively reinforcing because of the stress reduction that accompanies intoxication. Indeed, reduction in physiological stress is one clear effect of alcohol's action on the GABA neurotransmitter. Furthermore, this stress reduction response is one of a small number of genetically linked predictors of vulnerability to alcohol dependence (Schuckit, 1988, 1994). However, the stress reduction hypothesis does not adequately explain the intense craving of those with severe alcohol dependence, nor does it provide us with a cogent explanation of drug-seeking behavior in other varieties of drug abuse.

Positive Reinforcement

People also use substances for their rewarding effects. In his operant model of learning, Skinner (2002) observed that positive reinforcement increased the probability that people would engage in similar behavior. Cognitive behavioral and social learning models later emphasized the importance of beliefs and expectations (in addition to actual consequences) in the operant

response–reinforcement paradigm. Such real and perceived positive consequences do explain the initiation of drinking and may be a principal motivator for nondependent "problem" drinkers. For instance, positive expectancies of alcohol, tobacco, and other drugs serve as powerful moderators
of initiation of substance abuse, especially during adolescence and young
adulthood (Miller, Smith, & Goldman, 1990). Most children have developed firm positive expectancies about alcohol by age 6 and the intensity of
these beliefs predicts age of onset of alcohol use. In addition, people who
present with mild-to-moderate levels of substance abuse often report that
they continue to use for the sake of the consequent positive physiological
and mental states. Interestingly, in the case of alcohol and some drug use,
many of these reported positive consequences may be a function of positive
expectancies rather than the actual pharmacological effects of the drug
(Marlatt & Rohsenow, 1980). In studies where drinkers were given placebo
beverages, but told that they contained alcohol, they experienced many of
the same rewarding effects.

"Wanting" and "Liking"

The limitation of the positive and negative reinforcement models lies in the
assumed connection between liking and wanting. But it is more complicated to explain the behavior of people with advanced alcoholism and drug
addiction, where intense cravings are sometimes experienced in the absence
of any positive appraisals. That is, more experienced users may use *despite*
the consequences rather than *because* of them.

Berridge et al. (2009) suggest that affective response ("liking") and
motivational salience ("wanting") are mediated by different brain systems.
During the early stages of addiction, there is a clear connection between
affect (pleasure experienced and pain relieved) and urges to use. Much of
this evaluative and motivational process is clearly understood by the individual (i.e., is explicit). As the addiction progresses, something interesting
happens: First, the pleasure component of the drug experience tends to
become less important, even as the emotional valence increases; users may
like the drug less but feel that they *need* it more. Second, the motivational
component changes from explicit to implicit; the cognitive representation
of the drug effect decreases at the same time that users experience increased
urges to use. People with advanced addiction may feel like their actions are
simply beyond their control. These changes begin in the midstages of the
addiction process, when alcohol and drug use is only loosely associated
with the anticipation of pleasure, and are most salient during the advanced
stages of addiction, when urges to use are experienced apart from any
clear cognitive attributions of desire or pleasure. Advanced-stage addicts
frequently report simply being overwhelmed by an "irresistible urge" to
use without any strong positive or negative outcome expectancies. In the

language of Berridge and colleagues (2009), their motivation is determined by implicit motivational processes closely tied to the neurophysiology of drug abuse, a process they call "incentive sensitization."

Incentive Sensitization

One of the major drawbacks of the opponent process model was its failure to explain addiction to stimulants such as cocaine. Whereas users of opiates, alcohol, or barbiturates might indeed continue to abuse these substances to avoid withdrawal symptoms, this is less true with stimulant abuse because users of these drugs rarely develop the classic symptoms of pharmacodynamic tolerance and withdrawal. Rather, the symptoms of tolerance to cocaine are more related to changes in metabolism and the symptoms of withdrawal are more likely to be a consequence of changes in levels of neurotransmitters rather than a physiological accommodative process. This inadequacy of the opponent process model, in the face of rampant cocaine addiction, led to the development of the incentive sensitization model of addiction, a theory broad enough to explain the motivational processes of all major classes of addictive drugs.

The incentive sensitization model asserts that although drugs of abuse vary considerably with regard to their impact on the neurobiological system, they all elevate levels of the neurotransmitter dopamine in the midbrain and prefrontal cortex. Dopamine functions as a neurochemical marker of motivational salience; it tells the brain that something is important. Dopamine is elevated by natural processes essential to survival, including satiation of hunger and thirst, procreation, and other survival activities. Many drugs of abuse, including cocaine, alcohol, opiates, and amphetamines, have a neurochemical footprint that is similar to these survival processes, and thus literally can fake the brain into thinking that it needs the drug to survive. Importantly, substances that elevate dopamine trigger cravings that are independent of sensations of pleasure. These urges to use often lack any cognitive labeling, that is, they are "implicit." This cognitive "invisibility" is a function of the site of dopamine neurotransmission in the brain, which is outside the cerebral cortex and therefore unaccompanied by higher order mental processes.

Drugs use dopamine to get the brain's attention. The degree of sensitivity to this effect varies across individuals and likely has a genetic component, resulting in differing degrees of susceptibility to addiction that are only loosely related to quantity and frequency of use. However, once the process begins it tends to snowball because the brain becomes sensitized to the drug reward effect. Essentially the opposite of tolerance, this suggests that with continued use, the reward value of the substance increases; smaller doses yield higher reward value, with consequent increases in urges to use. This process of incentive sensitization often develops quickly and is slow to extinguish after a person has stopped using. This is why many long-term abstinent cocaine-, amphetamine-, alcohol-, opiate-, or nicotine-dependent individuals experience "out of the blue" relapses. Cross-sensitization also occurs, such that individuals who have been addicted to one substance are at risk of rapid dependence upon another addictive substance or behavior. Thus, the connection between substances of abuse and behavioral addictions may be through this common pathway.

The incentive sensitization model helps to clarify the role of motivation in addiction. It provides a common neurobiological pathway for substances of abuse and addictive behaviors; explains the phenomenon of craving and relapse absent any cognitive or affective appraisals; provides a rationale for long-term treatment and support, particularly for those who have abused cocaine and amphetamines; and opens up new avenues for the investigation of psychopharmacological treatments for addictive disorders.

Motivation and Change

The first part of this chapter has covered theories of motivation related to the acquisition and maintenance of addictive behaviors. We now turn to motivational theories of behavior change. In examining motivation to change, it's fair to say that the "currency" of motivation is not fixed. Although it may seem to people that they make choices as a result of a rational decision-making process, social psychologists find that choice can be readily affected by changing characteristics of the message or messenger. Thus, the currency of motivation depends not only on the product, but also on what other things are for sale, how one perceives the marketplace, and what one thinks of the seller.

Decision Making

There is a long history of explaining motivation in terms of decision-making strategies. Benjamin Franklin made difficult decisions by listing his competing motivations in a sort of algebraic equation. After listing the likely pros and cons of an outcome and giving weights to the importance of each item, he added up the two lists and acted accordingly. Thus, Franklin had developed a comparative model of decision making in which it was not the total number of gains or losses but the value of gains and losses *in relation to each other* that influenced his decisions.

During the early stages of addiction, decisions to use a substance are often associated with a weighing of the pros and cons of use, relative to other available options (Herrnstein & Prelec, 1992). As addiction develops, rational decision making seems to take a back seat to neurobiological processes. However, there is still a clear role for decision making with regard to the pros and cons of committing to treatment. Janis and Mann (1968, 1977) introduced the use of the decisional balance in modern psychology as a means of structuring the decision maker's "vigilant" consideration of the pros and cons of each available alternative. Asserting that attention needed to be given to both the utilitarian and the core value-based gains and losses to the self and to others, Janis and Mann designed an eight-cell table to be used in the examination of each possible decisional choice. If one considers two alternatives, such as continuing to use a drug versus quitting, then the table expands to 16 cells, quite an eyeful of information.

Velicer, DiClemente, Prochaska, and Brandenburg (1985) presented a simplified four-cell decisional balance that queried the pros and cons of the status quo versus the pros and cons of change. This four-cell matrix has become the conventional means of graphically representing the decisional balance sheet in addictions treatment protocols such as motivational interviewing (MI; Miller & Rollnick, 1991) and guided self-change (Sobell & Sobell, 1993).

Miller and Rollnick (2002) use the decisional balance to both clarify the issues at stake and to help the person resolve ambivalence toward change. By carefully querying the client about the "good and not so good" aspects of both options, they are able to use decisional conflict to "tip" the balance towards change. For a drinker considering abstinence, the conflict might be thus: "If I continue to drink, I will continue to enjoy the benefits of being with friends [benefit of staying the same]. However, my family relationships and health will continue to deteriorate [costs of staying the same]. On the other hand, if I quit drinking, I will feel better physically [benefit of change], but I won't be able to spend the evenings with my friends and will probably feel more stressed [costs of change]."

The decisional balance points to the complex nature of decision-making processes and the intricate interplay of forces for and against change. However, decision making rarely occurs in a vacuum; it is most often part of an interpersonal process and, as such, requires a thorough understanding of the social factors that impede or facilitate motivation.

Self-Determination Theory

We have all experienced teachers and coaches whose students give them every inch of performance and mentors of all type who inspire confidence and creativity in their protégés. What do these individuals have in common? What is the secret to their success as motivators of others?

Self-determination theory (SDT; Deci & Ryan, 1985; Ryan & Deci, 2000; Ryan, Sheldon, Kasser, & Deci, 1996) is a broad-based theory of motivation that specifies the causes, processes, and outcomes of "optimal" thriving. SDT grew out of work examining the relative contributions of intrinsic and extrinsic motivation to human performance. Research using the SDT framework has found that two factors—the degree of self-determined motivation and the perceived locus of causality (the extent to which an individual believes that he or she is the active agent in the change process)—determine the extent to which an individual will persist in a target behavior. Comparisons between people whose motivation is self-determined and those who have been externally coerced generally show that those in the former group are more excited and confident about their behavior, which translates into enhanced performance, more creativity, and better overall well-being. Because of the large functional differences between internal and external motivators on behavioral outcome, SDT first asks *what kind* of motivation is operating at any particular time.

Organismic integration theory (Ryan et al., 1996) identifies four modes of self-regulation, varying in the degree to which behavior is regulated from the outside versus the inside. At the extreme end of the continuum, the *externally regulated* individual behaves only to gain reward or avoid penalty. There is very little generalization of effort when these contingencies are delayed or removed. For example, people may avoid alcohol or drug use while being monitored by breathalyzer or urine test; however, the old behavior usually returns in full force once the external monitoring ceases. *Introjected regulation*, the next point on the continuum, refers to motivation that is based on the affective or evaluative responses of others and, as such, is still an example of externally derived regulation. Behavior that is motivated to please a spouse, parent, or employer tends to be fraught with anxiety, and is quite unstable over time.

Identified regulation describes people who execute the desirable behavior or curtail the undesirable behavior because they appreciate the rationale for the behavior change and sincerely want the outcome. A smoker who ceases smoking following a heart attack because of the connection between tobacco and heart disease is displaying the identified level of regulation. This type of internal motivation is generally sufficient to explain most health behavior changes that are easy to implement, do not entail the giving up of pleasurable activities, and where persistence over time is not a big challenge. Unfortunately, when it comes to addictive behaviors, the initiation of change is often difficult, the addictive substance is still reinforcing, and the maintenance of change may be quite challenging. For most people, this requires *integrated regulation*, the highest level of internal motivation. At this level of regulation, the reasons for change are not only clearly understood and embraced by the individual, but, in addition, they reflect an instantiation of the person's core values and sense of personal identity. The individual who abstains from alcohol because it helps him or her move closer to strongly held personal values is embracing change at this deep level. Approaches to addictions treatment as disparate as Alcoholics Anonymous (AA), motivational interviewing, and humanistic psychotherapies all promote the integrated level of regulation.

Although the four modes of self-regulation are in part determined by the nature of the behavior change at hand, they are also influenced by the individual's ability to satisfy basic psychological needs. When making choices, people attempt to satisfy three basic psychological needs: *autonomy, competence*, and *relatedness*. These three factors are the nutrients that predict what things people will choose and which changes will flourish. The first basic need, *autonomy*, involves the perception that what one does is by one's own choice. Autonomy is closely related to self-efficacy (Bandura, 1994). However, "self-efficacy" refers to outcome expectations, whereas "autonomy" is more connected to an individual's perception of him- or herself as the determining agent of an action (Ryan & Connell, 1989). In this theory, threats, deadlines, punitive evaluations, and imposed goals all undermine self-determination because they communicate that the change is out of the person's hands. An individual's perception of his or her behavior as freely chosen also affects the way he or she perceives external contingencies. For instance, an individual who perceives his or her recovery behaviors (e.g., attending support meetings, avoiding alcohol, reducing stress) as freely chosen is more likely to report that he or she engages in those behaviors because they "feel right" rather than for the external rewards they provide (e.g., family support, continued employment, avoiding legal difficulties).

The second basic need is for *competence*, the perception that one is a capable, effective person. Like self-efficacy, competence is enhanced by positive feedback and "optimal" challenges. Individuals who receive positive feedback enjoy the behavior and try harder because they believe that they are good at the behavior.

Finally, SDT postulates a need for *relatedness*, a feeling of belonging and participation in social groups. Because much behavior is not, strictly speaking, internally motivated, it is also important to understand how autonomy and competence are promoted within the context of *externally* motivated behavior. One reason people engage in externally motivated behavior is because the behaviors are modeled or prompted by others to whom they feel attached. Thus, a woman might work two jobs, save money, or give up drinking because it is meaningful to her sister or makes a better life for her children. Autonomy is supported in social contexts when people in the environment "take that person's perspective, provide choice, encourage self-initiation, and minimize controls" (Ryan et al., 1996, p. 14). People judge their attitudes, in part, through the social context, which may explain why people are more likely to respond favorably to difficult messages if delivered by a trusted partner or friend, and more likely to buy a product from a salesman they view as likeable (Dennis, 2006; Homans, 1958).

In sum, SDT proposes that individuals who are internally motivated, who feel that they have freely chosen their behaviors, and who are immersed in contexts that support feelings of competence will demonstrate persistently healthy, self-determined behaviors. Conversely, for those individuals who are externally motivated, feel that they are not the determining agent in their behavior, and encounter an environment that is controlling, change will be brief, and relapse to old behaviors will occur rapidly once the external contingencies are removed.

SDT shows promise as a theoretical base for clinical techniques such as MI (Markland, Ryan, Tobin, & Rollnick, 2005; Vansteenkiste & Sheldon, 2006) (see Figure 1.1). From the SDT framework, MI is effective because it increases the client's perception of choice, enhances feelings of competence, and stresses a positive working relationship between the client and the counselor. In this way, MI is thought to enhance the quality, and not just the quantity, of client motivation. For example, Miller and Rollnick (2002) state that motivation is best when there is a high intrinsic value to the change (willingness), the individual feels capable of making the change (ability), and values the immediacy of change over other priorities (readiness). MI supports the need for competence by presenting clear information about outcomes contingencies, by helping clients to develop their own realistic goals, and by providing positive feedback. Autonomy support is

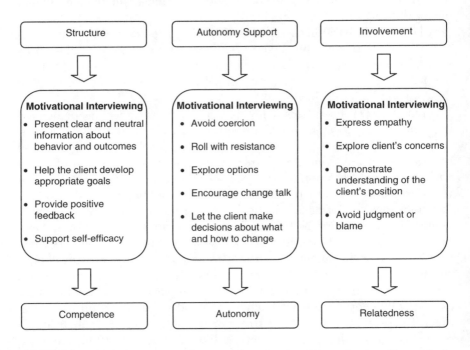

FIGURE 1.1. Self-determination theory and motivational interviewing. From Markland, Ryan, Tobin, and Rollnick (2005). Copyright 2005 by the Guilford Press. Reprinted by permission.

evident through MI techniques such as the avoidance of confrontation, encouraging change talk, and allowing clients to come to their own conclusions. Finally, relatedness is enhanced by a specific emphasis on rapport building and careful empathic listening.

Reactance

Self-determination can be undermined by interpersonal reactance, a troubling consequence of poorly executed attempts at persuasion. In his theory of psychological reactance, Brehm (1966, 1968) asserted that, at any point in time, people have an array of "free behaviors" that they take for granted; when loss of these freedoms is threatened, their value to the individual increases. For example, in a series of studies by Worchel, Lee, and Adewole (1975), people were asked to rate the taste and quality of cookies pulled from a jar. Cookies that were pulled from a jar that contained just a few were rated as significantly more tasty than cookies pulled from a full jar. The finding was even more pronounced when participants saw the experimenter pull out scarce cookies to give to other participants. Those cookies were rated the tastiest of all.

From cookies to cars, there is strong evidence that the desirability of a product can be influenced by perceptions of diminished personal choice. Retail stores commonly use message-framing strategies like this to increase the desirability of a product: "For a limited time only!" Only three left at this price!" When considering political attitudes, Worchel and Brehm (1970) found that people reported a greater desire to hear a speech, and more attitude change after hearing it, when told that it had been previously censured. Studying consumer behavior, Bushman (1998) observed that warning labels regarding the fat content of cream cheese were associated with *increased* frequency of choosing high-fat products. This kind of reactance can be an unintended consequence of strongly worded messages that ask people to give up a high-risk behavior (e.g., "Just say no!" "Tobacco is killing you!"). If not carefully phrased, such messages can be understood as limiting personal choice. Such messages not only impinge on personal perceptions of autonomy, but also may inadvertently communicate that the behavior is more desirable because it is being prohibited. Indeed, many theorists suggest that self-destructive behaviors, such as severe eating disorders and self-mutilation, are maintained because they allow a person to assert autonomy and control. If you take away freedom of choice, those behaviors may become more important to the individual.

Recently, reactance considerations have been incorporated into the design and evaluation of health communications. Quick (2005) notes that public health messages can vary on three important dimensions: threat to choice (e.g., "Just say no!"), vividness (e.g., "Unprotected exposure to the sun results in severe skin blisters that ooze and become crusty"), and explicitness (e.g., "No more than three drinks per day"). Although each of these three dimensions impacts reactance, the most important variable seems, once again, to be threat to choice (Quick & Stephenson, 2007, 2008). For instance, health care messages that include high threat-to-choice language tend to increase anger and other negative thoughts, and lead to lower rates of medication adherence (Levav & Zhu, 2009; Quick & Kim, 2009; Quick & Stephenson, 2007).

Reactance has clear implications for conversations about alcohol and drug abuse. Communications that have high threat value, are confrontational and controlling, or that limit client choices are likely to engender a motivational state that defends against change, regardless of whether the change might actually be beneficial. Conversely, approaches that support autonomy, offer a menu of choices, and acknowledge the short-term losses associated with change are likely to engender a motivational state conducive to behavior change.

The Language of Motivation

The use of reactance theory to guide message framing is an example of the importance of language in interpersonal relations. Philosophers, linguists, and social scientists have for many years studied the role that language plays in an individual's understanding of him- or herself and his or her social world (Chomsky, 1979; Mead, 1934; Sullivan, 1953). The interplay between language, beliefs, intentions, and actions is particularly important when considering substance abuse counseling, which by in large uses a language-driven approach. Early on, psychology theory emphasized language as a way to gain insight, to discover something about oneself. However, more recent theory has focused on the way that language can change one's internal state rather than simply describe it.

Heider (1958) spent the better part of 50 years studying the language of motivation. He began by categorizing language during ordinary interactions. In doing so, Heider observed that humans have an innate capacity to interpret social relations through the lens of linguistically based categories. That is, language not only communicates motivation and intent, but also helps people to understand and predict social interactions (Malle, 2004). Moreover, because people use similar rules for categorizing people as they do for categorizing objects, many of the rules-of-thumb and errors people make in object perception (e.g., optical illusions) also apply to social perception (e.g., making inappropriate attributions about the causes of behavior). According to Heider, *intentionality* is one of the most important attributions people make: Are an individual's actions intentional or unintentional? If deemed intentional, then the perceiver searches for an internal explanation, such as the beliefs or values of the person (Malle, 2004). On the other hand, if the behavior is deemed unintentional, then the perceiver looks to situational factors, such as external pressure, accidents, or random chance to explain the behavior. Malle and Knobe (1997) found that people judged that a behavior was intentional if the agent (1) desired the outcome, (2) believed that his or her action would lead to the outcome, (3) intended to perform the action, (4) had the skill to perform the action, and (5) was aware that he or she was performing it. The first two factors (belief and desire) reflect intention, while the factors that follow (skill and awareness) reflect intentionality. Thus, intentionality includes desire, awareness, and action.

Interestingly, the words we use to describe our own intent can also change behavior. The linguist J. L. Austin (1962) said that language is not just used to describe reality, but can also be used to *create* reality. In his aptly titled book, *How to Do Things with Words*, he refutes the view that the primary use of language is to describe reality in terms of being "true" or "false." In fact, he argues that "truth value" utterances actually constitute a very small part of ordinary language. In his most striking example, he describes performative utterances that actually complete an action. For instance, if I say, "I promise to love you" or "I'll bet you a dollar it rains tomorrow," I am not describing something, but rather doing a kind of action with my words.

There is evidence that language can affect other behaviors as well. Self-perception theory (Bem, 1967, 1972) suggests that people form attitudes by carefully observing their own behavior, including the language they use to describe reality. Rather than attitude informing behavior, Bem holds that people use behavior to generate conclusions about their own attitudes. That is, people make guesses about their own internal states by watching their own behavior. Although the theory is counterintuitive, there is evidence to suggest that emotions and attitudes do in fact follow behavior, particularly when people are less certain about how they feel about something (Laird, 2007). In fact, self-perception theory is the basis for marketing techniques such as the "foot-in-the-door," which suggests that a person is more likely to comply with a large request (e.g., to donate money) if he or she has first complied with a small request (e.g., fill out a short questionnaire). The idea is that the initial behavior changes the person's perception of him- or herself (e.g., "I am altruistic. I care about this cause."), which in turn increases the likelihood that he or she will act consistently with this perception in submitting to the second request. To a great extent, this process happens outside explicit awareness. People are more likely to attribute their decisions to their newfound altruism than to any characteristic of the salesman, which is why it is such an effective sales technique. Self-perception is also a key, if poorly understood, component of AA and the other 12-step programs. The many AA slogans are often chanted aloud, allowing the words that are uttered to sink into the speaker's head. Furthermore, beliefs such as "fake it 'til you make it" suggest that behavior change often precedes attitude change.

As a logical extension of Heider's theory of intentionality, self-perception theory suggests that not only must we carefully listen to words used by our clients, but we must also provide opportunities for them to utter words that are valenced toward change. If clients talk about problem recognition, confidence, or the benefits of change, they are more likely to commit to and adhere to a plan of action. Clients are describing themselves both to the therapist and to themselves. (The opposite also holds true. If clients hear themselves voice reasons against change or pessimism about change, they are more likely to commit to remaining in the status quo.) In either case, "change talk" and "sustain talk" are more likely to be followed by similar statements, in part because they change a person's implicit perception of him- or herself.

Heider's ideas have spawned programs of research on the nature of intentionality (Knobe, 2006; Malle, 2004) and behavioral commitment (Amrhein, 2004; Searle, 1989). Building upon Heider's initial focus on the parsing of intentionality, psycholinguists have developed different lexicons of self-motivational utterances (Gale, 1991; Russell, 1987; Siegfried, 1995). However, most of these systems have been limited to describing the nature of language within the therapy session; most have failed to reliably predict client outcome.

One promising exception to this trend is the work of Amrhein and colleagues (Amrhein, 2004; Amrhein, Miller, Yahne, Palmer, & Fulcher, 2003; Moyers et al., 2007). Amrhein (Amrhein et al., 2003) parsed self-motivational language into five categories: *Desire, Ability, Reasons, Need,* and *Commitment* (DARN-C). The first four categories (DARN) signify preparation, while the last category (C) indicates commitment to change. (More recent versions have added "Taking Steps" as a separate category; see Table 1.1). Within each of these categories, Amrhein proposed that

---

TABLE 1.1. Linguistic Categories from the Motivational Interviewing Skills Code 2.1

- Desire: Affective valence in support of change. *Want, Desire, Like*
- Ability: Efficacy related to change. *Can, Possible, Willpower*
- Reasons: Benefits of, or rationale for, change. *If, Then*
- Need: Strong desire in the absence of any particular reason. *Need, Must*
- Taking Steps: Specific steps that the client has already taken toward change. *I did, I went, I worked*
- Commitment: Agreement, intention, or obligation to change. *I will, I swear, I'm going to*

Note. Data from Miller, Moyers, Ernst, and Amrhein (2008).

language varies by strength. Thus, "I'll definitely stop using" expresses stronger commitment than "I'll probably stop using."

Statements of desire, ability, reasons, and need may reflect *intention* to change. They also may provide a way to try out motivational ideas, without having to commit to a course of action. Commitment statements indicate *intentionality*, the conjoining of intention and opportunity. Commitment statements *obligate* the speaker to take an action, such as when a person says something he or she has to "live up" to. Self-determination theory suggests that, once a person has made a verbal obligation, he or she is more likely to follow through with the action in order to assert his or her autonomy and competence. At the same time, self-perception theory suggests that commitment statements will become more likely as a person hears him- or herself voice the reasons, benefits, and optimism for change.

In their analysis of treatment sessions for drug-using clients, Amrhein and colleagues (2003) found support for this language chain. The strength of client commitment language (but not the other categories) directly predicted drug use at 12 months. The other categories predicted commitment language, and thus were *indirectly* related to change. Moreover, the strongest predictor of behavior change was client speech at the end of the counseling session, when clients were asked to discuss a change plan. Commitment language at the beginning of the session, when clients were discussing their reasons for presenting to treatment, did not predict behavior change. Some subsequent research (Moyers, Martin, Houck, Christopher, & Tonigan, 2009; Vader, Walters, Prabhu, Houck, & Field, 2010) has found that the overall strength of change language (rather than just commitment) predicts outcome, but this pattern from preparatory to commitment speech remains a guide for MI interactions. It may be that all kinds of "change talk" predict outcome, but DARN talk probably influences behavior directly, as well as indirectly through commitment talk.

Conclusion

Every crime has a motive if you know where to look. On the surface, addicted persons act despite countermotives. However, looking closely we see that substances of abuse are powerful short-term reinforcers that eventually "hijack" brain reward systems, often generating a seemingly blind compulsion that is matched only by survival drives such as fight-or-flight, hunger, and procreation. This is the paradoxical situation in which addicted persons find themselves: engaging in destructive behavior despite their best interests. This also explains why experienced users may *like* the drug less, but feel that they *need* it more.

But people with addictive disorders are people first and, as such, are privy to all the usual processes of influence that increase or decrease motivation. As change agents, we can facilitate or hinder this process. If we undermine autonomy, relatedness, and competence, the consequent behavior change will be unstable and ungrounded in the individual's core sense of self. If we argue too passionately for change, offer few choices, and nag clients about the likely negative consequences, the individual is likely to dig in his or her heels, defending the "priceless" freedom of personal choice.

Furthermore, there are the complexities of the language of motivation. People use language to make sense of their own behavior and the behavior of others. Words give motivational significance to behavior: "He relapsed because his disease took over"; "She drinks to self-medicate"; "He's just an old stoner who lives and breathes for weed." These sentences not only describe behavior, but attribute causality and responsibility, which in turn changes our behavior.

How can clinicians become better wordsmiths for change? We must appreciate that verbal behavior not only predicts behavior change, but also is the in-session proxy for change. Words not only precurse change, they *are* change. They carry behavioral significance in and of themselves because they are the in-session component of the targeted change. Counseling that supports self-determination and invites clients to voice their reasons for and optimism about change creates a conversation that sequences from intention to planning to commitment. In-session commitment, when paired with postsession opportunity, yields change. Words lead to action, and action over time changes addictive behaviors.

References

Amrhein, P. C. (2004). How does motivational interviewing work?: What client talk reveals. *Journal of Cognitive Psychotherapy, 18*(4), 323–336.

Amrhein, P. C., Miller, W. R., Yahne, C. E., Palmer, M., & Fulcher, L. (2003). Client commitment language during motivational interviewing predicts drug use outcomes. *Journal of Consulting and Clinical Psychology, 71*(5), 862–878.

Austin, J. L. (1962). *How to do things with words.* Oxford, UK: Oxford University Press.

Bandura, A. (1994). *Self-efficacy: The exercise of control.* New York: Freeman.

Bem, D. J. (1967). Self-perception: An alternative interpretation of cognitive dissonance phenomena. *Psychological Review, 74*(3), 183–200.

Bem, D. J. (1972). Self-perception theory. In L. Berkowitz (Ed.), *Advances in experimental social psychology* (Vol. 6, pp. 1–62). New York: Academic Press.

Berridge, K. C. (2009). Wanting and liking: Observations from the neuroscience and psychology laboratory. *Inquiry (Oslo), 52*(4), 378.

Berridge, K. C., Robinson, T. E., & Aldridge, J. W. (2009). Dissecting components of reward: "Liking," "wanting," and learning. *Current Opinions in Pharmacology, 9*(1), 65–73.

Brehm, J. W. (1966). *A theory of psychological reactance.* New York: Academic Press.

Brehm, J. W. (1968). Attitude change from threat to attitudinal freedom. In A. G. Greenwald, T. C. Brock, & T. M. Ostrom (Eds.), *Psychological foundations of attitudes* *pp. 277–296). New York: Academic Press.

Bushman, B. J. (1998). Effects of warning and information labels of full-fat, reduced-fat, and no-fat products. *Journal of Applied Psychology, 83*, 97–101.

Chomsky, N. (1979). *Language and responsibility.* New York: Pantheon Books.

Deci, E. L., & Ryan, R. M. (1985). *Intrinsic motivation and self-determination in human behavior.* New York: Plenum Press.

Dennis, M. R. (2006). Compliance and intimacy: Young adults' attempts to motivate health-promoting behaviors by romantic partners. *Health Communication, 19*(3), 259–267.

Gale, J. E. (1991). *Conversation analysis of therapeutic discourse: The pursuit of a therapeutic agenda.* Norwood, NJ: Ablex.

Heider, F. (1958). *The psychology of interpersonal relations.* New York: Wiley.

Herrnstein, R. J., & Prelec, D. (1992). A theory of addiction. In G. Loewenstein & J. Elster (Eds.), *Choice over time* (pp. 331–358). New York: Russel Sage Press.

Homans, G. C. (1958). Social behavior as exchange. *American Journal of Sociology, 63*, 597–606.

Janis, I. L., & Mann, L. (1968). A conflict theory approach to attitude change and decision making. In A. G. Greenwald, T. C. Brock, & T. M. Ostrom (Eds.), *Psychological foundations of attitudes* (pp. 327–360). New York: Academic Press.

Janis, I. L., & Mann, L. (1977). *Decision making.* New Haven, CT: Yale University Press.

Knobe, J. (2006). The concept of intentional action: A case study in the uses of folk psychology. *Philosophical Studies, 130*, 203–231.

Laird, J. D. (2007). *Feelings: The perceptions of self.* New York: Oxford University Press.

Levav, J., & Zhu, R. (2009). Seeking freedom through variety. *Journal of Consumer Research, 36*, 600–610.

Lyvers, M. (1998). Drug addiction as a physical disease: The role of physical dependence and other chronic drug-induced neurophysiological changes in compulsive drug self-administration. *Experimental and Clinical Psychopharmacology, 6*(1), 107–125.

Lyvers, M. (2000). "Loss of control" in alcoholism and drug addiction: A neuroscientific interpretation. *Experimental and Clinical Psychopharmacology, 8*(2), 225–249.

Malle, B. F. (2004). *How the mind explains behavior: Folk explanations, meaning, and social interaction.* Cambridge, MA: MIT Press.

Malle, B. F., & Knobe, J. (1997). The folk concept of intentionality. *Journal of Experimental Social Psychology, 33*, 101–121.

Markland, D., Ryan, R. M., Tobin, V. J., & Rollnick, S. (2005). Motivational interviewing and self-determination theory. *Journal of Social and Clinical Psychology, 24*(6), 811–831.

Marlatt, G. A., & Rohsenow, D. J. (1980). Cognitive processes in alcohol use: Expectancy and the balanced placebo design. In N. K. Mello (Ed.), *Advances in substance abuse* (Vol. 1, pp. 159–199). Greenwich, CT: JAI Press.

Mead, G. H. (1934). *Mind, self, and society*. Chicago: University of Chicago Press.

Miller, P. M., Smith, G. T., & Goldman, M. S. (1990). Emergence of alcohol expectancies in childhood: A possible critical period. *Journal of Studies on Alcohol, 51*, 343–349.

Miller, W. R., Moyers, T. B., Ernst, D., & Amrhein, P. (2008). *Manual for the motivational interviewing skill code (MISC), version 2.1* [Electronic version]. Retrieved January 20, 2009, from *casaa.unm.edu/download/misc.pdf*.

Miller, W. R., & Rollnick, S. (1991). *Motivational interviewing: Preparing people to change addictive behavior*. New York: Guilford Press.

Miller, W. R., & Rollnick, S. (2002). *Motivational interviewing: Preparing people for change* (2nd ed.). New York: Guilford Press.

Moyers, T. B., Martin, T., Christopher, P. J., Houck, J. M., Tonigan, J. S., & Amrhein, P. C. (2007). Client language as a mediator of motivational interviewing efficacy: Where is the evidence? *Alcoholism: Clinical and Experimental Research, 31*(10 Suppl.), 40s–47s.

Moyers, T. B., Martin, T., Houck, J. M., Christopher, P. J., & Tonigan, J. S. (2009). From in-session behaviors to drinking outcomes: A causal chain for motivational interviewing. *Journal of Consulting and Clinical Psychology, 77*(6), 1113–1124.

Quick, B. L. (2005). *An explication of the reactance processing model*. Unpublished doctoral dissertation, Texas A&M University.

Quick, B. L., & Kim, D. K. (2009). Examining reactance and reactance restoration with South Korean adolescents: A test of psychological reactance within a collectivist culture. *Communication Research, 36*, 765–783.

Quick, B. L., & Stephenson, M. T. (2007). Further evidence that psychological reactance can be modeled as a combination of anger and negative cognitions. *Communication Research, 34*, 255–276.

Quick, B. L., & Stephenson, M. T. (2008). Examining the role of trait reactance and sensation seeking on perceived threat, state reactance, and reactance restoration. *Human Communication Research, 34*, 448–476.

Robinson, T. E., & Berridge, K. C. (2001). Incentive-sensitization and addiction. *Addiction, 96*, 103–114.

Robinson, T. E., & Berridge, K. C. (2008). The incentive sensitization theory of addiction: Some current issues. *Philosophical Transactions of the Royal Society, 363*, 3137–3146.

Russell, R. L. (1987). Introduction. In *Language in psychotherapy: Strategies of discovery* (pp. 1–9). New York: Plenum Press.

Ryan, R. M., & Connell, J. P. (1989). Perceived locus of causality and internalization: Examining reasons for acting in two domains. *Journal of Personality and Social Psychology 57*(5), 749–761.

Ryan, R. M., & Deci, E. L. (2000). Self-determination theory and the facilitation of intrinsic motivation, social development, and well-being. *American Psychologist, 55*(1), 68–78.

Ryan, R. M., Sheldon, K. M., Kasser, T., & Deci, E. L. (1996). All goals are not created equal: An organismic perspective on the nature of goals and their regulation. In P. M. Gollwitzer & J. A. Bargh (Eds.), *The psychology of action: Linking cognition and motivation to behavior* (pp. 7–26). New York: Guilford Press.

Schuckit, M. A. (1988). Reactions to alcohol in sons of alcoholics and controls. *Alcoholism: Clinical and Experimental Research, 12*(4), 465–470.

Schuckit, M. A. (1994). Low level of response to alcohol as a predictor of future alcoholism. *American Journal of Psychiatry, 151*(2), 184–189.

Searle, J. R. (1989). How performatives work. *Linguistics and Philosophy, 12*, 535–558.

Siegfried, J. (1995). Introduction. In *Therapeutic and everyday discourse: Towards a microanalysis in psychotherapy process research* (pp. 1–25). Norwood, NJ: Ablex.

Skinner, B. F. (2002). The experimental analysis of behavior. In R. W. Reiber & K. Salzinger (Eds.), *Psychology: Theoretical-historical perspectives* (2nd ed., pp. 374–385). Washington, DC: APA Press.

Sobell, M. B., & Sobell, L. C. (1993). *Problem drinkers: Guided-self change treatment*. New York: Guilford Press.

Solomon, R. L., & Corbit, J. D. (1974). An opponent-process theory of motivation: I. Temporal dynamics of affect. *Psychological Review, 81*(2), 119–145.

Sullivan, H. S. (1953). *Interpersonal psychiatry*. New York: Norton.

Vader, A. M., Walters, S. T., Prabhu, G. C., Houck, J. M., & Field, C. A. (2010). The language of motivational interviewing and feedback: Counselor language, client language, and client drinking outcomes. *Psychology of Addictive Behaviors, 24*(2), 190–197.

Vansteenkiste, M., & Sheldon, K. M. (2006). There's nothing more practical than a good theory: Integrating motivational interviewing and self-determination theory. *British Journal of Clinical Psychology, 45*, 63–82.

Velicer, W. F., DiClemente, C. C., Prochaska, J. O., & Brandenburg, N. (1985). Decisional balance measure for assessing and predicting smoking status. *Journal of Personality and Social Psychology, 48*, 1279–1289.

Worchel, S., & Brehm, J. W. (1970). Effects of threats to attitudinal freedom as a function of agreement with the communicator. *Journal of Personality and Social Psychology, 14*, 18–22.

Worchel, S., Lee., J., & Adewole, A. (1975). Effects of supply and demand on rating of object value. *Journal of Personality and Social Psychology, 32*, 906–914.

Chapter 2

Motivational Interviewing in Practice

Erin M. Tooley
Theresa B. Moyers

Motivational interviewing (MI) originated in the 1980s as a treatment for substance abuse patients. At the time, it stood in stark contrast to many contemporary treatments that emphasized confrontation in response to client resistance or "denial" (Walters, Rotgers, Saunders, Wilkinson, & Towers, 2003). In contrast to this approach, Miller and Rollnick (2002) conceptualized client resistance and motivation as the product of an interaction between therapist and client. A therapist using MI influences the interaction by seeking to minimize the client's natural resistance to change (Miller, Benefield, & Tonigan, 1993). Miller and Rollnick (2002, p. 25) define "MI" as a "client-centered, directive method for enhancing intrinsic motivation to change by exploring and resolving client ambivalence." MI is effective with a variety of behaviors including addiction behaviors such as alcohol abuse, illicit drug use, and gambling; health-promotion behaviors such as exercise and healthy eating; and risky behaviors such as unsafe sex practices (Hettema, Steele, & Miller, 2005; Lundahl, Kunz, Brownell, Tollefson, & Burke, 2010). A single session of MI has also been found to be effective as an introduction to other types of substance abuse treatment in terms of enhancing client motivation, treatment retention, and outcome (Bien, Miller, & Boroughs, 1993; Brown & Miller, 1993).

Research on MI has focused increasingly on potential mechanisms of change that might lead to more favorable client outcomes. One candidate is a client's verbalization of "change talk," defined as language that expresses movement toward changing a particular problematic behavior (Miller & Rollnick, 2002). An assumption of MI is that clients feel some degree of ambivalence about their behavior, even if they subscribe more strongly to one side of the ambivalence (e.g., not changing) than the other.

An ambivalent client will express arguments both for and against change. Recent research has focused on ways to elicit change talk from the client and how it may influence outcome. For instance, Amrhein, Miller, Yahne, Palmer, and Fulcher (2003) found that certain kinds of change talk, specifically talk about desire, ability, reason, and need to change, predicted strength-of-commitment talk. This commitment language, in turn, predicted behavior change. They also found a particular pattern of change talk that predicted behavior change most strongly. Increasing commitment language across the treatment session was associated with greater rates of abstinence 1 year later (Amrhein et al., 2003). In contrast, Moyers, Martin, Houck, Christopher, and Tonigan (2009) found that commitment language itself did not predict subsequent alcohol use any better than a general category-of-change talk. They found that both commitment language and "preparatory language" (i.e., desire, ability, reasons, and need) together predicted outcomes. Despite these differences in the relative importance of commitment versus preparatory language, change talk has emerged as a potential mediator of behavior change. On the other side, client "sustain talk," or a client's verbalizations of desire, reasons, need, ability, or commitment to maintaining the status quo, has been found to be inversely related to behavior change (Miller et al., 1993).

A Theory of MI

Although MI was not developed upon a particular theory, many researchers and clinicians have attempted to develop a more concrete understanding of how and why MI is effective in changing behavior. Nigg, Allegrante, and Ory (2002) explain that theory provides the framework necessary to understand the mechanisms of behavior change, understand why the mechanisms worked or failed, identify mediators that are important to target in an intervention, and determine why or how an intervention was or was not effective. Based on research spanning the last 30 years, Miller and Rose (2009) propose a theory that highlights both relational and technical components of MI. The relational component involves an interpersonal bond between the client and the therapist, sometimes referred to as "common factors" in therapy, which is referred to as "the spirit of MI" (Rollnick & Miller, 1995). The technical component involves the use of MI techniques to differentially evoke change talk and minimize sustain talk. Both of these components are thought to be important in the behavior change process (Miller & Rose, 2009). The technical and relational components are thought to influence client outcome directly, as well as through increased change talk and diminished resistance (Miller & Rose, 2009).

Relational Components

Miller and Rose's (2009) theory predicts both direct and indirect relationships between therapist factors and client behavior change. They theorize that both therapist empathy and MI style, which includes endorsement of collaboration, evocation, and client autonomy, play a role in predicting client change talk and subsequent behavior change.

Empathy

Empathy may be one of the most studied "common" therapist factors examined in psychotherapy outcome research. Miller and Rollnick (2002) describe Carl Roger's concept of accurate empathy as the pillar upon which therapist skillfulness in MI rests. Often, therapists mistakenly feel that they must either have had the same experiences as the client or agree with the client in order to communicate empathy. Instead, Rogers's definition of accurate empathy refers to a therapist's ability to communicate *understanding* of the client through reflections of explicit content and the underlying meaning of the client's words (Miller & Rollnick, 2002). A skilled MI therapist offers reflections with the goal of trying to understand what the client is saying, his or her feelings, and the meaning of his or her words. Although information gathering can be an important part of any substance use treatment, MI requires a shift in priorities from gathering information to communicating understanding and acceptance of the client. A therapist high in accurate empathy will respond to clients with more reflections than questions; will provide more complex reflections that emphasize the client's underlying thoughts, ideas, emotions, and meaning; and will encourage the client to provide more detail in order to gain a greater understanding of his or her perspective.

The Spirit of MI

A therapist's MI style comes from a set of underlying beliefs, referred to as the "spirit" of MI, that are differentiated from specific therapeutic techniques (Rollnick & Miller, 1995). Collaboration is one important core belief underlying the spirit of MI (Miller & Rollnick, 2002). It is important for the counselor to assume the role of a partner or collaborator, rather than an expert, with his or her client. This involves eliciting and respecting the client's personal reasons for change and ideas about how that change might occur. The therapist tries to elicit the perspectives and ideas of the client with the assumption that some of them will prove favorable to a desired change. This can be difficult for some therapists who believe that their most important role is to provide expert information. Therapists must be aware of their own assumptions to avoid inadvertently assuming this kind of expert role. Similarly, therapists who are highly collaborative will actively encourage the sharing of power in a session. As a result, these therapists allow the client's ideas to influence the direction and outcome of the session, will actively seek client input regarding behavior change, will carefully and minimally give advice and information, and will explicitly identify the client, rather than themselves, as the expert.

A related belief is that the goal of the counseling session is to evoke the client's existing internal motivation and personal resources for change (Miller & Rollnick, 2002). Rather than relying on advice-giving strategies, the therapist uses MI techniques to draw out the client's own ideas about the target behavior. A therapist practicing MI will evoke the reasons for change and enhance the client's self-efficacy by, for example, eliciting the client's most important values, his or her resources for change, and his or her previous success stories. Persuading and convincing are not part of an MI approach; ideally, a client should be talking him- or herself into change.

A therapist who endorses the spirit of MI also believes in a client's autonomy regarding change (Miller & Rollnick, 2002). MI therapists support the client's right to make his or her own decisions, even if that means maintaining the status quo. To this end, a therapist may help the client to explore his or her options genuinely, explicitly acknowledge the client's choice to maintain the status quo, and explore in a nonjudgmental manner the client's personal ideas about how change might occur.

Technical Components

Miller and Rose's (2009) theory also predicts direct and indirect relationships between therapist use of MI-consistent (or -inconsistent) methods and subsequent client behavior change. These technical skills include a variety of methods that influence client outcomes directly, as well as indirectly through the evocation of change talk and minimization of sustain talk.

Differential Evocation and Reinforcement of Change Talk

In MI, a therapist takes an active, directive role. A therapist creates opportunities for a client to offer change language and decreases opportunities for a client to offer sustain language. A therapist then works to reinforce and elicit further change language (Miller & Moyers, 2006). Research indicates that client change talk is more likely to occur when therapist MI-consistent behaviors are frequent and MI-inconsistent behaviors are less frequent (Moyers et al., 2009). Further, the therapist's general clinical skills, or microskills, such as questions, reflections, and summaries, create the opportunity for a client's discussion of change.

MI-Consistent Behaviors

The Motivational Interviewing Skill Code, Version 2.1, is a coding system designed to evaluate therapist competence in MI (Miller, Moyers, Ernst, & Amrhein, 2008). In this coding system, several in-session therapist behaviors are considered MI-consistent. The first is *asking permission*, both directly, by asking permission before giving advice or information, and indirectly, by asking a client what he or she already knows about a topic before giving information. This enhances the collaborative atmosphere of the session by equalizing the power between the client and the therapist. The client is explicitly free to decline the information or advice.

Affirmations are also MI-consistent behaviors. Affirming includes saying something complimentary about the client's personal characteristics or efforts. When genuinely offered by the therapist, these comments communicate respect and appreciation. Our experience is that skilled therapists can almost always find something that they appreciate in their clients and can explicitly convey this appreciation.

Finally, therapists can enhance a client's sense of autonomy by *emphasizing the client's control* or freedom to make his or her own decisions. This may include agreeing with the client who says he or she does not have to change, exploring options (including sustaining the behavior) genuinely, and verbalizing that the client has the freedom to choose change or to maintain the status quo.

MI-Inconsistent Behaviors

The avoidance of behaviors that are inconsistent with the spirit of MI may be even more important than maximizing the use of MI-consistent behaviors. Gaume, Gmel, Faouzi, and Daeppen (2009) found that the percentage of MI-inconsistent and MI-consistent skills used in session were better predictors of drinking outcomes than the overall use of MI-consistent skills. This is consistent with the findings of Miller et al. (1993), which indicated that a therapist's use of confrontation predicted higher levels of client drinking at follow-up. Therefore, an MI therapist not only seeks to increase the use of MI-consistent behaviors, but also seeks to avoid the use of MI-inconsistent behaviors. These include advising without permission, confronting, and directing (Moyers, Martin, Manuel, Hendrickson, & Miller, 2005). However, there may be exceptions to this rule; there is some evidence that confronting, warning, and directing clients within an empathic and accepting therapeutic context may actually enhance a client's participation in treatment (Moyers, Miller, & Hendrickson, 2005). It may be that the manner in which MI-inconsistent behaviors are offered by the therapist is critical to their impact on the client. That is, a confrontation might not always function as a confrontation if it is offered in an empathic, genuine manner.

Miller and Rollnick (2002) describe client resistance and sustain talk as natural reactions to a therapist's attempts to confront and coerce him or her into changing behavior. Therefore, it is important to avoid the use of *confrontation* to evoke client change talk. A therapist confronts when he or she "directly disagrees, argues, corrects, shames, blames, seeks to persuade, criticizes, judges, labels, moralizes, ridicules, or questions the client's honesty" (Miller et al., 2008, p. 6). These behaviors tend to evoke guilt or shame and enhance a sense of parental authority over the client. This throws off the balance of power in the session and will likely evoke more sustain talk than change talk.

Advising without permission is another example of an MI-inconsistent behavior (Miller et al., 2008). When a therapist offers advice, suggestions, or solutions without first obtaining permission, this detracts from the collaborative spirit and also may reduce the client's perception of choice. Sometimes a client may ask a therapist for advice, in which case permission has indirectly been obtained by the therapist. Rather than give advice, a skilled MI therapist will focus on eliciting from the client his or her own ideas about the target behavior and how change might occur.

Directing is defined as giving the client orders, imperatives, or demands (Miller et al., 2008). This can include telling the client to try a new behavior, telling the client what he or she needs to do with respect to treatment, or explaining what the client must do in order to change his or her behavior. The result may be to minimize the client's sense of autonomy and diminish the overall spirit of collaboration between the therapist and the client.

Microskills: A Means toward an End

Microskills, or general clinical skills related to most types of therapy, that are important in MI include open-ended questions, affirmations, reflections, and summaries. These methods can be easily remembered with the acronym OARS. Because affirmations have been discussed previously, this section will focus on questions, reflections, and summary statements.

Therapist questions are a relatively common part of any psychosocial intervention. In MI, it is important for a therapist to encourage the client's expression so that he or she exhibits speech that may be shaped by the therapist (Miller & Rollnick, 2002). One way that this is accomplished is by the asking of open-ended, rather than closed-ended, questions. A *closed-ended question* is one that can be answered with a yes or no or a limited set of potential responses. For example, "Do you want to change your drinking?" is a closed-ended question because it pulls for a yes-or-no response from the client. An *open-ended question*, in contrast, invites an infinite set of potential responses. "What do you want to do about your drinking?" is an open-ended question because the client could respond in many different ways. Particularly skillful open-ended questions will seek to directly elicit change talk by asking for reasons for change, potential avenues for change, consequences of the behavior, or ability to change the behavior. An MI therapist should attempt to use a majority of open-ended questions with clients and minimize his or her use of closed-ended questions.

Miller and Rollnick (2002) define a *reflection* as a guess at the meaning of what the client has verbalized. Because a reflective statement merely makes an observation or guess about what the client is thinking, it is less likely to pull resistance from the client. A therapist may offer simple reflections by stating back exactly what the client has just said or paraphrasing the content. For example, if a client says, "I don't think I can change my drinking," a simple reflection would be "You feel unsure about your ability to change your drinking." A complex reflection, however, adds more meaning to the client's statement by drawing a conclusion, emphasizing emotion, or highlighting an important insight. For example, a complex reflection of the previous client statement could be "The thought of changing your drinking scares you." A skilled MI therapist uses reflections to highlight and reinforce change talk. Using a *double-sided reflection*, or a reflection of both sides of the client's ambivalence, can be a useful way to invite further exploration of a client's change talk. For example, "You really enjoy the feeling using marijuana gives you but you are worried about failing a drug test at work" would be an example of a double-sided reflection. Ending the reflection with the change talk statement invites the client to say more about his or her reasons for change. Often, when a therapist differentially responds to change talk, the client will respond by providing more or stronger change talk.

Summaries are a special kind of reflection that pull together the client's important points in a clear and coherent way. A summary statement can reinforce something a client has said, provide direction for where to go next, show the client that the therapist has understood what has been said so far, and set the stage for the client to further elaborate (Miller & Rollnick, 2002). A skilled MI therapist will summarize client statements about change in order to reinforce and elicit further change statements. A summary can also be a useful way to bring the conversation back to the target behavior when the focus has wandered elsewhere.

Putting Together the Technical and Relational Components

Often therapists new to MI will focus specifically on increasing their use of the microskills without an eye toward the bigger picture of evoking client change talk. However, in Miller and Rose's (2009) theory, both the relational and the technical components of MI are important. A therapist's empathy and MI spirit will lead both directly to client behavior change and indirectly through evocation of change talk. A therapist who uses accurate empathy and who fosters an environment of collaboration, evocation, and autonomy will create a context in which the client is free to explore his or her personal motivation for change without the fear of persecution or judgment. As a result, a client in this context will likely exhibit less resistance and more change talk.

The technical component involves maximizing MI-consistent behaviors, such as open-ended questions and accurate reflections, and minimizing MI-inconsistent behaviors, such as directing and advising without permission. Like the relational component, these MI-consistent methods both directly predict client behavior change and indirectly predict outcome through the elicitation of change talk (Miller & Rose, 2009). A skilled MI therapist uses these methods to differentially elicit and reinforce the client's desire, ability, reasons, and need to change the target behavior. These technical skills are used as a means toward an end of client change talk. This directive skill comes with training and experience.

A Word about Training

Learning MI is more complicated than it may seem. In one study by Miller and Mount (2001), therapists left a 2-day training workshop feeling proficient about their MI skills. However, recordings of work samples, when coded for MI competence, showed little-to-modest improvement in MI skill and little change in client change talk. Thus, it is important for those learning MI to keep in mind that one workshop is usually not enough to gain proficiency. Therapists learning MI are encouraged to seek additional supervision and feedback, just as they would for any other complex psychosocial treatment. Feedback of a therapist's MI skills and additional coaching by an expert supervisor have been found to improve MI competence beyond the effects of the usual workshop-only learning format (Miller, Yahne, Moyers, Martinez, & Pirritano, 2004). Further, therapist competence translates into client outcomes. Gaume et al. (2009) found that therapists who were more skillful in MI, as judged by independent ratings of MI competence, achieved better client outcomes than therapists who were less skillful.

Developing Discrepancy in Favor of Change

Sustain talk may be a part of client resistance to change. In MI, resistance is seen as a natural part of ambivalence when considering change. Miller and Rollnick (2002) emphasize the importance of "rolling with resistance" as a way to minimize client defensiveness. This may involve affirming or supporting the client's effort or using reflections to indicate understanding of the client's situation or feelings. However, according to Miller and Rose's (2009) theory, sustain talk should not be evoked and reinforced in the same way as change talk. A skilled MI therapist will recognize and validate a client's reasons for maintaining the status quo when the *client* brings them up but will then shift the focus back toward arguments for change.

Values Clarification

Another way a therapist might develop discrepancy between goals and behavior is by discussing the client's personal values. Miller and Rollnick (2002, p. 285) define *values* as "behavioral ideals or preferences for experiences." A therapist might simply ask a client about his or her personal values or use a structured task such as a card sort to elicit this information (Miller, C'de Baca, Matthews, & Wilbourne, 2001). A therapist might then explore with the client how his or her current behavior is related to these values or how his or her behavior is helping or hindering his or her work in important life areas. A similar activity is the exploration of the client's short- and long-term goals. A therapist might elicit this information from the client and then explore how his or her behavior is assisting in the attainment of these goals. Further discrepancy can be developed by asking the client to imagine his or her ideal life and how his or her behavior fits in with that image.

Giving Feedback and Information

Though MI does not rely on education as a primary means of eliciting motivation, certain information and relevant feedback can be useful in developing discrepancy between current behavior and future goals. When giving information, there is a risk of enhancing the view of the therapist as an expert. One way to avoid this risk is by asking the client first what he or she knows about the topic of interest (e.g., side effects of prescription medications). Then the therapist will provide information and ask for a response from the client. This is referred to as the "elicit–provide–elicit" formula (Rollnick, Mason, & Butler, 1999). This system can be especially useful when a therapist feels ethically compelled to give information. A therapist may also ask permission directly before giving the information or indirectly by indicating that the client should feel free to refuse the information.

A major component of many types of substance abuse treatment is a detailed assessment. The information that results from this assessment can be very useful in developing discrepancy. A therapist must tread lightly, however, as a client may respond with resistance when facing difficult information. It is useful to ask permission to go over the feedback, provide it in a neutral fashion, and then pay careful attention to the client's response. If the client dismisses it, the therapist should avoid arguing and move on to the next topic.

Putting It Together

In a typical MI session, a therapist might begin by working to foster an atmosphere that exemplifies the MI spirit. A therapist will explore both sides of the client's ambivalence regarding a specific target behavior while enhancing the client's autonomy and perception of collaboration. The therapist will use the technical skills and relational skills described above, along with specific MI methods, to develop discrepancy and evoke client change talk. The therapist may then begin to be more selective and directive regarding the evocation and reinforcement of change talk. As the session continues, the therapist will seek to strengthen a client's change talk and elicit commitment language regarding changing the behavior. If a client seems sufficiently motivated to change, the therapist and the client may decide to develop a collaborative change plan. Alternatively, a therapist may determine that a client is not ready to make a commitment to change and will in this case accept the client's decision in a nonjudgmental and supportive manner.

When Should a Therapist Use MI?

No treatment is effective for every client. There are situations in which MI will likely be helpful with clients and others when perhaps another form of treatment should be used. An assumption of MI is that it is most suited to clients who are ambivalent about their behavior. When a client is genuinely not ambivalent about making a change, MI will probably not be a useful approach. This happens at times when clients are comfortable with the costs of their behavior, when they are coerced into treatment, or when their behavior is costing them nothing. Alternatively, when a client has reached the action phase where he or she is fully ready to change, a therapist may transition into an action-oriented treatment rather than engage in further exploration with MI. MI is often used as a prelude to other types of psychosocial treatment; there is evidence that several sessions of MI preceding another type of treatment may enhance treatment retention and the strength and endurance in behavior change (Brown & Miller, 1993; Burke, Arkowitz, & Menchola, 2003; Hettema et al., 2005).

Another important assumption in MI is that the client must have some intrinsic motivation to change his or her behavior. This intrinsic motivation can certainly originate in the form of consequences from others. It is relatively common, in our experience, that ambivalence about a behavior can come from a consequence such as an arrest, a health problem, or difficulties with a partner or job performance. Nevertheless, in situations where the client is mandated to treatment or the client's autonomy is somehow compromised, MI may not be appropriate if the client carries no genuine ambivalence to the treatment session. Because the client's autonomy and freedom of choice are important to the spirit of MI, it may compromise a therapist's ability to use this treatment if the client does not have freedom of choice. A client may feel pressured to say what he or she thinks the therapist may want to hear or provide disingenuous change talk. Amhrein et al. (2003) found that clients who provided more change talk at the beginning of the session and clients whose level of change talk did not change throughout a session were less likely to maintain abstinence. However, many clients who are initially mandated to substance abuse treatment through the court system do find treatment helpful in reducing their using behavior. Negative consequences in this context are more apparent; thus ambivalence may be more likely when strong negative consequences are experienced.

Selecting a Target Behavior

Certain target behaviors seem more suited for MI than others. A target for treatment in MI should be a behavior of which both the client and therapist have an accurate understanding. A clear target allows the therapist to appropriately direct the session and evoke, reinforce, and strengthen change talk related to that target behavior. Change talk, by definition, is speech related to the desire, ability, reason, need, or commitment to change a specific target behavior. A more controversial question within the literature is how many behavioral targets should be addressed at once. Particularly within behavioral medicine, clients may be interested in changing multiple health behaviors. For example, a diagnosis of diabetes points to several target behaviors that could be a focus of treatment including diet, exercise, medication adherence, blood sugar monitoring, and stress management. Rollnick et al. (2008) recommend exploring each of these potential targets with the client and initially targeting the one in which the client is most interested. Most research suggests that the focus should be on one behavior at a time.

Selecting an MI Therapist

Because accurate empathy and the MI spirit are likely to vary naturally from therapist to therapist, it may be desirable to select potential MI therapists based on initial levels of these qualities (Miller, Moyers, Arciniega, Ernst, & Forcehimes, 2005). Also, a therapist's baseline level of counseling skills predicts better posttraining MI skill level (Moyers et al., 2008). Therefore, those clinicians with better basic counseling skills may be better able to learn MI and use it more competently in practice. Gaume et al. (2009) examined a series of therapist characteristics they referred to as "MI attitude," which included therapist acceptance, MI spirit, use of complex reflections, using more reflections than questions, and avoidance of warning and confronting that predicted more beneficial client outcomes. Similarly, Moyers et al. (2005) found that therapists' interpersonal skills, as measured by global ratings of therapist acceptance, egalitarianism, empathy, warmth, and MI spirit, were associated with higher levels of client involvement in treatment, further supporting the value of the MI spirit. Therefore, a focus on the development of this MI spirit, or "attitude," and/or a preselection of therapists on initial levels of these qualities may facilitate the development of the most effective MI therapists.

Case Example

Here is an example of how MI might work with a hypothetical, ambivalent client named Abby. Abby is a college student who was recently charged with possession of marijuana and has been mandated to treatment as part of her probation. For brevity, the illustration presents a relatively low-risk client.

(1) INTERVIEWER: Hi, Abby. Thanks so much for coming in today. Can you tell me a little bit about what brought you here? [closed question, evocation]

(2) ABBY: Well, to be honest, I'm not really happy about being here. I got caught at a party with a little pot and it's like it's the end of the world or something.

(3) INTERVIEWER: So you're here because you had some pot on you at a party and everyone seems to be overreacting to it. I can understand why you don't want to be here. [simple reflection, rolling with resistance]

(4) ABBY: Well, it just seems like people are taking it too far. My parents aren't even speaking to me, I might be kicked out of school, and now I have all this legal stuff to deal with.

(5) INTERVIEWER: It feels pretty overwhelming for you right now with all of these problems coming up with the courts, school, and your parents. That's a lot for anyone to deal with! I want you to know that my purpose here isn't to judge you but to have a conversation with you about your marijuana use so that you can make the choice that's right for you. [support, collaboration, evocation]

(6) ABBY: I don't want to quit smoking weed, but the idea of getting kicked out of school is terrifying.

(7) INTERVIEWER: After this legal problem, it seems that the negatives might be outweighing the positives. [complex reflection of change talk]

(8) ABBY: It was so embarrassing having to go to court, I could have just screamed. I mean, I don't belong there. I'm a good person, I work hard in school, I'm smart. Now everyone just sees me as this slacker pothead. I mean, sure, weed helps me relax, especially after exams or on the weekends, but it never affects school.

(9) INTERVIEWER: As a college student you deal with a lot of stress. The weed helps you wind down but it never affects your performance in your classes. Doing well in school and working hard is really important to you. [support, complex reflection of sustain talk]

(10) ABBY: Well, actually, I guess in the last semester, I've started smoking more often during the week. There have been a few times where I haven't made it to class or just couldn't get my homework done. But I work hard, I deserve to slack off every once in a while. It's normal for people to miss class occasionally.

(11) INTERVIEWER: Weed is almost like an escape for you, it helps you cope with all of the demands. You said you've noticed though that smoking weed has influenced school a little more recently. Tell me more about that. [complex reflection of sustain talk, open-ended question]

(12) ABBY: Exactly—it's like a minivacation. This last semester has been hell! I never should have taken 18 credits. There are times when I feel so overwhelmed, all I can do is cry. Smoking pot helps to calm me down and make me feel normal again for a little while.

(13) INTERVIEWER: So you were already overwhelmed with school and now, with all of these possession charges and everything that's come along with it, you're faced with even more stress you don't need. That's got to be tough to deal with. [complex reflection of change talk, support]

(14) ABBY: Yeah, it really doesn't seem fair. All of my friends smoke

and they aren't having to deal with all of this drama. All of this over a little bit of pot. The stuff should be legal anyway.

(15) INTERVIEWER: It almost doesn't seem worth it. [complex reflection of change talk]

(16) ABBY: Yeah, for all of the drama it's caused in my life. But it just makes me feel so much better. There were times in the past few weeks that all I wanted to do was smoke. The only thing that stopped me was the stupid drug test I have to take for my probation officer.

(17) INTERVIEWER: On the one hand, you're feeling like you want to smoke even more because of all of the stress you're under and, on the other hand, you feel like it's not worth all of the issues that have come up around it. [double-sided complex reflection of both sustain and change talk]

(18) ABBY: I'm not sure what to do.

(19) INTERVIEWER: You want something to change but you aren't sure what yet. I know you're feeling pressured but I want you to know that the choice with what you do with your marijuana use is completely up to you. The goals we make in here will be goals that are important to you. [simple reflection of change talk, affirm, support autonomy, support collaboration]

(20) ABBY: Okay, that sounds good. My parents sure want me to stop.

So far, the therapist has focused on building rapport and evoking the client's ideas about her marijuana use and her feelings about the consequences that have arisen. Initially, Abby verbalized some resistance (in comment 2) to coming in for treatment. However, the therapist reflected it and rolled with resistance, rather than arguing with her. The therapist also asked an open-ended question to elicit both sides of Abby's ambivalence regarding her marijuana use (comment 5). Even though the statement the therapist used was a reflection (and not a question), it elicited Abby's ideas about the pros and cons of her behavior. There were several points where the therapist offered statements of support (comments 3, 5, 9, 13, and 19). This enhances the collaborative atmosphere of the session. The therapist also fostered collaboration with Abby in line 5 by explaining that she wasn't going to judge her, that she wanted to hear her ideas about her using, and in comment 19 by explaining that the goals made in treatment would reflect what she was interested in working on. The therapist avoided a debate about legality (comment 14) and explicitly pointed out that Abby had the freedom to choose whether or not she changed her behavior (comment 19) which supported her autonomy. The therapist also enhanced the spirit of evocation in the session and elicited change talk by proactively eliciting Abby's experiences and ideas regarding the target behavior (comments 5 and 11) by asking open-ended questions. The therapist used many accurate complex reflections (comments 5, 7, 9, 11, 13, 15, and 17) to both enhance accurate empathy and elicit change talk. In fact, there were many more reflections offered than questions. As a result, Abby is verbalizing quite a bit of change talk. There were many instances in which she offered both change and sustain talk in the same sentence. This demonstrates Abby's ambivalence about changing her marijuana use. Here is where the therapist can begin to direct the discussion more toward the change talk by using the technical MI skills. A specific technique that can be helpful is the double-sided reflection (comment 17). This reflection highlights both sides of the ambivalence, which develops discrepancy. Ending the reflection with the change talk statement pulls for more change talk from the client.

(21) INTERVIEWER: Your parents are pretty upset about your marijuana use. [simple reflection]

(22) ABBY: Yeah, it all seems so crazy. I just don't understand how a little weed could be this big of a deal. I mean, they really should legalize it. It helps with all kinds of medical conditions.

(23) INTERVIEWER: It seems to you like you've paid a high price for something that should be legal anyway. It's hard to understand how weed can be bad when it can help people with all kinds of problems. It helps you with your stress. [rolls with resistance, complex reflection of sustain talk]

(24) ABBY: I should probably be able to deal with it on my own.

(25) INTERVIEWER: You don't want to have to use weed to be able to lower your stress. It's important to you to be able to handle it on your own. [complex reflection of change talk]

(26) ABBY: Kinda. But weed is just so easy.

(27) INTERVIEWER: You've mentioned several benefits of using marijuana for you: it helps you manage your stress pretty easily, it helps you feel "normal" when you're feeling really anxious, and it's almost like a minivacation. What else do you like about marijuana? [simple reflection of sustain talk, open-ended question]

(28) ABBY: Well, I like the smell of it. Sometimes it helps me just be silly and laugh and have a good time with my friends.

(29) INTERVIEWER: So the smell and the fact that you have fun with your friends when you do it. [simple reflection of sustain talk]

(30) ABBY: Sometimes it's so nice to be able to just laugh with your friends, you know?

(31) INTERVIEWER: That's almost like the minivacation you were

talking about. It can help you escape the drudgery of studying and helps you just be silly for a little while. [complex reflection of sustain talk]

(32) ABBY: Yeah, exactly.

(33) INTERVIEWER: There's a lot that you enjoy about smoking marijuana but right now you're facing even more stress because of it. Tell me more about some of the downsides of your marijuana use. [double-sided reflection; open-ended question]

Abby backpedaled a bit at the beginning of this exchange so the therapist elected to explore the benefits of maintaining the status quo as a way to roll with resistance. However, the therapist brought the conversation back to her reasons for change in comment 33.

(34) ABBY: Now all I can think about is my mom's face when I told her that I had been arrested.

(35) INTERVIEWER: Your parents took it pretty hard. [simple reflection]

(36) ABBY: Yeah, they are pretty disappointed in me. I feel awful. I want them to be proud of me, you know?

(37) INTERVIEWER: Definitely. It's important that your parents see you for who you are, not just for the weed. [complex reflection of change talk]

(38) ABBY: And now I'm just the kid who might flunk out of school because she's a pothead.

(39) INTERVIEWER: I can see how this must be hard for you, especially since you are so hard working and dedicated to school. Tell me about your goals with respect to school. How do you see your life once you graduate? [support, affirm, open-ended question]

(40) ABBY: Well I'm pre-med now. My goal is to do well in my classes and then go to med school once I'm done with my bachelor's degree. But now I wonder if that's going to happen.

(41) INTERVIEWER: You're afraid your legal problems due to the marijuana might influence your future goals. [complex reflection]

In this exchange, the therapist evoked change talk from Abby by using open-ended questions and reflections. The therapist helped to highlight a discrepancy between Abby's future goals (med school), her values (hard work), and her behavior (using marijuana). The therapist also supported and affirmed her, which enhanced the accepting and empathic atmosphere of the session. Exploring the negative aspects of marijuana use without arguing, persuading, or giving information might be difficult for some therapists. The most important thing is to evoke *Abby's* ideas about the costs of using marijuana. The therapist might continue on this line of thought for a while, eliciting change talk and attempting to elicit stronger and stronger statements.

> (42) INTERVIEWER: Okay, I feel like I have a pretty good grasp of the things you like about marijuana and the things that aren't so good. Thanks so much for sharing all of this with me! It sounds like the main things you like about marijuana are that it helps you relax, it helps you cope when you feel stressed, it's like a minivacation away from schoolwork, and you have a lot of fun when you smoke with your friends. The things you don't like are the fact that you got in trouble for having it, you noticed that it affected your motivation to go to class or do homework occasionally, and your parents are disappointed that you use marijuana. What do you make of all that? [simple reflection, open-ended question; summary]
>
> (43) ABBY: Well, I just won't smoke right now. I'm on probation.
>
> (44) INTERVIEWER: I think that's a sensible plan. How do you feel about talking about your plan in more detail? [affirm, open-ended question]

The therapist heard a shift in Abby's language while weighing the pros and cons of smoking. The therapist provided a detailed summary of both sides of the ambivalence and then asked Abby what she wanted to do. At this point, three different things could happen. Abby may feel ready to commit to a change and she and the therapist could begin to develop a collaborative change plan. On the flip side, Abby may resolve her ambivalence the other way and decide that it is more important to continue using marijuana. If this occurs, the therapist would accept her right to make this decision. It is important to remember that a therapist does not have to agree with the client's decision. The third option is that Abby may still be unsure about what she wants to do. The therapist should carefully avoid pushing her into making a change when she is not ready. If this is the case, the therapist might continue to explore Abby's ambivalence and elicit change talk. In our example, Abby seems ready to talk about changing her marijuana use. Up until this point, the therapist has focused on eliciting change talk. Now the therapist will want to transition to a focus on evoking stronger change talk and commitment statements.

> (45) ABBY: That sounds good. I'm just not sure how to do it.
>
> (46) INTERVIEWER: It's time to change, but you aren't sure where to start. [complex reflection]

Abby seems to be feeling somewhat unsure of herself so the therapist may choose to explore how she thinks change might happen. It may also be useful to explore Abby's past successes or use more affirmation statements to enhance her confidence in her own ability to change. One particularly useful tool is the confidence ruler, as demonstrated below.

> (47) INTERVIEWER: So Abby, if you had to say how confident you were in the ability to decrease your pot use on a scale from 1 to 10, with 10 being completely confident and 1 being completely unable to do so, where do you feel you are? [closed question]
>
> (48) ABBY: I guess maybe a 4.
>
> (49) INTERVIEWER: Okay, a 4. About in the midrange. What makes you a 4 and not a 2? [simple reflection, open question]

This may be a somewhat unexpected response from the therapist. However, asking why she is not a lower number on the scale will actually encourage more change talk, particularly ability statements that will enhance the client's confidence in her ability to make changes. This tool can also be used to elicit change talk regarding a client's perceived *importance* of or *readiness* to change a behavior.

From here, the interviewer will want to further strengthen Abby's commitment to change her marijuana use. If MI is being used as a stand-alone treatment, the therapist may help the client develop a change plan. In developing the plan, it will be important to continue to respect Abby's choice and autonomy and incorporate her perspective and ideas about how to change. If MI is being used as a prelude to another form of substance use treatment, the therapist may refer Abby or transition into the other treatment approach. Again, the illustration presents a relatively low-risk client. MI has been used effectively, both alone and in combination with other treatments, with much more dependent and high-risk clients.

Conclusion

MI is a flexible treatment in terms of the types of target behaviors it treats and duration of treatment. MI has been shown to be effective as a brief one-session intervention, a prelude to another form of treatment, or a stand-alone treatment for behavior change. However, it is important to remember that MI will not be useful for every client, for every therapist, or in every context. It is important to pay close attention to each client's outcomes. If MI does not move clients toward change, even with methods in keeping with the MI spirit, supervision, and coaching, switching to another form of treatment may be warranted. This flexibility and ability to monitor client outcomes is important in translating treatments that have been found effective in research studies into everyday practice.

References

Amrhein, P. C., Miller, W. R., Yahne, C. E., Palmer, M., & Fulcher, L. (2003). Client commitment language during motivational interviewing predicts drug use outcomes. *Journal of Consulting and Clinical Psychology, 71*, 862–878.

Bien, T. H., Miller, W. H., & Boroughs, J. M. (1993). Motivational interviewing with alcohol outpatients. *Behavioural and Cognitive Psychotherapy, 21*(4), 347–356.

Brown, J. M., & Miller, W. R. (1993). Impact of motivational interviewing on participation and outcome in residential alcoholism treatment. *Psychology of Addictive Behaviors, 7*, 211–218.

Burke, B. L., Arkowitz, H., & Menchola, M. (2003). The efficacy of motivational interviewing: A meta-analysis of controlled clinical trials. *Journal of Consulting and Clinical Psychology, 71*, 843–861.

Gaume, J., Gmel, G., Faouzi, M., & Daeppen, J. B. (2009). Counselor skill influences outcomes of brief motivational interventions. *Journal of Substance Abuse Treatment, 37*, 151–159.

Hettema, J., Steele, J., & Miller, W. R. (2005). Motivational interviewing. *Annual Review of Clinical Psychology, 1*, 91–111.

Lundahl, B. W., Kunz, C., Brownell, C., Tollefson, D., & Burke, B. L. (2010). A meta-analysis of motivational interviewing: Twenty-five years of empirical studies. *Research on Social Work Practice, 20*, 137–160.

Miller, W. R., Benefield, R. G., & Tonigan, J. S. (1993). Enhancing motivation for change in problem drinking: A controlled comparison of two therapist styles. *Journal of Consulting and Clinical Psychology, 61*, 455–461.

Miller, W. R., C'de Baca, J., Matthews, D. B., & Wilbourne, P. L. (2001). Personal values card sort. Retrieved from *www.motivationalinterview.org/library/valuesinstructions.pdf*.

Miller, W. R., & Mount, K. A. (2001). A small study of training in motivational interviewing: Does one workshop change clinician and client behavior? *Behavioural and Cognitive Psychotherapy, 29*, 457–471.

Miller, W. R., & Moyers, T. B. (2006). Eight stages in learning motivational interviewing. *Journal of Teaching in the Addictions, 5*, 3–17.

Miller, W. R., Moyers, T. B., Arciniega, L., Ernst, D., & Forcehimes, A. (2005). Training, supervision and quality monitoring of the COMBINE study behavioral interventions. *Journal of Studies on Alcohol, 66*(Suppl. 15), 188–195.

Miller, W. R., Moyers, T. B., Ernst, D., & Amrhein, P. (2008). *Manual for the Motivational Interviewing Skill Code (MISC), Version 2.1*. Unpublished manual, University of New Mexico. Retrieved from *casaa.unm.edu/mimanuals.html*.

Miller, W. R., & Rollnick, S. (2002). *Motivational interviewing: Preparing people for change* (2nd ed.). New York: Guilford Press.

Miller, W. R., & Rose, G. S. (2009). Toward a theory of motivational interviewing. *American Psychologist, 64*, 527–537.

Miller, W. R., Yahne, C. E., Moyers, T. B., Martinez, J., & Pirritano, M. (2004). A randomized trial of methods to help clinicians learn motivational interviewing. *Journal of Consulting and Clinical Psychology, 72,* 1050–1062.

Moyers, T. B., Manuel, J. K., Wilson, P. G., Hendrickson, S. M. L., Talcott, W., & Durand, P. (2008). A randomized trial investigating training in motivational interviewing for behavioral health providers. *Behavioural and Cognitive Psychotherapy, 36,* 149–162.

Moyers, T. B., Martin, T., Houck, J.M., Christopher, P. J., & Tonigan, J. S. (2009). From in-session behaviors to drinking outcomes: A causal chain for motivational interviewing. *Journal of Consulting and Clinical Psychology, 77,* 1113–1124.

Moyers, T. B., Martin, T., Manuel, J. K., Hendrickson, S. M. L., & Miller, W. R. (2005). Assessing competence in the use of motivational interviewing. *Journal of Substance Abuse Treatment, 28,* 19–26.

Moyers, T. B., Miller, W. R., & Hendrickson, S. M. L. (2005). How does motivational interviewing work?: Therapist interpersonal skill predicts client involvement within motivational interviewing sessions. *Journal of Consulting and Clinical Psychology, 73,* 590–598.

Nigg, C., Allegrante, J. P., & Ory, M. (2002). Theory-comparison and multiple-behavior research: Common themes advancing health behavior research. *Health Education Research, 17,* 670–679.

Rollnick, S. P., Mason, P., & Butler, C. (1999). *Health behavior change: A guide for practitioners.* London, UK: Churchill Livingstone.

Rollnick, S. P., & Miller, W. R. (1995). What is motivational interviewing? *Behavioural and Cognitive Psychotherapy, 23,* 325–334.

Rollnick, S. P., Miller, W. R., & Butler, C. C. (2008). *Motivational interviewing in health care: Helping patients change behavior.* New York: Guilford Press.

Walters, S. T., Rotgers, F., Saunders, B., Wilkinson, C., & Towers, T. (2003). Theoretical perspectives on motivation and addictive behavior. In F. Rotgers, J. Morgenstern, & S. T. Walters (Eds.), *Treating substance abuse: Theory and technique* (2nd ed., pp. 279–297). New York: Guilford Press.

Chapter 3

The Behavioral Economics of Substance Abuse

James G. Murphy
James MacKillop
Rudy E. Vuchinich
Jalie A. Tucker

This chapter explores the basic theory and research that underlies behavioral treatment approaches such as the community reinforcement approach (CRA) and contingency management (CM). These treatments attempt to reduce substance abuse by manipulating one or more basic behavioral mechanisms (e.g., response cost or drug price, alternative reinforcement, or alternative reward delay) that have been shown to influence substance use in laboratory research. Among substance abuse treatments, CM is somewhat unique in that it originated from experimental psychology rather than from the psychotherapy literature or from cultural and spiritual ideas about addictive behavior. In this chapter, we show how the underlying "matching law" theory developed, discuss some of the conceptual innovations produced by this theory, and present some ways that these innovations connect with behavioral economics. We then present the basic concepts and empirical relations in the behavioral economics of substance abuse, with an emphasis on the role of drug price, alternative reinforcement, and temporal discounting on individuals' drug use patterns. We highlight several recent studies that suggest that these variables may be critically related to the process of changing addictive behavior patterns. We conclude with a brief introduction to neuroeconomics, an emerging field that bridges behavioral economics and cognitive neuroscience.

The Matching Law

The original behavioral theory of choice was called the "matching law" (Herrnstein, 1970). The theory began with tests of the way that animals made choices in laboratory settings (Rachlin, 1987). In a typical scenario, animals were exposed to two schedules of reinforcement (the choice alternatives) simultaneously. The dependent variable was the frequency of responding to the two alternatives. Herrnstein's (1961) original study varied the frequency of reinforcement for each alternative. That is, more frequent reinforcement was provided by one alternative and then by the other.

The critical issue in Herrnstein's experiment was how the relative frequency of responding was distributed across the two choice alternatives. The result was surprisingly simple, as shown in Equation 1.

$$B_1/B_2 = FR_1/FR_2 \qquad (1)$$

In Equation 1, B_1 and B_2 represent the number of responses allocated to alternatives 1 and 2, respectively, and FR_1 and FR_2 represent the frequency or number of reinforcements received from alternatives 1 and 2, respectively. Thus, the animals' behavior was distributed over the response options in direct proportion to the frequency of reinforcement received from those options. The more frequent the reinforcement, the greater the rate of responding. For example, if one-third of the total reinforcements were received from alternative 1, then one-third of responding was allocated to alternative 1, and so on for different distributions of responding and reinforcement across the alternatives. Subsequent research investigated how variations in dimensions of reinforcement other than frequency would affect relative behavioral allocation. Catania (1963) studied schedules in which the frequency of reinforcement was held constant and *the amount of food per reinforcement* was manipulated. He found that behavioral allocation matched relative reinforcement amounts, as reflected in Equation 2.

$$B_1/B_2 = AR_1/AR_2 \qquad (2)$$

In Equation 2, B_1 and B_2 are the same as in Equation 1, and AR_1 and AR_2 represent the amounts of food received per reinforcement from options 1 and 2, respectively. Thus, relative behavioral allocation was directly proportional to relative reinforcement amount; the greater the amount of food given per reinforcement, the greater the rate of responding. So, for example, if the amount of food received per reinforcement from option 1 was twice that of option 2, then twice as many responses were allocated to option 1 than to option 2.

As a further extension, Chung and Herrnstein (1967) studied the effects of *delay of reinforcement* on behavioral allocation. They found a matching relation in which relative behavioral allocation matched the inverse of the relative delays of reinforcement, as depicted in Equation 3.

$$B_1/B_2 = DR_2/DR_1 \tag{3}$$

In Equation 3, B_1 and B_2 are as before, and DR_1 and DR_2 represent the delays of receipt of reinforcement from options 1 and 2, respectively. Thus, behavioral allocation was inversely proportional to the relative delays of reinforcement; the longer the wait, the lower the response. So, if reinforcement for option 1 was delayed twice as long as that for option 2, then half as many responses would be allocated to option 1 than to option 2. Research on behavioral allocation in choice situations involving different amounts and delays of reinforcement (e.g., Rachlin & Green, 1972) has had significant implications for understanding impulsiveness and self-control. We return to this topic later in the chapter in the context of understanding addictive behavior.

These early empirical results were sufficiently general for Herrnstein (1970) to propose the matching law as an overall framework for describing behavioral allocation to any particular response option. This general version of the matching law is expressed in Equation 4.

$$B_1/B_0 = R_1/R_0 \tag{4}$$

In Equation 4, B_1 and R_1 refer to behavior allocated to and reinforcement received from a particular response option, respectively. B_0 and R_0 refer to behavior allocated to and reinforcement received from all other response options in that situation. Thus, Equation 4 states that the proportion of behavior allocated to any given response option (B_1) will be a joint function of reinforcement received from that option (R_1) and reinforcement received from all other sources (R_0). In other words, any reinforcement is relative to other reinforcement available in the environment.

Relativism of the Matching Law

The relativism of the matching law was a significant departure from the ideas that dominated learning theory at the time (cf. Rachlin & Laibson, 1997). The principle of the reflex was the prevailing concept, in which each response was thought to correspond to a particular environmental or internal stimulus. Thus, the stream of behavior was decomposed into a series of *reflexes*, that is, individual responses as a reaction to external stimuli.

The theory was concerned with understanding the strength of individual stimulus–response connections (e.g., Hull, 1943) or of individual responses (e.g., Skinner, 1938). Given this focus on individual responses directed by the reflex concept, the determinants of any particular response were thought to reside in the positive or negative stimuli that immediately preceded or immediately followed it. Little attention was paid to the more general context of other behavior and other consequences that surrounded a particular response. But Herrnstein's (1970) research and equations clearly indicated that behavior allocated to a particular response option could be altered by modifying the reinforcement for other options. This finding did not accord well with an account based on reflexes.

Assume, for example, that we want to increase the frequency of B_1 in Equation 4, which we could easily do by enriching R_1. An account based on individual responses would argue that the enriched R_1 strengthened the reflex of which B_1 is a part, and thereby increased its occurrence. This is fine as far as it goes, but it ignores the more general context in which B_1 and R_1 are occurring. Because the matching law focuses on that context, Equation 4 provides a somewhat different interpretation of such a change: enriching R_1 would increase the reinforcement ratio on the right side of the equation, which would realign the behavior ratio on the left side of the equation so that B_1 constituted a larger fraction of behavioral output. Thus, according to the matching law, enriching R_1 increases B_1 because R_1 is now relatively more valuable in this context. Moreover, in Equation 4, B_1 and B_0 exhaust the response possibilities, and total behavioral output cannot exceed their sum. Thus, a decrease in B_0 necessarily involves an increase in B_1. So, the matching law states that we also could increase the frequency of B_1 by decreasing R_0, the reinforcement for behavior other than B_1. Decreasing R_0, like increasing R_1, also would increase the reinforcement ratio (i.e., make R_1 relatively more valuable) on the right side of Equation 4. This, in turn, would realign the behavior ratio on the left side of the equation so that a larger fraction of behavioral output would consist of B_1. Such indirect behavior modification due to the relativism inherent in the matching law was not easily handled by accounts that focused on individual responses (Rachlin & Laibson, 1997).

Molarity of the Matching Law

The matching law is a *molar* account of behavior in that it relates aggregates of behavior (e.g., patterns of drinking and exercise over time) to aggregates of reinforcement as measured over some interval (cf. Vuchinich, 1995). It cannot and does not attempt to account for the occurrence of particular B_1 or B_0 responses (the decision to drink vs. exercise on a particular day or moment), which would be the goal of a *molecular* account of behavior. Abandoning the focus of particular responses was a significant departure from what was regarded as an acceptable explanation for behavior at the time (Lacey & Rachlin, 1978). Other influential behavioral theories in that era (e.g., Hull, 1943; Skinner, 1938) were molecular and were designed, at least in principle, to explain the occurrence of particular responses. In contrast, the matching law is concerned with understanding the distribution of behavior to response alternatives in relation to the contextually determined value of the consequences of those alternatives.

The Economic Connection

Given this shift in orientation, the field became concerned with understanding the manner in which behavioral allocation entrains with the availability of valued consequences over time. As this choice literature developed, several scientists (e.g., Hursh, 1980; Rachlin, Green, Kagel, & Battalio, 1976) recognized that this type of question was very similar to the questions addressed by consumer demand theory in economics. The basic scenarios were the same; animals in laboratory experiments and human consumers in the economy both allocate limited resources (e.g., time, behavior, money) to gain access to activities of variable value (e.g., eating, drinking, leisure) under conditions of variable environmental constraint. Recognizing this commonality led to a merger of the behavioral analysis of choice and of microeconomic theory, now known as "behavioral economics" (e.g., Hursh, 1980; Kagel, Battalio, & Green, 1995).

Behavioral Economics of Substance Use: Basic Concepts and Empirical Relations

The relevance of behavioral economics in substance abuse was recognized early in its development (e.g., Vuchinich, 1982), and research applications to human substance abuse are growing (e.g., Bickel, Yi, Landes, Hill, & Baxter, 2011; Mackillop & Murphy, 2007; Tucker, Roth, Vignolo, & Westfall, 2009). Behavioral economics applies the general principles of relativism and molarity to understanding substance abuse. As such, behavioral economics has focused on studying patterns of substance abuse as they develop and change over time in the context of changes in access to substance use and to other activities.

In general, the *value* a person places on a substance is a function of the benefit/cost ratio of substance use in relation to the benefit/cost ratios of other available activities. This section summarizes behavioral economic research on substance abuse in terms of three broad topics: (1) substance use as a function of its own benefit/cost ratio (e.g., constraints on access to the abused substance, such as price), (2) substance use as a function of the benefit/cost ratio of other activities (e.g., constraints on access to and price of valuable activities other than substance use), and (3) intertemporal choice situations, in which an individual must choose between outcomes that vary in amount and delay of reinforcement.

Substance Use as a Function of Its Own Benefit/Cost Ratio

Demand, the amount of a commodity that is purchased, is the primary dependent variable in microeconomics (Kagel et al., 1995). Because excessive consumption is the crux of the problem in substance abuse, the focus on demand renders behavioral economics immediately relevant (Hursh, 1993). Early laboratory research demonstrated that consumption of abused substances varies inversely with their cost (cf. Vuchinich & Tucker, 1988); in general, the greater the cost, the lower the use. This relation has been expanded through the analysis of demand curves, which plot consumption of a commodity as a function of its price.

This relation is shown by the solid line in Figure 3.1, a demand curve for a hypothetical commodity A. One key concept for describing this consumption–price relation is *own-price elasticity of demand*, which is the ratio of changes in price to changes in consumption (cf. Hursh, 1993). Thus, own-price elasticity of demand shows how consumption changes as price changes. The dotted line in Figure 3.1 shows "unit elasticity" (–1.0), wherein demand decreases by the same proportion that price increases. Demand elasticities fall along a continuum from *inelastic* demand (e > –1.0), which shows little or no changes in consumption as price changes (the left part of the curve in Figure 3.1), to elastic demand (e < –1.0), which shows substantial changes in consumption as price changes (the right part of the demand curve in Figure 3.1). Demand typically shows mixed elasticity across a range of price changes, being more inelastic at low prices and more elastic at high prices, as depicted by the solid line in Figure 3.1. Most products follow a similar curve. For example, rising gas prices will not produce substantial changes in gas purchases and driving until they get quite high.

Behavioral economic research in this area initially focused on two questions: (1) Does demand for abused substances show an inverse relation with price? (2) Do the quantitative properties of demand curves (i.e., own-price elasticity) aid in the description of the determinants of substance consumption? The answer to both of these questions is yes. DeGrandpre, Bickel, Hughes, Layng, and Badger (1993) analyzed data from numerous drug self-administration experiments using demand curve analyses (including studies of cocaine, *d*-amphetemine, ethanol, morphine, and other drugs). Arranging the data into demand curves revealed mixed elasticity for all drugs studied: demand was inelastic at lower prices and elastic at higher prices.

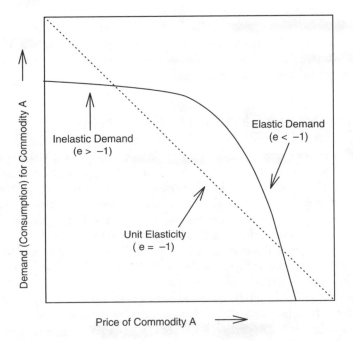

FIGURE 3.1. Demand for hypothetical Commodity *A* as a function of its own price (solid line). Own-price elasticity of demand (*e*) is defined as the ratio of proportional changes in consumption of *A* to proportional changes in the price of *A*. The dotted line shows unit elasticity, in which consumption decreases by the same proportion as price increases. The demand curve for *A* shows the typical mixed elasticity, with relatively inelastic demand at low prices and relatively elastic demand at high prices.

Recently, time- and cost-efficient demand curve measures have been developed and administered in clinical settings to measure both (1) the impact of drug price on reported consumption, and (2) individual differences in demand for drugs (Little & Correia, 2006; Jacobs & Bickel, 1999; MacKillop et al., 2010; Murphy, Correia, & Barnett, 2007; Murphy, MacKillop, Skidmore, & Pederson, 2009; Murphy, MacKillop, Tidey, Brazil, & Colby, 2011; Skidmore & Murphy, 2011). These studies have asked participants to report their hypothetical choices regarding alcohol and drug purchases at varying prices during a fixed period of time (one evening or one day). These reports help generate "demand curves" that show participants' hypothetical consumption at each price (e.g., the standard drinks a participant would purchase across a range of drink prices (e.g., free to $10 per drink). Expenditure curves plot expenditures at each price (i.e., number of drinks purchased multiplied by drink price). These demand and expenditure curves have been used to generate reliable and valid (Murphy et al., 2009) estimates of substance-related reinforcement including demand intensity (i.e., peak consumption at lowest price), elasticity (i.e., changes in the rate of consumption as a function of changes in price), maximum inelastic price (P_{max}), greatest expenditure on alcohol (O_{max}), and breakpoint (i.e., the first price that completely suppresses consumption). Figure 3.2 shows demand and expenditure curves, along with the resulting reinforcement indices. Although demand almost always decreases in response to price increases, there are individual differences in the relative value of these parameters that might measure an important element of substance abuse severity not captured by existing measures of problems or DSM symptoms (MacKillop et al., 2010; Murphy et al., 2009; Tucker et al., 2009), such as the relative behavioral allocation to substance use or elasticity of demand for a particular substance.

As an example, Murphy and MacKillop (2006) used a simulated (hypothetical) alcohol purchase task to generate alcohol demand in a sample of young adult drinkers. They found that the average number of standard drinks consumed was approximately seven when the price was $0.25 or less per drink. Consumption remained at or above five drinks at prices up to $1.50 per drink, and then became more elastic and showed a steady linear decrease as prices increased beyond that. Not surprisingly, participants with a history of engaging in heavy episodic drinking reported more consumption and expenditures, and more inelastic demand. Two other studies that examined individual difference in demand suggested that intensity of demand accounted for unique variance in alcohol problems and dependence symptoms (MacKillop et al., 2010; Murphy et al., 2009). Similar results were found in demand curve analyses of hypothetical cigarette purchases among teen smokers; cigarette purchases varied inversely with price, and more dependent smokers reported greater and more inelastic demand (MacKillop et al., 2008; Murphy et al., 2011).

Importantly, individual differences in demand curve measures of alcohol reinforcement have also been associated with *changes* in drinking following a single motivational intervention for heavy drinking college students. Specifically, drinkers with higher maximum expenditure (i.e., O_{max}) for alcohol and lower price sensitivity (i.e., high breakpoint, P_{max}, and elasticity) at baseline reported greater drinking 6 months following an intervention (MacKillop & Murphy, 2007). Hence, demand curves may measure strength of preference for drugs in a way that predicts responsiveness to interventions. It is possible that participants might actually be matched to interventions using these behavioral economic measures of problem severity.

Another study among 200 heavy drinking college students found that students' hypothetical drinking decreased across the entire range of drink prices if they were instructed to imagine that they had a college class the next morning. Drinking decreased further if they were instructed to

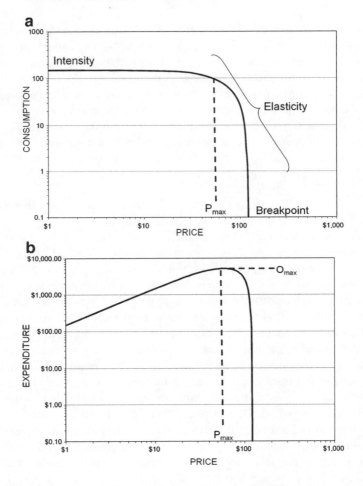

FIGURE 3.2. Prototypical behavioral economic demand and expenditure curves. (a) The demand curve and the following associated facets of demand: intensity (i.e., consumption at minimal price), elasticity (i.e., slope of the demand curve), P_{max} (i.e., maximum inelastic price), and breakpoint (i.e., price at which consumption is reduced to zero). (b) The expenditure curve and O_{max} (i.e., maximum expenditure), with the accompanying P_{max}, which is also the price at which O_{max} takes place. From MacKillop et al. (2009). Copyright 2009. Reprinted with kind permission from Springer Science + Business Media.

imagine that the morning class was going to include a test (Skidmore & Murphy, 2011). In this study, the next morning class can be viewed as an indirect method of increasing the "cost" of drinking or as providing a valued alternative to drinking. The results are consistent with survey research indicating that students drink less when they have class the next morning (Wood, Sher, & Rutledge, 2007). The results also provide support for the behavioral economic view that decisions to drink or use drugs are sensitive both to price and alternative reinforcement contingencies.

Substance Use as a Function of the Benefit/Cost Ratio of Other Activities

Behavioral economic theory assumes that the value of substance use will depend on other available activities and on their benefit/cost ratios. This more general context is a key issue in substance abuse research because decisions to use substances occur in natural environments that presumably contain opportunities to engage in a variety of other activities. Understanding the conditions under which substance consumption emerges as a preferred activity from an array of other activities is a basic problem for substance abuse research (Bickel et al., 2007; Loewenstein, 1996; Redish, 2004; Vuchinich & Heather, 2003). In general, the choice perspective suggests that demand for abused substances will vary inversely with the benefit/cost ratios of other activities. Numerous laboratory studies with animals and humans have demonstrated this important qualitative relationship (reviewed by Higgins, Heil, & Plebani-Lussier, 2004).

Quantifying how drug demand interacts with the availability of and demand for other reinforcers can be explained using the economic concept of *cross-price elasticity of demand*. This concept refers to how demand for one commodity changes when the price for another commodity changes (Hursh, 1993; Kagel et al., 1995). This is represented in Figure 3.3, which shows two possible ways that demand for commodity *B* may change as a function of the price of commodity *A*. If demand varies inversely (positive cross-price), the commodities are *substitutes* (the solid line in Figure 3.3). If demand varies directly (negative cross-price), they are *complements* (the dashed line). For instance, Coke and Pepsi serve as ready substitutes for each other, while flour and sugar are complements.

Bickel, DeGrandpre, and Higgins (1995) evaluated this concept in a reanalysis of 16 drug self-administration studies that looked at substitutability relations between drugs (including caffeine, nicotine, cocaine, alcohol, heroin, and other drugs) and alternative drug and nondrug reinforcers (e.g., food, sucrose, water). Demand for the drugs was related with other reinforcers at all points along the substitutability continuum. In separate studies, for example, substitute relations were found between sucrose and alcohol (when the price of sucrose was low alcohol consumption was low),

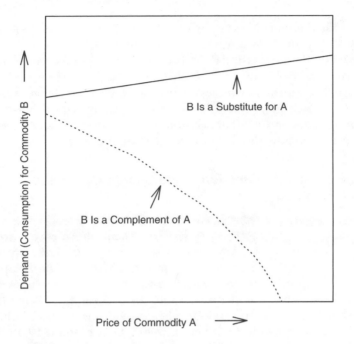

FIGURE 3.3. Demand for hypothetical Commodity *B* as a function of the price of Commodity *A*. Cross-price elasticity of demand is defined as the ratio of proportional changes in consumption of *B* to proportional changes in the price of *A*. Positive cross-price elasticity (solid line) indicates that *B* is a substitute for *A* (consumption of *B* increases as consumption of *A* decreases). Negative cross-price elasticity (dotted line) indicates that *B* is a complement of *A* (consumption of *B* decreases as consumption of *A* decreases).

whereas complement relations were found between alcohol and cigarettes (when the price of alcohol was low cigarette consumption was high). Thus, behavioral economic concepts concerning cross-price elasticity relations are useful for describing how demand for drugs interacts with demand for other types of things.

Benefit/cost ratios of activities other than substance use are also important in understanding substance abuse in the natural environment. In laboratory settings, *positive reinforcement* is defined as a process whereby a behavior increases following the presentation of a reinforcing stimulus (food, drugs, etc.); in naturalistic studies of humans, reinforcement is usually measured by some combination of activity participation and enjoyment ratings (Correia, Carey, Simons, & Borsari, 2003; Correia, Simons, Carey, & Borsari, 1998). Reinforcement surveys, for example, measure the frequency of engagement in, and subjective pleasure associated with, a variety of activities (e.g., socializing, watching TV, exercising, and reading). For instance, jogging would be considered a high-value reinforcer for an individual who jogs frequently and enjoys running. Reinforcement surveys such as the Pleasant Events Schedule (PES; MacPhillamy & Lewinsohn, 1982) have been modified to differentiate substance-related and substance-free reinforcement. Correia et al. (1998) found an inverse relationship between substance-free reinforcement and the frequency of drug and alcohol use. As you might expect, lower participation in and enjoyment of substance-free activities are associated with increased substance use. Other research has suggested that heavy drinkers (Correia et al., 2003) and cocaine users (van Etten, Higgins, Budney, & Badger, 1998) report less reinforcement from a variety of nonsocial activities compared to control participants without a history of heavy drinking or cocaine use. Interestingly, a recent study of college students found that frequent heavy drinkers reported *greater* substance-free reinforcement from peer and sexual activities (Skidmore & Murphy, 2010). So although many categories of substance-free activities may serve as substitutes for substance use, among young adults social activity and substance use may be complements.

Temporal Discounting, Impulsiveness, and Substance Abuse

In everyday life, outcomes of choices typically do not occur immediately. Most often, people make choices to influence future outcomes. Behavioral allocation in these conditions is called *intertemporal choice* because the outcomes of the choice alternatives are spread out in time. Intertemporal choice behavior is especially important for understanding substance abuse, since individuals presumably are repeatedly choosing between a readily available but relatively small reward (substance use) and activities that will produce delayed but more valuable rewards (e.g., positive intimate, family, or social relations; vocational or academic success).

If the smaller reinforcer is available relatively sooner, then intertemporal choice in this situation can be described as either impulsive or self-controlled. Choice of the smaller, sooner reinforcer (SSR) is labeled "impulsive," and choice of the larger, later reinforcer (LLR) is labeled "self-controlled." As an example from the animal laboratory (e.g., Rachlin & Green, 1972), say alternative 1 (the LLR) is 6 seconds of food ($A_1 = 6$) and alternative 2 (the SSR) is 2 seconds of food ($A_2 = 2$), and that the LLR is available 8 seconds after the SSR. These relations are shown in Figure 3.4, with time along the x-axis, reward value along the y-axis, and the rewards represented as vertical boxes at the times they are available. In Figure 3.4, the 2-second food reward (A_2) is available at time 14, and the 6-second food reward (A_1) is available at time 22.

This decision-making process is well described by the hyperbolic temporal discounting function shown in Equation 5 (Mazur, 1987).

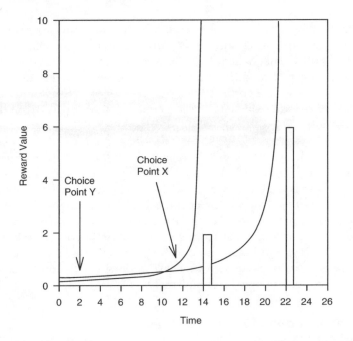

FIGURE 3.4. Intertemporal choice between 2 seconds of food available at time 14 and 6 seconds of food available at time 22. Value curves to the left of the rewards were drawn from Equation 7.

hyperbolic temporal discounting function [handwritten annotation]

$$v_i = A_i / 1 + kD_i \tag{5}$$

In Equation 5, v_i is the present value of a reward of amount A_i that is available after a delay of D_i. The k parameter is a constant that is proportional to the degree of temporal discounting, with higher and lower k values describing greater and lesser degrees of discounting, respectively. This discount function is in the form of a hyperbola; hence it is termed "hyperbolic temporal discounting."

Ainslie (1975, 1992), Rachlin (1995), and others (e.g., Bickel et al., 2007; Loewenstein, 1996) have written extensively on the general implications of hyperbolic discounting for understanding impulsiveness and self-control. These intertemporal choice dynamics also are important for understanding substance abuse. In Figure 3.5, the SSR is analogous to an alcohol or drug consumption episode, and the LLR is analogous to a more valuable but delayed nondrinking or nondrug activity. The choice dynamics that result from hyperbolic discounting are consistent with two general and important aspects of substance abuse patterns. First, even when reward availability does not change, individuals often display ambivalence in that their preference for substance use will vary depending on the amount of time between

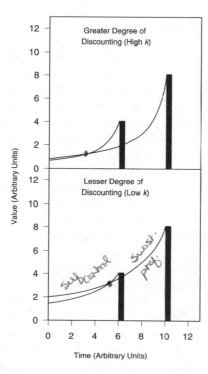

FIGURE 3.5. Both panels show an intertemporal choice between a smaller and a larger reward available at time 6 and time 10, respectively. The upper and lower panels show greater and lesser degrees of hyperbolic temporal discounting, respectively.

the substance use and the alternative activity. The LLRs will be preferred before the point where the reward value curves cross (often at the point that substance use become immediately available), and substance use will be preferred after that point. For example, an individual might prefer the longer delayed rewards associated with sobriety throughout the day (and thus choose to abstain), but switch preferences upon driving past a bar (a signal for immediately available alcohol) on the way home from work. But once the substance is no longer immediately available (the next morning), preference will revert back to the LLRs, and the individual may regret the substance use episode. Such ambivalence is a key feature of substance use problems (e.g., Miller, 1998). Second, the LLRs that enter into these choice dynamics will likely differ across individuals and across time for the same individual (Vuchinich & Tucker, 1996a, 1996b). Such variability is consistent with the diverse life-health problems associated with substance abuse.

This behavioral economic theoretical framework also makes a straightforward prediction regarding differences in the degree of temporal discounting between substance-abusing and normal populations. This prediction is displayed graphically in Figure 3.5, which again shows an intertemporal choice between an SSR that is available at time 6 and an LLR that is available at time 10. The reward value curves in both panels of Figure 3.5 were drawn using the hyperbolic function in Equation 7, with the top and bottom panels showing the curves for relatively high and relatively low values of k, respectively. The higher k used in the top panel produces steeper value curves than the lower k used in the bottom panel. Preference between the SSR and the LLR reverses with the passage of time in both panels, with higher and lower discounting producing sooner and later preference shifts, respectively. As suggested by Figure 3.5, an individual with a high degree of temporal discounting (top panel) would spend more time preferring the SSR (i.e., substance use) than an individual with a low degree of discounting (bottom panel). This leads to the prediction that k values would be larger among substance-abusing persons.

The general hypothesis that discounting is a model of self-control and may contribute to substance abuse was first proposed over 35 years ago (Ainslie, 1975; Rachlin & Green, 1972), and it has been supported in numerous empirical studies. The majority of studies have examined its role using an experimental psychopathology approach that compared criterion groups comprised of substance-abusing individuals to control groups without a substance misuse history. These studies have consistently found more precipitous discounting among alcohol-dependent persons (MacKillop et al., 2010; Mitchell, Fields, D'Esposito, & Boettiger, 2005; Petry, 2001a; Vuchinich & Simpson, 1998), smokers (Bickel, Odum, & Madden, 1999; Mitchell, 1999; Reynolds, 2006), stimulant-dependent individuals (Coffey, Gudleski, Saladin, & Brady, 2003; Hoffman et al., 2008; Kirby & Petry, 2004), opiate-dependent individuals (Kirby & Petry, 2004; Kirby, Petry, & Bickel, 1999), and individuals engaging in mixed patterns of substance abuse (Kirby & Petry, 2004; Petry, 2002, 2003). In addition, significantly greater discounting has been evident in pathological gamblers (MacKillop, Anderson, Castelda, Mattson, & Donovick, 2006; Petry, 2001b) and obese individuals (Weller, Cook, Avsar, & Cox, 2008), and high rates of discounting are inversely associated with the probability of engaging in an array of health behaviors, including exercise, cholesterol testing, dental visits, influenza vaccinations, mammogram screenings, Pap smears, and prostate exams (Bradford, 2010). Although a few studies have not found this association between discounting and healthy behavior (e.g., Johnson et al., 2010; MacKillop, Mattson, Anderson MacKillop, Castelda, & Donovick, 2007; Nederkoorn, Smulders, Havermans, Roefs, & Jansen, 2006), the majority of studies have been supportive (for reviews, see de Wit, 2009; Reynolds, 2006). Indeed, highly impulsive discounting has been proposed to be a core feature of self-regulation failures in general (Bickel & Mueller, 2009).

Although there is substantial evidence of a link between temporal discounting and substance abuse, it is unclear whether excessively impulsive temporal discounting is an antecedent or a consequence of persistent excessive drug use. Two studies found lower levels of discounting in individuals who successfully stopped using alcohol or tobacco (Bickel et al., 1999; Petry, 2001a). This suggests either that people who abuse substances may have relatively intact self-control mechanisms that allow them to choose (or benefit from) treatment or that successful treatment (or drug abstinence) increases self-control capacity.

Although relatively few studies have been conducted on this topic, there is evidence that highly impulsive discounting does play an etiological role and is associated with a negative treatment prognosis. With regard to the development of substance abuse, a 6-year longitudinal study on discounting and smoking in adolescents by Audrain-McGovern et al. (2009) found that impulsive discounting prospectively predicted the onset of smoking, and that discounting was stable over the course of adolescence. Another study conducted with preschoolers found that their degree of discounting predicted adult drug use 20 years later (Ayduk et al., 2000). Finally, a number of studies using animal models have found that level of temporal discounting is positively associated with speed of drug use acquisition (Anker, Perry, Gliddon, & Carroll, 2009; Marusich & Bardo, 2009; Perry, Larson, German, Madden, & Carroll, 2005). This further supports the idea that greater discounting contributes to the etiology of substance abuse.

There is also evidence that experimental manipulations can alter discounting. More specifically, studies have revealed that acute withdrawal symptoms, a core feature of substance dependence, significantly increases SSR preferences (Badger et al., 2007; Carroll, Mach, La Nasa, & Newman; Field, Santarcangelo, Sumnall, Goudie, & Cole, 2006; Mitchell, 2004). In addition, a recent study of heavy drinkers and individuals with alcohol use disorders found that the participants' overall levels of craving for alcohol and discounting both predicted the level of alcohol use disorder severity and that the two variables were also significantly associated with each other (MacKillop et al., 2010). Thus, self-control violations may be especially likely when a person is experiencing negative affective states such as craving. Finally, although the evidence suggests that discounting is an etiological variable, it may nonetheless be a viable treatment target. Although little work has been done in this area, one recent promising study found that an intervention focused on executive functioning may increase self-control preferences for LLRs (Bickel et al., 2011).

More generally, the literature on delay discounting and substance abuse indicates that people who abuse substances are relatively impervious to the delayed negative outcomes associated with drug use (e.g., physical, occupational, psychological, and social impairment; legal repercussions) or the delayed positive outcomes associated with abstinence (e.g., improved health, financial, or relationship functioning), especially in the face of visceral states such as withdrawal, craving, or negative affect (Loewenstein, 1996; MacKillop et al., 2010). These results explain why people with severe substance abuse problems may benefit from interventions such as CM or CRA that provide a tangible and immediate reward for abstinence (e.g., opportunities for employment, money, or vouchers for goods or services) that "compete" with the immediate reinforcement associated with drug use.

Objects of Choice: Particular Acts or Temporally Extended Patterns of Acts

The preceding discussion of intertemporal choice and temporal discounting characterized the objects of choice (i.e., SSRs and LLRs) as discrete events that occur at a particular time, much like food reinforcement for an animal in the laboratory. In this conception, if an individual prefers the LLR, he or she forgoes the SSR and then the LLR arrives later at a given point in time (as in Figures 3.4 and 3.5). Many SSRs in the natural environment, like a drug- or alcohol-consumption episode, may reasonably be viewed as discrete, tangible, and temporally circumscribed events. However, most naturally occurring LLRs, like vocational success, are not so reasonably viewed in this way (Rachlin, 1995; Vuchinich & Tucker, 1996b). Real-life LLRs (e.g., "vocational success," "marital happiness," "health") are not discrete, tangible, and temporally circumscribed events. Rather, they are more like abstractions that consist of many smaller rewards that occur over an extended temporal interval in a complex but coherent pattern. An individual's behavior is allocated over time to activities that produce a series of relatively small but immediate gratifications (e.g., SSRs associated with alcohol consumption), or that may produce a more temporally extended but more valuable gratification (e.g., the LLR associated with "vocational success"). But even if an individual lets every discrete drinking opportunity (the SSR) pass by, "vocational success" (the LLR) would not suddenly arrive fully formed at a specific future time. Rather, vocational success takes time to develop and maintain. As more acts are emitted that are consistent with the molar pattern of vocational success (e.g., continuously improving work products), and as less behavior is devoted to activities that may undermine vocational success (e.g., excessive drinking), then more of the constituent parts of the overall LLR will be accrued over an extended interval.

Rachlin (1995) proposed a shift in the view of intertemporal choice situations that attempts to accommodate these considerations. Hyperbolic discounting produces temporal inconsistencies between short-term and long-term preferences, but perhaps the key distinction is between the value of *discrete acts* and the value of *patterns of acts*, rather than between the value of a discrete SSR and the value of a discrete LLR. Rachlin argued that the temporal inconsistencies often found between individuals' preferences at different points in time are better characterized as differences between the value of discrete acts that determine short-term preferences and the value of temporally extended patterns of acts that determine long-term preferences. In this view, obtaining the higher valued, long-term preferences entails temporally extended patterns of behavior. But the development and maintenance of such patterns may be undermined because their component acts often are relatively less valuable than alternative particular acts that are inconsistent with the pattern. Thus, a key issue becomes whether the objects of choice are perceived as discrete acts or as patterns of acts.

For example, suppose that the long-term, higher valued Pattern A in Figure 3.6 represents a satisfying family life, and that some of the particular acts (X) that constitute that pattern are quiet but mildly enjoyable evenings at home with family members. Further suppose that the long-term, lower valued Pattern B represents alcohol abuse, and that some of the particular acts (Y) that constitute that pattern are raucous and highly enjoyable evenings out of the home that involve heavy drinking with friends. In

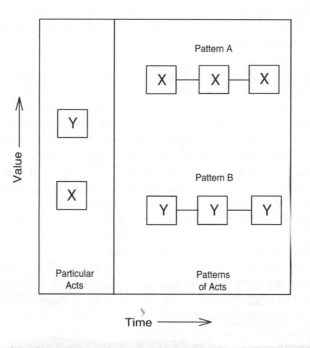

FIGURE 3.6. The relative value of particular acts (X and Y) when considered in isolation (left side), and the relative value of temporally extended patterns of behavior (A and B) that contain Acts X and Y as components (right side).

a discrete choice between Act X and Act Y, the value of an evening out with friends (Act Y) may be much higher than the value of an evening at home with the family (Act X). However, over an extended interval, the pattern that produces a satisfying family life (Pattern A) would almost certainly be preferred to the pattern of alcohol abuse (Pattern B) and all its resulting problems. Thus, if the choice is between temporally extended patterns of behavior A or B, then Pattern A would likely be preferred because it has greater value over an extended temporal horizon. On the other hand, if the choice is between individual acts (X and Y), then Act Y would likely be preferred because it has more immediate value. The degree of temporal extension with which the objects of choice are perceived may thus be critically important in the allocation of behavior that leads to patterns of substance abuse or to the realization of more valuable LLRs.

Viewing the primary unit of analysis as *patterns* of acts, rather than as a *particular* act, is a recent development. There is, however, some evidence relevant to the value of behavior patterns. In laboratory studies using both humans and animals, Rachlin (1995) found that, if contingencies were established that generated cohesive patterns in participants' behavior, then behavioral allocation was more consistent with long-term preferences. Other studies (e.g., Loewenstein & Prelec, 1992, 1993) showed that, if future events were part of a temporally extended sequence or pattern, then their value was greater than if they were independent events in separate, discrete choices.

One clinical implication of this research is that interventions should encourage people who abuse substances to view their day-to-day behavior as part of a pattern leading toward long-term outcomes, rather than as a series of discrete decisions (to use drugs vs. engaging in another activity on a given day). Personalized feedback on drug use patterns, expenditures, and consequences may help to accomplish this perspective shift. Indeed, personalized feedback appears to be one of the key ingredients of successful brief interventions for substance abuse (Lewis & Neighbors, 2006; Walters, Vader, Harris, Field, & Jouriles, 2009). The goals of feedback-based interventions are consistent with basic behavioral economic research suggesting that self-control choices are more likely when behavior is seen as part of a cohesive pattern, rather than as a discrete choice (Heyman & Dunn, 2002; Rachlin, 1995; Simpson & Vuchinich, 2000). For example, after receiving feedback that you spent $2,000 on marijuana in the past year, the decision to purchase and smoke marijuana might become part of a general pattern of behavior related to the goal of saving money rather than a discrete decision related to preference. CM interventions also encourage a more molar approach to understanding behavior by employing escalating schedules of monetary or voucher-based reinforcement that create an explicit and temporally extended connection between daily decisions about drug use.

Whereas an individual day of abstinence might result in a small-magnitude voucher (e.g., $5), after 2 weeks of continuous abstinence, a participant might receive a $50 voucher for a negative drug test result.

The Progression and Cessation of Addiction

The key challenge to any theory of addiction is explaining why some individuals continue to use substances despite experiencing negative consequences. There are several formal behavioral economic theories of addiction including (1) melioration addiction theory (Herrnstein & Prelec, 1992), (2) relative addiction theory (Rachlin, 1997), and (3) rational addiction theory (Becker & Murphy, 1988). Although a full review of these theories is beyond the scope of this chapter, they share several important commonalities.

A key assumption of behavioral economic theories of addiction is that the cost/benefit ratio of drug consumption versus engagement in other activities changes over time as a function of the amount of engagement in these respective activities (Rachlin, 1997). The nature of the change in the cost/benefit ratio is markedly different for drugs versus other substitute activities. Drugs are generally "price-habituated" activities, which means that as the amount of consumption increases over time, the derived benefit from a consumption episode lessens. This is consistent with the observation that tolerance reduces the rewarding effects of a given drug dose in experienced drug users. In contrast, many substance-free activities are "price-sensitized," which means that there is a positive relationship between participation and the benefits derived from the activity. For instance, interpersonal relationships, exercise/sports, and hobbies generally result in increased benefits over time, as the skills required for these activities develop. Conversely, if these activities are neglected, their cost/benefit ratio will decrease (e.g., running after an extended sedentary period, attempting to access social support after a period of social isolation, attending a calculus class after missing the previous three classes).

Behavioral economic theories suggest that the central dynamic of addiction is the relative distribution of behavior over time to constructive price-sensitized activities versus drug use. Because drug use is price-habituated, it is generally self-limiting. Whereas moderate substance use (e.g., a glass of wine with dinner) typically results in reliable benefits (e.g., relaxation, social facilitation), regular heavy drug use will generally diminish those benefits. This may be due to increasing tolerance or to negative consequences that tip the cost/benefit ratio. Indeed, the fact that the number of moderate drinkers and drug users far exceeds the number of heavy users and the fact that many people who abuse substances have periods of moderate use are consistent with this self-limiting prediction.

Behavioral economic theory predicts that there are several conditions that could lead to increased drug use. First, drug use may increase after an event wherein there was a reduction in substance-free substitutes, such as the loss of a friend, family member, or job; moving to a new environment; or an injury or illness. Second, use may increase after an event or situation that leads to a reduction in the monetary or behavioral price of drug use. For example, moving to a neighborhood with numerous bars or easy access to drugs, or beginning a relationship with a heavy drinker or drug user, would reduce the real price of drugs. Because drug use and many substance-free activities are mutually substitutable, an increase in drug use related to these price reductions will often result in decreased engagement in substance-free activities. This decrease will, in turn, reduce the -alue of these price-sensitized substance-free activities, resulting in greater substance use (Rachlin, 1997).

Thus, although the value of any drug use episode will continue to decrease as use escalates, the concurrent reduction in the value of price-sensitized substance-free substitutes will often make drug use the option with the greatest immediate benefit (Koob, 2006; Redish, 2004). This is especially true for drugs of abuse that produce strong withdrawal effects (e.g., sedatives and opiates), which result in negatively reinforced patterns of use. This progression toward greater drug use is exacerbated by the fact that drug use often has a negative impact on other activities (e.g., hangover or withdrawal-related impairment, substance-related arguments, social stigma, legal fines/sanctions) in addition to diminishing engagement in substance-free activities. Moreover, many drugs of abuse have direct neurochemical effects that further narrow the behavioral repertoire toward drug use (Koob, 2006). Acute drug use can reduce the dopamine reward threshold such that dopamine firing occurs in response to milder rewarding stimuli. This may lead to greater pleasure or reinforcing efficacy associated with activities that occur during intoxication (e.g., creative activities, socializing, sexual activity). Chronic drug use, conversely, *raises* the dopamine reward threshold, making substance-free activities less reinforcing and less likely to effectively substitute for drug use (Koob, 2006).

It is also possible, however, for contextual events—such as an increase in the price of drugs or a decrease in the price of substance-free activities—to increase the cost/benefit ratio of substance-free activities, leading to reduced drug use (Tucker, Vuchinich, & Gladsjo, 1994; Tucker, Vuchinich, & Pukish, 1995). Ending a relationship with a partner who abuses substances, getting a job, or beginning a family might generate such a change in the cost/benefit ratio. As mentioned previously, CM and CRA interventions provide immediate reinforcement and thus attempt to alter the cost/benefit ratio by creating a concrete loss of reinforcement following a positive drug test. The success of these interventions suggests that even people with severe substance abuse problems are sensitive to changes in the cost/benefit ratio of drug and alternative reinforcers (Higgins et al., 2004).

Behavioral Economics of Addictive Behavior Change

Several recent studies have investigated the relevance of behavioral economic variables in the process of changing addictive behaviors. One study found that college students who were instructed to increase two specific categories of substance-free behaviors—exercise and creative activities –also reported a small, but statistically significant reduction in drinking (Correia, Benson, & Carey, 2005). Control participants who were not instructed to change their participation in substance-free activities did not report changes in drinking. Another study found that students who reduced their drinking following a brief intervention increased their engagement in academic activities. This suggests that academics may be a key substitute for drinking (Murphy, Correia, Colby, & Vuchinich, 2005). This study also found that a baseline measure of the ratio of substance-related reinforcement to overall reinforcement (derived from the matching law) predicted drinking at a 6-month follow-up, even after controlling for baseline drinking. Thus, individuals who, prior to treatment, have a number of enjoyable alternatives to drinking are more likely to reduce their drinking following an intervention. This behavioral economic index of relative substance-related reinforcement, like the demand curve indices described earlier, may provide a novel measure of problem severity that predicts response to treatment.

Vuchinich and Tucker (1996b) explored the association between reinforcement and relapse among alcohol-dependent males who had completed inpatient treatment. Relapses occurred more often and tended to be more severe when nondrinking rewards were less available. In later research that compared active problem drinkers with former problem drinkers, Tucker, Vuchinich, and colleagues (Tucker et al., 1994, 1995; Tucker, Vuchinich, & Rippens, 2002a) investigated the environmental contexts surrounding successful long-term resolutions achieved with and without treatment. Resolution is the reverse process compared to relapse, wherein the reward structure in the natural environment shifts toward greater availability of nondrinking rewards. Such relationships were observed between stable resolution and increased access to valued nondrinking rewards in the natural environments of former problem drinkers. Treatment tended to enhance this pattern of improved circumstances during the postresolution period. The pattern was not found for active problem drinkers, whose life circumstances tended to worsen over time.

In general, the aforementioned studies suggest that alternative drug-free reinforcement is critically related to the development, progression, and cessation of substance abuse. These studies provide strong support for the utility of intervention approaches such as CM and CRA that attempt to explicitly increase engagement in substance-free activities.

Similarly, clinical and real-world studies have found that measures of behavioral impulsivity, including temporal discounting, can predict outcomes of attempts to stop or reduce substance misuse. The earliest work in this area examined the utility of a behavioral economic index of the monetary value of rewards across time in predicting success in abstinence or moderation both assisted and unassisted with treatment. In a series of prospective studies of recently resolved problem drinkers recruited from the community (Tucker, Foushee, & Black, 2008; Tucker, Vuchinich, Black, & Rippens, 2006; Tucker, Vuchinich, & Rippens, 2002b), participants' personal spending on different commodities, including alcoholic beverages, was assessed retrospectively over the year prior to initial resolution, and drinking outcomes were assessed prospectively over 1- to 2-year follow-up periods. A measure of relative monetary allocation to short-term versus longer term objectives (e.g., drinking vs. saving for the future) derived from spending patterns during the year prior to initial resolution was a significant predictor of stable resolution. *Stability* was defined as either continuous abstinence or moderate drinking without problems throughout the follow-up period. Those participants who reported a higher proportion of preresolution spending on savings than on alcoholic beverages were more likely to remain continuously resolved compared to those who relapsed. The relationship held across participants with different help-seeking experiences (e.g., treatment, Alcoholics Anonymous, or unassisted).

A subsequent analysis further evaluated the utility of this Alcohol-Savings Discretionary Expenditure (ASDE) index to distinguish stable moderation resolutions from stable abstinent resolutions and unstable resolutions that involved problem drinking at some point during the follow-up period (Tucker et al., 2009). Abstinence and relapse reflect discrete success or failure of behavioral regulation of drinking, whereas moderation involves a repetitive pattern of drinking that can reflect either complete restraint or loss-of-control (Marlatt, 1985). Consistent with this differential regulation process, stable moderation resolutions were predicted by relatively lower baseline ASDE values compared to abstinent and unstable resolutions. Moderation was thus associated with greater relative allocation to saving for the future during the year prior to resolution onset, suggesting that the temporal intervals over which problem drinkers organize their behavior, even while drinking heavily, may help identify those who are best able to make a transition from problem drinking to stable moderate use. Furthermore, the index independently predicted moderation in complex models that included other established predictors, such as alcohol dependence, drinking problem duration, and age.

This differential allocation pattern appears to measure the relative reinforcement value of alcohol in the context of resource allocation to commodities available over time. It is conceptually similar to a discounting process and provides a comprehensive benchmark based on behavior patterns in the natural environment which can help evaluate the utility of brief measures of relative preferences, such as laboratory discounting tasks.

Thus, the relationship between substance abuse and temporal discounting appears to have considerable generality across substance-abusing populations and across laboratory and natural environments. Converging with these findings, several recent studies found that impulsive discounting also predicted smoking cessation treatment failure in different clinical samples (Krishnan-Sarin et al., 2007; MacKillop & Kahler, 2009). For instance, Yoon et al. (2007) found that pregnant smokers who scored higher on a pretreatment measure of delayed reward discounting were less likely to respond to a CM intervention intended to reduce smoking. Although there is a need for more longitudinal research, these studies provide evidence that the high preferences for SSRs observed in people who abuse substances reflects a decision-making orientation that both predates substance abuse and predicts poor treatment outcome.

Behavioral Economics and Neuroeconomics: Integrating Brain and Behavior

The field of neuroeconomics, the integration of behavioral economics and cognitive neuroscience, represents a new frontier for applying behavioral economics to understand substance abuse. This approach seeks to characterize the underlying neurobiological substrates associated with behavioral economic phenomena and, reciprocally, to understand better neurocognitive functioning using novel paradigms. To date, the most common approach has been the use of functional magnetic resonance imaging (fMRI) to identify the neuroanatomical structures exhibiting greater metabolic activity during decision-making tasks. For example, an fMRI study of individuals engaging in a behavioral economic game found that unfair divisions of resources elicited activity in expected brain regions, such as the dorsolateral prefrontal cortex, which is associated with cognitive processing, and also in unexpected regions, such as the anterior insula, a region associated with emotion and processing visceral body states (Sanfey, Rilling, Aronson, Nystrom, & Cohen, 2003). Thus, the brain's deliberative and affective faculties worked together to determine the observed behavior, which may explain why decision-making preferences are economically irrational, but nonetheless normative in humans. This study is representative of the burgeoning number of investigations in this area that have begun to elucidate the neural basis for several fundamental processes in behavioral economics, such as attributions of incentive value (for a review, see Knutson & Bossaerts, 2007).

Most relevant to the behavioral economics of substance abuse are neuroeconomic studies of delay discounting. Here, fMRI studies have identified a number of brain regions that are consistently activated during temporal discounting tasks (Bickel, Pitcock, Yi, & Angtuaco, 2009; McClure,

Laibson, Loewenstein, & Cohen, 2004; Monterosso et al., 2007). Despite relatively different methodologies, a recent meta-analysis of 13 studies found 25 regions of common activation (Carter, Meyer, & Huettel, 2010). These included cortical structures, such as the medial and inferior prefrontal cortex (PFC), the anterior insular cortex, the posterior parietal cortex and posterior cingulate, and subcortical structures, such as the ventral striatum and midbrain. Taken together, these findings show a neurocognitive "tug-of-war" between subcortical motivational circuits and cortical inhibitory control circuits (Bechara, 2005; Bickel et al., 2007; also see Kable & Glimcher, 2007; Monterosso & Luo, 2010), with the observed behavior being determined by the relative balance between motivational drive and self-control.

Despite recent progress, the neuroanatomical differences that are associated with substance misuse have not been extensively studied. Only three fMRI studies of discounting and addictive behavior have been conducted (reviewed below) and, although they revealed some differences between people with and without substance abuse problems, research in this area remains preliminary. Two studies compared temporal discounting between individuals with and without stimulant dependence. Monterosso et al. (2007) found that stimulant-dependent individuals exhibited less prefrontal and parietal cortex activity relative to controls when making easy choices, and Hoffman et al. (2008) identified similar patterns, with reduced activity in the dorsolateral PFC, precuneus, and ventral striatum. Applying the same design and a similar approach to alcohol dependence, Boetigger et al. (2009) found differential activation in the PFC and posterior parietal cortex, among other regions. In particular, individuals with alcohol dependence exhibited greater dorsolateral PFC activity compared to controls, but attenuated lateral orbitofrontal cortex activity. Thus, these studies suggest meaningful differences in cortical regions responsible for inhibition and consideration of the future between people with and without substance abuse problems, but limited differences in motivational neurocircuitry. This, of course, may be because the commodity in play is money, which is a general reward that may be less differentially salient compared to an individual's drug of choice.

Conclusion

Behavioral economic researchers have made considerable progress in describing the individual differences and contextual variables that influence the development, progression, and cessation of a variety of addictive behavior patterns. Key strengths of behavioral economic research include (1) a strong theoretical foundation in economic and learning theory, (2) a clear translation of concepts and measures from basic laboratory research to clinical settings, (3) a tradition of applying quantitative models to the description and prediction of substance abuse and associated decision-making processes, (4) decision-making tasks and paradigms that are amenable to both clinical translation (e.g., predicting treatment outcome) and to basic science translation (e.g., identifying genetic and fMR correlates of discounting), and (5) concepts and experimental paradigms that have lead to the development of efficacious treatments such as contingency management.

In addition to supporting a contextualist perspective on substance abuse, behavioral economics has shifted our views of reinforcement, has made rich connections with economic theory and neuroscience, and has yielded concepts that are applicable across clinical, public health, economic, and policy arenas. Although the methods and tools of these perspectives differ greatly, sharing a common scientific language should facilitate multidisciplinary interchange that is critical to address a complex behavioral health problem like substance abuse. The promise of behavioral economics as an organizing framework that can span multiple levels of application is beginning to emerge in the substance abuse intervention field and in behavioral health generally (Bickel et al., 2007; Bickel & Vuchinich, 2000). Although there is little doubt that variables such as price, alternatives, and reward delay influence decisions about drug use, an important goal for future research is to translate these basic concepts into efforts to understand and treat addiction.

Acknowledgments

Preparation of this chapter was supported in part by National Institutes of Health/National Institute on Alcohol Abuse and Alcoholism Grant Nos. 1 R01 AA017880-01A1 and 1R21 AA016304-01A2.

References

Ainslie, G. (1975). Specious reward: A behavioral theory of impulsiveness and self-control. *Psychological Bulletin, 82*, 463–496.

Ainslie, G. (1992). *Picoeconomics: The strategic interaction of successive motivational states within the person.* Cambridge, UK: Cambridge University Press.

Anker, J. J., Perry, J. L., Gliddon, L. A., & Carroll, M. E. (2009). Impulsivity predicts the escalation of cocaine self-administration in rats. *Pharmacology Biochemistry and Behaviour, 93*(3), 343–348.

Audrain-McGovern, J., Rodriguez, D., Epstein, L. H., Cuevas, J., Rodgers, K., & Wileyto, E. P. (2009). Does delay discounting play an etiological role in smoking or is it a consequence of smoking? *Drug and Alcohol Dependence, 103*(3), 99–106.

Ayduk, O., Mendoza-Denton, R., Mischel, W., Downey, G., Peake, P., & Rodriguez, M. (2000). Regulating the interpersonal self: Strategic self-regulation for coping with rejection sensitivity. *Journal of Personality and Social Psychology, 79*, 776–792.

Badger, G. J., Bickel, W. K., Giordano, L. A., Jacobs, E. A., Loewenstein, G., & Marsch, L. (2007). Altered states: The impact of immediate craving on the valuation of current and future opioids. *Journal of Health Economics, 26*(5), 865–876.

Bechara, A. (2005). Decision making, impulse control and loss of willpower to resist drugs: A neurocognitive perspective. *Nature Neuroscience, 8*(11), 1458–1463.

Becker, G. S., & Murphy, K. M. (1988). A theory of rational addiction. *Journal of Political Economy, 96*, 675–700.

Bickel, W. K., DeGrandpre, R. J., & Higgins, S. T. (1995). The behavioral economics of concurrent drug reinforcers: A review and reanalysis of drug self-administration research. *Psychopharmacology, 118*, 250–259.

Bickel, W. K., Miller, M. L., Yi, R., Kowal, B. P., Lindquist, D. M., & Pitcock, J. A. (2007). Behavioral and neuroeconomics of drug addiction: Competing neural systems and temporal discounting processes. *Drug and Alcohol Dependence, 90*(Suppl. 1), S85–S91.

Bickel, W. K., & Mueller, E. T. (2009). Toward the study of trans-disease processes: A novel approach with special reference to the study of co-morbidity. *Journal of Dual Diagnosis, 5*(2), 131–138.

Bickel, W. K., Odum, A. L., & Madden, G. J. (1999). Impulsivity and cigarette smoking: Delay discounting in current, never, and ex-smokers. *Psychopharmacology (Berlin), 146*(4), 447–454.

Bickel, W. K., Pitcock, J. A., Yi, R., & Angtuaco, E. J. (2009). Congruence of BOLD response across intertemporal choice conditions: Fictive and real money gains and losses. *Journal of Neuroscience, 29*(27), 8839–8846.

Bickel, W. K., & Vuchinich, R. E. (Eds.). (2000). *Reframing health behavior change with behavioral economics*. Mahwah, NJ: Erlbaum.

Bickel, W. K., Yi, R., Landes, R. D., Hill, P. F., & Baxter, C. (2011). Remember the future: Working memory training decreases delay discounting among stimulant addicts. *Biological Psychiatry, 69*(3), 260–265.

Boettiger, C. A., Kelley, E. A., Mitchell, J. M., D'Esposito, M., & Fields, H. L. (2009). Now or later?: An fMRI study of the effects of endogenous opioid blockade on a decision-making network. *Pharmacology Biochemistry and Behaviour, 93*(3), 291–299.

Bradford, W. D. (2010). The association between individual time preferences and health maintenance habits. *Journal of Medical Decision Making, 30*(1), 99–112.

Carroll, M. E., Mach, J. L., La Nasa, R. M., & Newman, J. L. (2009). Impulsivity as a behavioral measure of withdrawal of orally delivered PCP and nondrug rewards in male and female monkeys. *Psychopharmacology (Berlin), 207*(1), 85–98.

Carter, R. M., Meyer, J. R., & Huettel, S. A. (2010). Functional neuroimaging of intertemporal choice models: A review. *Journal of Neuroscience, Psychology, and Economics, 3*(1), 27–45.

Catania, A. C. (1963). Concurrent performances: A baseline for the study of reinforcement magnitude. *Journal of the Experimental Analysis of Behavior, 6,* 299–300.

Chung, S.H., & Herrnstein, R. J. (1967). Choice and delay of reinforcement. *Journal of the Experimental Analysis of Behavior, 10,* 67–74.

Coffey, S. F., Gudleski, G. D., Saladin, M. E., & Brady, K. T. (2003). Impulsivity and rapid discounting of delayed hypothetical rewards in cocaine-dependent individuals. *Experimental and Clinical Psychopharmacology, 11*(1), 18–25.

Correia, C. J., Benson, T., & Carey, K. B. (2005). Decreased substance use following increases in alternative behaviors: A preliminary investigation. *Addictive Behaviors, 30,* 19–27.

Correia, C. J., Carey, K. B., Simons, J., & Borsari, B. E. (2003). Relationships between binge drinking and substance-free reinforcement in a sample of college students: A preliminary investigation. *Addictive Behaviors, 28,* 361–368.

Correia, C. J., Simons, J., Carey, K. B., & Borsari, B. E. (1998). Predicting drug abuse: Application of behavioral theories of choice. *Addictive Behaviors, 23,* 705–709.

DeGrandpre, R. J., Bickel, W. K., Hughes, J. R., Layng, M. P., & Badger, G. (1993). Unit price as a useful metric in analyzing effects of reinforcer magnitude. *Journal of the Experimental Analysis of Behavior, 60,* 641–666.

de Wit, H. (2009). Impulsivity as a determinant and consequence of drug use: A review of underlying processes. *Addiction Biology, 14*(1), 22–31.

Field, M., Santarcangelo. M., Sumnall, H., Goudie, A., & Cole, J. (2006). Delay discounting and the behavioural economics of cigarette purchases in smokers: The effects of nicotine deprivation. *Psychopharmacology (Berlin), 186*(2), 255–263.

Herrnstein, R. J. (1961). Relative and absolute strength of response as a function of frequency of reinforcement. *Journal of the Experimental Analysis of Behavior, 4,* 267–272.

Herrnstein, R. J. (1970). On the law of effect. *Journal of the Experimental Analysis of Behavior, 13,* 243–266.

Herrnstein, R. J., & Prelec, D. (1992). A theory of addiction. In G. Loewenstein & J. Elster (Eds.), *Choice over time* (pp. 331–360). New York: Russell Sage Foundation.

Heyman, G. M., & Dunn, B. (2002). Decision biases and persistent illicit drug use: An experimental study of distributed choice and addiction. *Drug and Alcohol Dependence, 67,* 193–203.

Higgins, S. T., Heil, S. H., & Plebani-Lussier, J. (2004). Clinical implications of reinforcement as a determinant of substance use disorders. *Annual Review of Psychology, 55,* 431–461.

Hoffman, W. F., Schwartz, D. L., Huckans, M. S., McFarland, B. H., Meiri, G., Stevens, A. A., et al. (2008). Cortical activation during delay discounting in abstinent methamphetamine dependent individuals. *Psychopharmacology (Berlin), 201*(2), 183–193.

Hull, C. L. (1943). *Principles of behavior.* New York: Appleton-Century.

Hursh, S. R. (1980). Economic concepts for the analysis of behavior. *Journal of the Experimental Analysis of Behavior, 34,* 219–238.

Hursh, S. R. (1993). Behavioral economics of drug self-administration: An introduction. *Drug and Alcohol Dependence, 33*, 165–172.

Kable, J. W., & Glimcher, P. W. (2007). The neural correlates of subjective value during intertemporal choice. *Nature Neuroscience, 10*(12), 1625–1633.

Kagel, J. H., Battalio, R. C., & Green, L. (1995). *Economic choice theory: An experimental analysis of animal behavior.* New York: Cambridge University Press.

Kirby, K. N., & Petry, N. M. (2004). Heroin and cocaine abusers have higher discount rates for delayed rewards than alcoholics or non-drug-using controls. *Addiction, 99*(4), 461–471.

Kirby, K. N., Petry, N. M., & Bickel, W. K. (1999). Heroin addicts have higher discount rates for delayed rewards than non-drug-using controls. *Journal of Experimental Psychology: General, 128*, 78–87.

Knutson, B., & Bossaerts, P. (2007). Neural antecedents of financial decisions. *Journal of Neuroscience, 27*(31), 8174–8177.

Koob, G. F. (2006). The neurobiology of addiction: A neuroadaptational view relevant for diagnosis. *Addiction, 101*(Suppl. 1), 23–30.

Krishnan-Sarin, S., Reynolds, B., Duhig, A. M., Smith, A., Liss, T., McFetridge, A., et al. (2007). Behavioral impulsivity predicts treatment outcome in a smoking cessation program for adolescent smokers. *Drug and Alcohol Dependence, 88*(1), 79–82.

Jacobs, E. A., & Bickel, W. K. (1999). Modeling drug consumption in the clinic via simulation procedures: Demand for heroin and cigarettes in opioid-dependent outpatients. *Experimental and Clinical Psychopharmacology, 7*(4), 412–426.

Johnson, M. W., Bickel, W. K., Baker, F., Moore, B. A., Badger, Q. J., & Budney, A. J. (2010). Delay discounting in current and former marijuana-dependent individuals. *Experimental and Clinical Psychopharmacology, 18*(1), 99–107.

Lacey, H. M., & Rachlin, H. (1978). Behavior, cognition, and theories of choice. *Behaviorism, 6*, 177–202.

Lewis, M. A., & Neighbors, C. (2006). Social norms approaches using descriptive drinking norms education: A review of the research on personalized normative feedback. *Journal of American College Health, 54*(4), 213–218.

Little, C., & Correia, C. J. (2006). Use of a multiple-choice procedure with college student drinkers. *Psychology of Addictive Behaviors, 20*, 445–452.

Loewenstein, G. F. (1996). Out of control: Visceral influences on behavior. *Organizational Behavior and Human Decision Processes, 65*, 272–292.

Loewenstein, G. F., & Prelec, D. (1992). Anomalies in intertemporal choice: Evidence and an interpretation. *Quarterly Journal of Economics, 107*, 573–597.

Loewenstein, G. F., & Prelec, D. (1993). Preferences for sequences of outcomes. *Psychological Review, 100*(1), 91–108.

MacKillop, J., Anderson, E. J., Castelda, B. A., Mattson, R. E., & Donovick, P. J. (2006). Divergent validity of measures of cognitive distortions, impulsivity, and time perspective in pathological gambling. *Journal of Gambling Studies, 22*(3), 339–354.

MacKillop, J., & Kahler, C. W. (2009). Delayed reward discounting predicts treatment response for heavy drinkers receiving smoking cessation treatment. *Drug and Alcohol Dependence, 104*(3), 197–203.

MacKillop, J., Mattson, R. E., Anderson Mackillop, E. J., Castelda, B. A., & Donovick, P. J. (2007). Multidimensional assessment of impulsivity in undergraduate hazardous drinkers and controls. *Journal of Studies on Alcohol and Drugs, 68*(6), 785–788.

MacKillop, J., Miranda, R. Jr., Monti, P. M., Ray, L. A., Murphy, J. G., Rohsenow, D. J., et al. (2010). Alcohol demand, delayed reward discounting, and craving in relation to drinking and alcohol use disorders. *Journal of Abnormal Psychology, 119*(1), 106–114.

MacKillop, J., & Murphy, J. G. (2007). A behavioral economic measure of demand for alcohol predicts brief intervention outcomes. *Drug and Alcohol Dependence, 89*, 227–233.

MacKillop, J., Murphy, J. G., Ray, L., Eisenberg, D. T. A., Lisman, S. A., Lum, J. K., et al. (2008). Further validation of a cigarette purchase task for assessing the relative reinforcing efficacy of nicotine in smokers. *Experimental and Clinical Psychopharmacology, 16*, 57–65.

MacKillop, J., Murphy, J. G., Tidey, J. W., Kahler, C., Ray, L. A., Bickel, W. (2009). Latent structure of the facets of alcohol reinforcement from a behavioral economic demand curve. *Psychopharmacology, 203*, 33–40.

MacPhillamy, D. J., & Lewinsohn, P. M. (1982). The Pleasant Events Schedule: Studies on reliability, validity, and scale intercorrelation. *Journal of Consulting and Clinical Psychology, 50*, 363–380.

Marlatt, G. A (1985). Lifestyle modification. In G. A. Marlatt & J. R. Gordon (Eds.), *Relapse prevention: Maintenance strategies in the treatment of addictive behaviors* (pp. 280–348). New York: Guilford Press.

Marusich, J. A., & Bardo, M. T. (2009). Differences in impulsivity on a delay-discounting task predict self-administration of a low unit dose of methylphenidate in rats. *Behavioural Pharmacology, 20*(5–6), 447–454.

Mazur, J. (1987). An adjusting procedure for studying delayed reinforcement. In M. Commons, J. Mazur, J. A. Nevin, & H. Rachlin (Eds.), *Quantitative analysis of behavior: Vol. 5. The effect of delay and of intervening events on reinforcement value* (pp. 55–76). Hillsdale, NJ: Erlbaum.

McClure, S. M., Laibson, D. I., Loewenstein, G., & Cohen, J. D. (2004). Separate neural systems value immediate and delayed monetary rewards. *Science, 306*(5695), 503–507.

Miller, W. R. (1998). Enhancing motivation for change. In W. R. Miller & N. Heather (Eds.), *Treating addictive behaviors* (2nd ed., pp. 121–132). New York: Plenum Press.

Mitchell, J. M., Fields, H. L., D'Esposito, M., & Boettiger, C. A. (2005). Impulsive responding in alcoholics. *Alcoholism: Clinical and Experimental Research, 29*(12), 2158–2169.

Mitchell, S. H. (1999). Measures of impulsivity in cigarette smokers and non-smokers. *Psychopharmacology, 146*, 455–464.

Mitchell, S. H. (2004). Effects of short-term nicotine deprivation on decision-making: Delay, uncertainty and effort discounting. *Nicotine and Tobacco Research, 6*(5), 819–828.

Monterosso, J. R., Ainslie, G., Xu, J., Cordova, X., Domier, C. P., & London, E.

D. (2007). Frontoparietal cortical activity of methamphetamine-dependent and comparison subjects performing a delay discounting task. *Human Brain Mapping, 28*(5), 383–393.

Monterosso, J. R., & Luo, S. (2010). An argument against dual valuation system competition: Cognitive capacities supporting future orientation mediate rather than compete with visceral motivations. *Journal of Neuroscience, Psychology and Economics, 3*, 1–14.

Murphy, J. G., Correia, C. J., & Barnett, N. P. (2007). Behavioral economic approaches to reduce college student drinking. *Addictive Behaviors, 32*(11), 2573–2585.

Murphy, J. G., Correia, C. J., Colby, S. M., & Vuchinich, R. E. (2005). Using behavioral theories of choice to predict drinking outcomes following a brief intervention. *Experimental and Clinical Psychopharmacology, 13*, 93–101.

Murphy, J. G., & MacKillop, J. (2006). Relative reinforcing efficacy of alcohol among college student drinkers. *Experimental and Clinical Psychopharmacology, 14, 219–227.*

Murphy, J. G., MacKillop, J., Skidmore, J. R. & Pederson, A. A. (2009). Reliability and validity of a demand curve measure of alcohol reinforcement. *Experimental and Clinical Psychopharmacology, 17*, 396–404.

Murphy, J. G., MacKillop, J., Tidey, J. W., Brazil, L. A., & Colby, S. M. (2011). Validity of a demand curve measure of nicotine reinforcement with adolescent smokers. *Drug and Alcohol Dependence, 113*, 207–214.

Nederkoorn, C., Smulders, F. T., Havermans, R. C., Roefs, A., & Jansen, A. (2006). Impulsivity in obese women. *Appetite, 47*(2), 253–256.

Perry, J. L., Larson, E. B., German, J. P., Madden, G. J., & Carroll, M. E. (2005). Impulsivity (delay discounting) as a predictor of acquisition of IV cocaine self-administration in female rats. *Psychopharmacology (Berlin), 178*(2–3), 193–201.

Petry, N. M. (2001a). Delay discounting of money and alcohol in actively using alcoholics, currently abstinent alcoholics, and controls. *Psychopharmacology (Berlin), 154*(3), 243–250.

Petry, N. M. (2001b). Substance abuse, pathological gambling, and impulsiveness. *Drug and Alcohol Dependence, 63*(1), 29–38.

Petry, N. M. (2002). Discounting of delayed rewards in substance abusers: Relationship to antisocial personality disorder. *Psychopharmacology (Berlin), 162*(4), 425–432.

Petry, N. M. (2003). Discounting of money, health, and freedom in substance abusers and controls. *Drug and Alcohol Dependence, 71*(2), 133–141.

Rachlin, H. (1987). Animal choice and human choice. In L. Green & J. Kagel (Eds.), *Advances in behavioral economics* (Vol. 1, pp. 48–64). Norwood, NJ: Ablex.

Rachlin, H. (1995). Self-control: Beyond commitment. *Behavioral and Brain Sciences, 18*, 109–159.

Rachlin, H. (1997). Four teleological theories of addiction. *Psychonomic Bulletin and Review, 4*, 462–473.

Rachlin, H., & Green, L. (1972). Commitment, choice, and self-control. *Journal of the Experimental Analysis of Behavior, 17*, 15–22.

Rachlin, H., Green, L., Kagel, J., & Battalio, R. (1976). Economic demand theory and psychological studies of choice. In G. Bower (Ed.), *The psychology of learning and motivation* (pp. 129–154). New York: Academic Press.

Rachlin, H., & Laibson, D. I. (1997). *The matching law: Papers in psychology and economics by Richard Herrnstein.* Cambridge, MA: Harvard University Press.

Redish, A. D. (2004). Addiction as a computational process gone awry. *Science, 306,* 1944–1947.

Reynolds, B. (2006). A review of delay-discounting research with humans: Relations to drug use and gambling. *Behavioural Pharmacology, 17*(8), 651–667.

Sanfey, A. G., Rilling, J. K., Aronson, J. A., Nystrom, L. E., & Cohen, J. D. (2003). The neural basis of economic decision-making in the Ultimatum Game. *Science, 300*(5626), 1755–1758.

Simpson, C. A., & Vuchinich, R. E. (2000). Temporal changes in the value of objects of choice: Discounting, behavior patterns, and health behavior. In W. K. Bickel & R. E. Vuchinich (Eds.), *Reframing health behavior change with behavioral economics.* Englewood Cliffs, NJ: Prentice-Hall.

Skidmore, J. R., & Murphy, J. G. (2010). Relations between heavy drinking, gender, and substance-free reinforcement. *Experimental and Clinical Psychopharmacology, 18,* 156–166.

Skidmore, J. R., & Murphy, J. G. (2011). The effect of drink price and next-day responsibilities on college student drinking: A behavioral economic analysis. *Psychology of Addictive Behaviors, 25,* 57–68.

Skinner, B. F. (1938). *The behavior of organisms: An experimental analysis.* Englewood Cliffs, NJ: Prentice-Hall.

Tucker, J. A., Foushee, H. R., & Black, B. C. (2008). Behavioral economic analysis of natural resolution of drinking problems using IVR self-monitoring. *Experimental and Clinical Psychopharmacology, 16,* 332–340.

Tucker, J. A., Roth, D. L., Vignolo, M., & Westfall, A. O. (2009). A behavioral economic reward index predicts drinking resolutions: Moderation re-visited and compared with other outcomes. *Journal of Consulting and Clinical Psychology, 77,* 219–228.

Tucker, J. A., Vuchinich, R. E., Black, B. C., & Rippens, P. D. (2006). Significance of a behavioral economic index of reward value in predicting problem drinking resolutions. *Journal of Consulting and Clinical Psychology, 74,* 317–326.

Tucker, J. A., Vuchinich, R. E., & Gladsjo, J. A. (1994). Environmental events surrounding natural recovery from alcohol-related problems. *Journal of Studies on Alcohol, 55,* 401–411.

Tucker, J. A., Vuchinich, R. E., & Pukish, M. A. (1995). Molar environmental contexts surrounding recovery from alcohol problems by treated and untreated problem drinkers. *Experimental and Clinical Psychopharmacology, 3,* 195–204.

Tucker, J. A., Vuchinich, R. E., & Rippens, P. D. (2002a). Environmental contexts surrounding resolution of drinking problems among problem drinkers with different help-seeking experiences. *Journal of Studies on Alcohol, 63,* 334–341.

Tucker, J. A., Vuchinich, R. E., & Rippens, P. D. (2002b). Predicting natural resolution of alcohol-related problems: A prospective behavioral economic analysis. *Experimental and Clinical Psychopharmacology, 10,* 248–257.

Van Etten, M. L., Higgins, S. T., Budney, A. J., & Badger, G. J. (1998). Comparison of the frequency and enjoyability of pleasant events in cocaine abusers vs. non-abusers using a standardized behavioral inventory. *Addiction, 93,* 1669–1680.

Vuchinich, R. E. (1982). Have behavioral theories of alcohol abuse focused too much on alcohol consumption? *Bulletin of the Society of Psychologists in Substance Abuse, 1,* 151–154.

Vuchinich, R. E. (1995). Alcohol abuse as molar choice: An update of a 1982 proposal. *Psychology of Addictive Behaviors, 9,* 223–235.

Vuchinich, R. E., & Heather, B. N. (2003). *Choice, behavioral economics, and addiction.* Oxford, UK: Elsevier.

Vuchinich, R. E., & Simpson, C. A. (1998). Hyperbolic temporal discounting in social drinkers and problem drinkers. *Experimental and Clinical Psychopharmacology, 6,* 292–305.

Vuchinich, R. E., & Tucker, J. A. (1988). Contributions from behavioral theories of choice to an analysis of alcohol abuse. *Journal of Abnormal Psychology, 97,* 181–195.

Vuchinich, R. E., & Tucker, J. A. (1996a). The molar context of alcohol abuse. In L. Green & J. Kagel (Eds.), *Advances in behavioral economics: Vol. 3. Substance use and abuse* (pp. 133–162). Norwood, NJ: Ablex Press.

Vuchinich, R. E., & Tucker, J. A. (1996b). Alcoholic relapse, life events, and behavioral theories of choice: A prospective analysis. *Experimental and Clinical Psychopharmacology, 4,* 19–28.

Walters, S. T., Vader, A. M., & Harris, T. R., Field, C. A., & Jouriles, E. N. (2009). Dismantling motivational interviewing and feedback for college drinkers: A randomized clinical trial. *Journal of Consulting and Clinical Psychology, 77,* 64–73.

Weller, R. E., Cook, E. W. 3rd, Avsar, K. B., & Cox, J. E. (2008). Obese women show greater delay discounting than healthy-weight women. *Appetite, 51*(3), 563–569.

Wood, P. K., Sher, K. J., & Rutledge, P. C. (2007). College student alcohol consumption, day of the week, and class schedule. *Alcoholism: Clinical and Experimental Research, 31,* 1195–1207.

Yoon, J. H., Higgins, S. T., Heil, S. H., Sugarbaker, R. J., Thomas, C. S., & Badger, G. J. (2007). Delay discounting predicts postpartum relapse to cigarette smoking among pregnant women. *Experimental and Clinical Psychopharmacology, 15*(2), 176–186.

Chapter 4

Contingency Management in Substance Abuse Treatment

Jesse Dallery
Steven E. Meredith
Alan J. Budney

Individuals who seek treatment for substance abuse problems can be difficult to engage in treatment. Even when clients make initial progress, frequently their motivation wanes and relapse occurs. Contingency management (CM) can facilitate robust change in this challenging clinical population. A large body of literature examining CM across a range of drug classes and clinical populations provides compelling empirical support for the efficacy of this treatment (Higgins, Silverman, & Heil, 2008). A recent meta-analysis of CM effects on drug abstinence concluded that the data "provide strong support for CM as being among the more effective approaches to promoting abstinence during and after the treatment of drug dependence disorders" (Prendergast, Podus, Finney, Greenwell, & Roll, 2006, p. 1556). In this chapter, we describe how CM has been implemented in a variety of research and clinical settings. We also discuss innovations in CM and how these innovations can overcome some of the major obstacles associated with disseminating this evidence-based treatment. Finally, we provide guidelines and recommendations about delivering CM in the clinic.

Theoretical Foundations of CM

An Operant Model of Drug Use

CM capitalizes on the knowledge that drug use can be modified by changing environmental contingencies. The goal is to systematically weaken the influence of reinforcement derived from drug use and to increase the frequency and magnitude of reinforcement derived from healthier alternative activities, especially those that are incompatible with drug use. Achieving this goal is a challenging task: choosing to use drugs results in certain immediate consequences (e.g., drug high and relief from withdrawal), whereas choosing abstinence typically results in delayed, and often uncertain, consequences (e.g., improved health, better interpersonal relationships, more money). Under these conditions, the "motivational balance" favors drug use. CM tips this balance by reinforcing abstinence with immediate, highly desirable consequences, contingent on objective evidence of abstinence.

One of the most fundamental processes governing human behavior, including drug use, is reinforcement. Positive reinforcement of drug use can be derived from the pharmacological effects of the drug (Griffiths, Bigelow, & Henningfield, 1980), or it can be socially mediated by others in the context of drug use. The latter source may be particularly relevant during the acquisition phase of substance abuse, but it also plays a role in the maintenance of drug use. Negative reinforcement also plays a significant role in drug seeking. For example, drug use may result in escape from or avoidance of withdrawal or other aversive emotional states, or it may result in avoidance of social or occupational activities. Conceptualizing substance abuse as learned human behavior implies that it is amenable to change via the same processes and principles as other types of human behavior (Martin & Pear, 2010).

The operant view is highly compatible with a number of biological and psychosocial theories and interventions targeting substance abuse. For example, individual differences in sensitivity to reinforcement (to drug and/or social reinforcers), punishment, and delay to reinforcement contribute in important ways to the pathogenesis of substance abuse. All healthy humans are assumed to possess the necessary neurobiological systems to experience drug reward and to have the potential to develop patterns of use or abuse. Genetic or acquired characteristics (e.g., family history of substance dependence, other psychiatric disorders) can affect the probability of developing drug abuse, but the behavioral model assumes that such special characteristics are not necessary for drug abuse to develop. In addition, the view incorporates the complex role of verbal processes in how drug use may be acquired, maintained, and interpreted by the user (DeGrandpre, 2000; Wilson & Hayes, 2000). It is beyond the scope of this chapter to explore the interdependent relations among genetic, neurobiological, and behavioral (including verbal behavior) variables. Nevertheless, below we address how a number of evidence-based psychosocial interventions, many of which rely on verbally mediated processes, may be integrated with CM interventions.

Basic Principles of CM

CM interventions involve the use of *positive reinforcement, negative reinforcement, positive punishment*, or *negative punishment* to increase or decrease the frequency of a target behavior such as drug abstinence. Although reinforcement and punishment are each effective tools in substance abuse treatment programs, the former are preferred by both patients and clinicians, and are more common in the treatment clinic. An important limitation of punishment is that it can increase treatment dropout. This is less of an issue in some circumstances (e.g., court-mandated treatment) and may be offset by inclusion of reinforcement contingencies.

Regardless of the type of contingency, all procedures must first specify a measurable target behavior to be increased or decreased. The target behavior or therapeutic goal in most CM interventions is drug abstinence as verified by a biological marker such as a drug metabolite measured in urine. Other less frequently employed goals have been counseling attendance, achievement of a specific treatment goal or homework task, or medication adherence.

In the context of a CM intervention, *positive reinforcement* involves delivery of a desired consequence contingent on the target behavior. Examples of desired consequences might include vouchers that can be exchanged for goods and services, methadone take-home privileges, access to affordable housing, or increased opportunities to win prizes. *Negative reinforcement* involves removing an aversive or confining circumstance contingent on meeting a therapeutic goal. Examples might include a reduction in the intensity of criminal justice supervision or schedule of counseling.

Negative punishment involves removal of a positive circumstance or condition contingent on evidence of the occurrence of an undesirable behavior. Examples of positive conditions that could be removed might include the reduction in the monetary value of vouchers that could be earned for drug abstinence or removal of a preferred schedule of medication dosing or counseling sessions. *Positive punishment* involves delivery of an undesirable consequence contingent on evidence of undesirable behavior. Punishing consequences employed in some substance abuse treatment programs include increases in treatment participation requirements, termination of treatment, suspension of employment, or a specified period of incarceration.

Early Examples of the Utility and Efficacy of CM

One of the first examples of CM to appear in the substance abuse treatment literature addressed the problem of chronic public drunkenness among "skid row" alcoholics (Miller, 1975). Individuals who received shelter, employment, food, clothing, and other services from local social agencies contingent on sobriety verified via negative breath-alcohol tests and staff observation showed reduced alcohol use, increased employment, and fewer legal problems than those who received these services regardless of whether or not they had used alcohol.

Concurrent alcoholism among methadone-maintained, opiate-dependent patients is commonly regarded as one of the major factors associated with treatment failure. One early method to reduce alcohol use in this population was to require disulfiram ingestion prior to receiving a daily dose of methadone (Liebson, Tommaselo, & Bigelow, 1978; see also Azrin, Sisson, Meyers, & Godley, 1982). In this case, methadone was used to reinforce disulfiram ingestion. Patients who did not take the mandatory doses of disulfiram had their daily dose of methadone reduced until it reached zero and then were discontinued from the program.

There are a variety of ways to creatively and effectively employ contingencies to decrease drug use or increase other prosocial behaviors in the context of a daily methadone-dispensing clinic (Kidorf & Stitzer, 1999). For example, the methadone take-home privilege involves providing an extra daily dose of methadone for ingestion at home so that patients do not need to attend the clinic as frequently (Stitzer & Bigelow, 1978). Attending the clinic daily can be burdensome, sometimes interfering with vocational or family responsibilities. Take-home privileges are also desirable to patients because skipping a daily dose may result in adverse withdrawal symptoms and increased risk for using heroin or other opiates. Take-home doses are not provided to all patients because they have the potential for abuse either through the patient ingesting the take-home dose prior to the scheduled dosing time or by selling it on the street.

The most common use of "take-homes" has been to reinforce abstinence from other drug use among methadone-dependent patients, as multiple substance abuse is common in this population. Numerous studies have demonstrated that making take-home doses contingent on abstinence from secondary drug(s) is an effective method for reducing drug use in this difficult treatment population (Stitzer, Iguchi, & Felch, 1992). Take-home privileges have also been used to enhance attendance at counseling sessions; contingent take-home interventions can increase counseling attendance from two- to sixfold compared with conditions that have no contingencies on attendance (Iguchi et al., 1996; Stitzer et al., 1977). Additional studies have demonstrated that contingent take-home doses can also impact other treatment-related behaviors such as compliance with clinic regulations, pursuit of vocational training, and payment of clinic fees (Magura, Casriel, Goldsmith, & Lipton, 1987; Stitzer & Bigelow, 1984). The particular methadone dose provided to clients has also been employed as a positive reinforcer within a CM program, which has been referred to as the "dose alternation" procedure (Kidorf, Brooner, & King, 1997; Stitzer, Bickel, Bigelow, & Liebson, 1986). The methadone take-home and dose-alternation procedures show how treatment providers can creatively use CM strategies within existing clinic settings to positively influence treatment participation and outcomes.

Voucher-Based CM

Cocaine Abuse

In the early 1990s, Higgins and colleagues (1993, 1994) developed an effective 24-week behavioral treatment for cocaine dependence that integrated the community reinforcement approach (CRA; see below) with a voucher-based CM program that targeted cocaine abstinence (see Budney & Higgins, 1998, for a clinician manual detailing how to implement this treatment). Clients provided urine specimens on a thrice-weekly schedule and earned vouchers for each cocaine-negative urine specimen. Vouchers had monetary value that increased with each consecutive cocaine-negative specimen, beginning with S2.50 for the first cocaine-free sample. If a client had an unexcused absence from a scheduled urine test or a cocaine-positive test result, the value of the vouchers was reset to the initial low level. The intervention increased treatment retention, and the schedule of reinforcement promoted initial abstinence by providing frequent reinforcement for cocaine abstinence. The schedule also promoted continuous periods of abstinence by increasing the amount of reinforcement earned in direct relation to the number of consecutive cocaine-negative specimens submitted, and by resetting the value of the vouchers back to low amounts of reinforcement if cocaine use occurred.

Vouchers were exchangeable for retail goods or services in the community. Clinic staff only purchased items requested by clients if therapists deemed them to be consistent with treatment goals. During the first 12 weeks of the program, clients could earn a maximum of approximately $1,000 in vouchers if all scheduled urine specimens tested negative for cocaine. No vouchers were earned if a specimen was cocaine-positive or was not submitted. To give patients who slipped an incentive to keep working toward cocaine abstinence, submission of five consecutive cocaine-negative specimens following a positive specimen returned the voucher amount to the value prior to the reset.

The efficacy of CRA plus vouchers has been demonstrated in several randomized trials for cocaine dependence. In the first study, CRA plus vouchers resulted in greater treatment completion and longer periods of sustained abstinence than standard drug abuse counseling. Importantly, cocaine abstinence did not show a precipitous decrease following the end of the voucher program (Higgins et al., 1993). The second trial comparing CRA alone to CRA plus vouchers demonstrated that the contingent voucher component contributed to the positive effects of CRA (Higgins et al., 1994). The third trial demonstrated that the positive effects of the voucher program were due to its direct effects on cocaine abstinence rather than merely an effect of increasing treatment retention (Higgins et al., 2000). This positive effect was maintained posttreatment, and rates of relapse did not differ between the contingent voucher treatment and the comparison interventions.

The generality of this voucher program has also been demonstrated with inner-city intravenous cocaine abusers enrolled in a methadone maintenance program (Silverman et al., 1996, 1998). Moreover, these studies showed that this intervention also increased rates of abstinence from illicit opiates even though the vouchers were contingent on cocaine abstinence only.

Other Drugs of Abuse

The efficacy of the voucher program for cocaine dependence prompted investigations of similar programs for other types of drug abuse. For example, voucher programs can improve marijuana abstinence rates when combined with motivational enhancement therapy or cognitive-behavioral coping skills therapy for marijuana-dependent adults (Budney, Higgins, Radonovich, & Novy, 2000; Budney, Moore, Rocha, & Higgins, 2006; Carroll et al., 2006; Kadden, Litt, Kabela-Cormier, & Petry, 2007). The voucher programs used in these trials were similar to the original Higgins and colleagues (1993, 1994, 2000) program, except the total magnitude of vouchers was approximately 50% of that used in the cocaine studies, and urinalysis monitoring was reduced from thrice to once or twice weekly.

Voucher-based reinforcement has also been demonstrated to enhance treatment outcomes with opioid-dependent individuals (Bickel, Amass, Higgins, Badger, & Esch, 1997; Preston, Umbricht, & Epstein, 2000). One approach modified the voucher program such that half of the available vouchers could be earned by providing opiate-negative specimens and the other half by participating in therapeutic activities specified as part of CRA therapy (Bickel et al., 1997). A strong correlation between completion of the therapeutic activities and opioid abstinence ($r = .76$) was observed. Another study also demonstrated that voucher programs targeting completion of treatment plan activities can improve outcomes (Iguchi, Belding, Morral, Lamb, & Husband, 1997).

Voucher programs have also been used to promote abstinence from cigarette smoking. In voucher-based programs for cigarette smoking, objective evidence of smoking status can be obtained via breath carbon monoxide (Breath CO) or via cotinine detected in urine or saliva. There are costs and benefits associated with both methods. Breath CO is noninvasive, immediate, and relatively inexpensive, but Breath CO must be monitored on a frequent basis to provide a reliable index of abstinence (e.g., twice per day; see Sigmon, Lamb, & Dallery, 2008, for further discussion). Cotinine can detect smoking over a longer duration (e.g., up to about a week), but it is more invasive, especially when tested in urine. Regardless of the method, several studies have shown that voucher-based programs can be efficacious in promoting smoking abstinence in a variety of patient populations (Sigmon et al., 2008). For example, Dunn, Sigmon, Reimann, Heil, and Higgins (2009) found that voucher-based CM could be used to promote cessation in methadone-maintained patients. Because patients must attend the clinic on a frequent basis, the authors argued that a methadone clinic represents an excellent setting to deliver CM for cessation.

Because polydrug abuse is common among persons seeking treatment for cocaine or opiate dependence, several studies have examined the effects of targeting multiple drugs. An initial voucher study examined a sequential approach by first reinforcing abstinence from the primary drug of abuse, cocaine, with vouchers and then moving on to abstinence from a secondary drug, marijuana (Budney, Higgins, Delaney, & Kent, 1991). Abstinence from both drugs was achieved, with the initiation of marijuana abstinence coinciding with the initiation of the modified voucher program (see also Piotrowski & Hall, 1999). Studies that have used vouchers similar in magnitude to those used by Higgins et al. (1994), but that required simultaneous abstinence from multiple drugs of abuse in order for participants to earn the vouchers, have had limited success (Downey, Helmus, & Schuster, 2000; Iguchi et al., 1997). However, Dallery, Silverman, Chutuape, Bigelow, and Stitzer (2001) demonstrated that higher rates of simultaneous abstinence from cocaine and opioids in treatment-resistant methadone patients can be achieved if the magnitude of the incentive is increased.

Abstinence from all drugs of abuse is a very difficult goal for most polydrug abusers. Programs for this difficult treatment population may need to consider using sequential strategies that require progressively more difficult abstinence goals, providing higher magnitude reinforcers for more difficult goals, or enlisting adjunct treatment strategies such as medication, short-term hospitalization, or more intensive counseling (Chutuape, Silverman, & Stitzer, 1999).

Medication Adherence

Recent work has extended the CM approach to promote adherence to antagonist medications, such as naltrexone, for the treatment of opioid dependence (Carroll & Rounsaville, 2007). Similarly, a small number of recent studies have demonstrated that CM exerts robust effects on highly active antiretroviral therapy (HAART) adherence among drug users (Rigsby et al., 2000; Rosen et al., 2007; Sorensen et al., 2007). Rigsby et al. (2000) conducted a pilot study in a sample of HIV-infected patients with a history of cocaine and heroin abuse. They found that 4 weeks of CM resulted in an average of 92% of HAART taken on time, in comparison with 70% in the non-CM controls (measured by medication event monitoring systems; MEMs). Two larger, randomized controlled studies replicated these initial findings (Sorensen et al., 2007; Rosen et al., 2007). Rosen et al. (2007) also found that the differences in adherence were accompanied by significant changes in viral load. Notably, the observed effect sizes for HAART adherence in these studies are among the highest effect sizes produced by behavioral interventions to promote adherence among HIV-infected drug users.

Alternative Methods to Deliver CM

Prize-Based Contingency Management

In addition to the voucher-based CM model developed by Higgins and colleagues, researchers have developed and tested a number of variations of voucher-based CM and alternative incentive-based procedures. For example, Petry, Martin, Cooney, and Kranzler (2000) designed an innovative CM intervention that they termed "prize-based contingency management," whereby participants could draw a slip of paper from a fishbowl contingent on demonstrating abstinence from alcohol. In their initial study, the bowl contained 250 slips of paper, each of which represented one of four possible outcomes: (1) 50 slips contained no prize, (2) 169 slips resulted in a low magnitude prize valued at approximately $1.00 (e.g., food coupons, toiletries, or bus tokens), (3) 17 slips contained a medium prize valued at approximately $20.00 (e.g., CDs, phone cards), and (4) one slip contained a large prize valued at approximately $100.00 (e.g., stereo, DVD, television). Using this fishbowl method, participants achieved high levels of alcohol abstinence relative to standard care alcohol treatment. One rationale for the use of prized-based CM is that it entails an intermittent and unpredictable schedule of reinforcement, which has been shown to produce higher and more persistent response rates than continuous or predictable schedules of reinforcement.

The "fishbowl" method has also been combined with an escalating schedule of voucher earnings, whereby participants receive an increasing number of slips of paper contingent on consecutive weeks of abstinence (Petry et al., 2005; Stitzer, Petry, & Peirce, 2010). In addition to increasing alcohol abstinence, this method has been applied to cocaine and opioid abstinence (Petry et al., 2004), polydrug abstinence (Peirce et al., 2006; Stitzer et al., 2010), and even drug abstinence with individuals who have a history of gambling (Petry & Alessi, 2010). Individuals with a history of gambling did not engage in a higher rate of gambling when exposed to the fishbowl method, which could be a concern given that gambling is also maintained on an intermittent schedule of reinforcement.

A fishbowl incentive program was used to reinforce abstinence in two large-scale studies conducted in the context of the Clinical Trials Network (CTN). The CTN was created by the National Institute on Drug Abuse to increase collaboration between researchers and clinicians in an effort to disseminate effective evidence-based practices into the community. The motivational incentives for enhanced drug abuse recovery (MIEDAR) protocol was developed by CTN researchers and clinicians to test the effectiveness of CM on improving treatment outcomes of stimulant users in real-world community treatment programs (Kellogg et al., 2005; Stitzer et al., 2010).

In the first study (Petry et al., 2005), stimulant users beginning outpatient psychosocial treatment for substance abuse in eight community clinics were divided into two groups. Both groups received standard care; however, one group also received prize-based CM. Patients in the CM group who submitted substance-free urine samples earned draws from a fishbowl for chances to win prizes. By the end of the 12-week intervention, 49% of patients in the CM group remained in treatment versus 35% of patients in the standard care group. Additionally, patients receiving CM were four times more likely than patients receiving only standard care to demonstrate continuous abstinence for 12 weeks (18 vs. 4.9%; Petry et al., 2005). In the second MIEDAR study (Peirce et al., 2006), patients were stimulant users enrolled in a methadone maintenance program at one of six community clinics. Once again, patients receiving CM in addition to standard care were more likely to demonstrate abstinence relative to patients receiving standard care (Peirce et al., 2006).

Cash-Based Incentive Procedures

One reason for using vouchers or prizes, as opposed to cash, is that cash might be used to purchase drugs or other counterproductive goods or services. Several studies, however, suggest that cash does not increase drug use relative to alternative incentive methods. For example, Festinger et al. (2005) randomly assigned drug treatment patients to receive cash or gift certificate payments for completing a 6-month follow-up assessment. Rates of drug use during the week following receipt of the incentives did not significantly differ based on incentive type (7–14% for cash, 8–25% for gift certificates). Further, Vandrey, Bigelow, and Stitzer (2007) found no significant difference in cocaine abstinence rates after receipt of $100 in checks relative to control (no-incentive) conditions. More extensive, randomized, controlled trials will be necessary to verify these findings that cash does not increase drug use or other risky behavior.

There may be benefits to providing cash (or checks) rather than vouchers. First, cash-based procedures may reduce staff demand (Vandrey et al., 2007). When vouchers are used as consequences for abstinence, staff must purchase the items for participants, which can be time-consuming. Second, cash can reduce the delay to reinforcement (Roll, Reilly, & Johanson, 2000). CM is most effective when the consequences are delivered immediately following verification of abstinence (Petry, Bickel, & Arnett, 1998; Roll et al., 2000). Not only do drug users prefer cash when given the choice between cash and vouchers (Reilly, Roll, & Downey, 2000), they also have been shown to discount the monetary value of vouchers by approximately 10–20% of their face value for cash (Rosado, Sigmon, Jones, & Stitzer, 2005). Finally, and perhaps most significantly, several studies have found that cash-based consequences promote higher rates of behavior change than alternative voucher-based strategies (Festinger et al., 2005; Vandrey et al., 2007).

Deposit Contract Procedures

Another method to incentivize abstinence—one that has received less attention relative to the methods described above—is to require an up-front deposit by the participant. The deposit can be earned back based on evidence of abstinence. In this sense, the up-front financial allocation serves as the contract between the person trying to quit and the clinic staff. The main difference between this method and traditional CM is that the participant's own funds (or some valuable collateral) are used to incentivize abstinence instead of (or in addition to) external funds. There is a long history of using deposit contracting to reduce or eliminate a range of target behaviors, particularly cigarette smoking (Dallery, Meredith, & Glenn, 2008; Paxton, 1983; Winett, 1973). For example, Winett (1973) assessed the effects of reimbursing a $55 deposit for smoking reductions and then abstinence over a relatively brief period (2–4 weeks). After 6 months, 50% of the participants in the contingent group reported not smoking, compared to 23.5% in the noncontingent control group. Dallery et al. (2008) demonstrated that the deposit contract method can be used with voucher-based CM in which smoking status was verified via Breath CO. The use of deposit contracts could result in a more sustainable intervention with potentially substantial cost offsets. It would not be desirable, however, if the cost of the deposit unduly discouraged participation for lower income smokers (or other drug users). One potential solution would be to use a sliding deposit scale, and corresponding earnings rate, based on income.

CM in Special Populations

Pregnant Women

Pregnant drug abusers represent a particularly important and vulnerable patient population. Drug use poses multiple risks to fetuses not only from the direct pharmacological effects of the drugs on the fetus, but from the generally impoverished environment of the mother, including her poor adherence to prenatal care. The observation that pregnant drug abusers continue to use drugs despite knowledge of potential adverse consequences to the fetus suggests that the severity of their drug abuse and related problems pose a particularly difficult challenge to treatment providers. A number of projects have demonstrated that creative contingent incentive programs can decrease drug use and increase prenatal care in this important population (Jones, Haug, Silverman, Stitzer, & Svikis, 2001).

CM has also been applied to pregnant smokers (Donatelle et al., 2004). In one of the first studies involving pregnant smokers, abstinence rates were 32% and 9% in the voucher and control groups, respectively (Donatelle, Prows, Champeau, & Hudson, 2002). Smoking status was verified on a monthly basis during the pregnancy and 2 months postpartum, and incentives were contingent upon providing negative cotinine samples. Local businesses, foundations, and health care organizations provided funding for the incentives. Each smoker also nominated a "social supporter" to help her quit, with the recommendation that the individual be a female nonsmoker, and the social supporter also received vouchers if the smoker was abstinent. Thus, it should be noted that it is not clear to what extent the social support versus voucher reinforcement produced the relatively high rates of smoking abstinence. Higgins et al. (2004) also examined the effects of contingent versus noncontingent (i.e., vouchers were delivered regardless of smoking status) vouchers in pregnant smokers. At the end of pregnancy, abstinence rates were 37% and 9% in the contingent and noncontingent groups, respectively, and these rates were remarkably maintained at 12-weeks postpartum (33% and 0%). Follow-up at 24 weeks postpartum found that CM also produced long-term gains: 27% of participants in the contingent group were abstinent compared to 0% in the noncontingent group. These findings are consistent with more studies in terms of abstinence outcomes (Heil et al., 2008; Higgins et al., 2010). These recent studies also indicate that CM improves fetal health. For example, Heil et al. (2008) found that fetal health measured by serial ultrasound during the third trimester indicated significantly greater growth in terms of estimated fetal weight, femur length, and abdominal circumference in the CM group compared to the control group.

Individuals with Serious Mental Illness

Individuals suffering from serious mental illness represent another high-risk group. Drug abuse in this group is three to six times higher than among the general population, and has been associated with increased severity of psychiatric symptoms, poor psychosocial functioning, high rates of rehospitalization, and noncompliance with pharmacological and psychosocial treatment for their mental illness (Kinnaman, Slade, Bennett, & Bellack, 2007; Sigmon & Higgins, 2006). Shaner, Eckman, Roberts, and Wilkins (1995) documented a temporal relationship between arrival of disability payments and peaks in cocaine use, psychiatric symptoms, and hospital admissions among cocaine-dependent men with schizophrenia. Thus, the money intended to compensate for these patients' disability appeared to be contributing to the severity of their problems. This spawned an idea that making such payments contingent on drug abstinence might reduce misuse of funds. Indeed, feasibility studies have demonstrated that abstinence from cocaine, cigarette, and marijuana use among patients with schizophrenia can be increased with contingent positive reinforcement (Roll, Higgins, Steingard, & McGinley, 1998; Shaner, Roberts, Eckman, & Tucker, 1997; Tidey, O'Neill, & Higgins, 1999).

Several researchers have been testing a promising mechanism to apply CM on a larger scale to address the problem of seriously mentally ill patients using disability income to support drug use (Ries & Comtois, 1997; Ries & Dyck, 1997). A model for this approach currently exists in some mental health centers that use representative payees and a form of contingent disbursement of benefits for severely ill and dually diagnosed patients. Ries et al. (2004) found that contingent management of benefits, which meant management of the type and frequency of benefits (not amount), produced higher rates of drug and alcohol abstinence than a noncontingent management group. This model may have substantial promise in terms of dissemination potential.

Adolescent Drug Abusers

Recently, researchers and clinicians have evaluated the efficacy of CM in adolescent drug users (Henggeler et al., 2006; Stanger & Budney, 2010) and smokers (Reynolds, Dallery, Shroff, Patak, & Leraas, 2008; Roll, 2005). For example, Stanger, Budney, Kamon, and Thostensen (2009) applied an abstinence incentive program in marijuana-abusing adolescents. Adolescents in the treatment group received incentives only if they showed abstinence from all drugs (verified by urinalysis and breath alcohol). In addition to the usual incentive program administered through the clinic, this CM program also instructed parents on how to implement a home-based CM program through use of a contract that specified incentives that would be provided each time abstinence was documented (twice per week) or punishments that would occur each time substance use was detected. Adolescents in the control group received incentives for attending treatment appointments. Both groups received individualized motivational enhancement and cognitive-behavioral therapy (MET/CBT) and twice-weekly drug testing. The experimental group showed greater marijuana abstinence during treatment (7.6 vs. 5.1 continuous weeks) and 50% versus 18% achieved at least 10 weeks of abstinence. The study suggested that reinforcement-based treatment strategies have considerable promise in adolescent, drug-abusing populations.

Given the evidence base for CM, several studies have developed and tested adoption and implementation strategies for using CM with adolescents in public treatment systems (Henggeler et al., 2007; McCollister, French, Sheidow, Henggeler, & Halliday-Boykins, 2009). These studies suggest that clinical priorities and client resistance were the most frequently cited barriers to adopting CM, but that public-sector practitioners are favorably inclined to implement CM. Overall, the application of CM to adolescent drug users represents an important advance in light of this highly sensitive developmental period.

Expanding the Range of CM Applications

The Therapeutic Workplace

An innovative application of CM with excellent potential for application is the reinforcement-based Therapeutic Workplace, an intervention that uses the opportunity to participate in paid work to reinforce abstinence (DeFulio, Donlin, Wong, & Silverman, 2009; Donlin, Knealing, Needham, Wong, & Silverman, 2008; Knealing, Roebuck, Wong, & Silverman, 2008; Silverman, Svikis, Robles, Stitzer, & Bigelow, 2001). The efficacy of this approach was demonstrated in a study of methadone-maintained pregnant women enrolled in treatment that included group and individual therapy, ob/gyn medical services, family planning, transportation to appointments, child care, initial residential care, and day treatment during the 28 days following residential care. Therapeutic Workplace participants were invited to attend a workplace 3 hours per day in addition to receiving these other services. To gain access to this program, each day they were required to provide a urine specimen that tested negative for cocaine and opiates. If the specimen tested positive, they were not allowed to work that day. Those who gained entrance received basic skills education and job skills training. At the end of the shift they received a voucher. Pay was dictated by an escalating reinforcement schedule. Additional vouchers could be earned for professional demeanor, meeting daily learning goals, and data-entry productivity.

More recently, DeFulio et al. (2009) found that contingent access to a workplace in cocaine-abusing, methadone-maintained patients produced higher rates of cocaine-negative urine specimens (79.3%) compared to a condition in which access to the workplace was permitted regardless of cocaine use (50.7%). There are at least four noteworthy features of this study. First, participants included in this study were those who showed persistent cocaine use during treatment in a standard methadone community clinic. Second, employment-based CM continued for 1 year, which is a much longer period than the vast majority of CM interventions targeting cocaine use (Silverman, Robles, Mudric, Bigelow, & Stitzer, 2004). Third, participants were paid in the form of checks rather than vouchers. Fourth, the study indicated additional public health benefits by showing that CM significantly reduced rates of HIV risk behaviors. Specifically, participants reported significantly lower rates of trading sex for drugs or money. Another study by Silverman and colleagues (2002) showed that employment-based CM led to higher rates of abstinence over a 3-year period. This is among the longest sustained CM interventions reported in the literature. Overall, this study and others offer strong support for the utility of integrating CM into employment settings to promote long-term abstinence.

Contingent Housing and Work Therapy for the Homeless

A creative CM approach to treating homeless substance abusers demonstrated that a contingent housing and work therapy program combined with an intensive psychosocial treatment can decrease drug abuse and increase other important areas of functioning among homeless crack and other substance abusers (Milby et al., 2000, 2003; Schumacher et al., 2007). Cocaine-abusing homeless persons earned access to a rent-free furnished apartment if they provided two consecutive weeks of cocaine-negative urine tests. Once living in the apartment, a cocaine-positive urine test resulted in immediate eviction and transportation to a shelter. Two consecutive drug-negative tests following eviction earned renewed access to the apartment. During the second phase of this program, participants could also participate in a paid work therapy program that involved construction (refurbishing apartments for the program) or food service work. Access to work was again contingent on 2 weeks of documented drug abstinence; once employed, drug-positive urine tests resulted in suspension from work.

Technological Innovations

One feature of many CM programs is that frequent, continued monitoring of drug status is necessary. Thus, requiring participants to make in-person visits may not be feasible depending on the CM delivery model and the drug targeted (DeFulio et al., 2009). To solve some of the logistical challenges associated with frequent monitoring of smoking status, Dallery and colleagues (Dallery & Glenn, 2005; Dallery, Glenn, & Raiff, 2007; Dallery et al., 2008; Stoops et al., 2009) developed an Internet-based CM intervention to promote smoking cessation. Smoking status was verified via a web camera. The results showed that the voucher program produced high rates of abstinence and excellent adherence with the monitoring schedule. In one study, 97% of 1,120 total samples scheduled were provided (Dallery et al., 2007). Thus, the Internet-based system obviated many of the logistical problems entailed by frequent CO monitoring.

Whether and how similar technological solutions may be applied to monitoring for other drug abuse is underexplored. Yet novel and emerging technologies are increasingly being integrated into systems of health care. For example, ubiquitous computing technologies that "weave themselves into the fabric of everyday life until they are indistinguishable from it" (Weiser, 1991, p. 94) can be employed to gain real-time data of physiological, environmental factors that precede and follow drug use (or abstinence). Boyer, Smelson, Fletcher, Ziedonis, and Picard (2010) have argued that existing models of assessment and treatment are inadequate to the task of providing tailored, continuous interventions for substance abuse, and that new tools are necessary—tools such as ubiquitous computing and other emerging technologies—to meet treatment needs.

Integrating CM with Other Psychosocial Interventions

Although some studies have shown that CM alone or combined with other treatments produces better long-term treatment outcomes than standard care (Higgins et al., 2000), this finding is unreliable across studies. Thus, the sustainability of CM interventions has been questioned because drug use sometimes returns to preintervention levels after CM is withdrawn. This concern applies equally to all interventions for drug use, including psychosocial and pharmacological interventions (McLellan, O'Brien, Lewis, & Kleber, 2000). Nevertheless, researchers have sought to improve long-term treatment outcomes by combining CM with various evidence-based psychosocial interventions.

Early work combined voucher-based CM with CRA (Higgins et al., 1994). CRA and CM are founded on the same basic principles that substance abuse is maintained by substance-related reinforcers and a lack of alternative reinforcers. Like CM, CRA increases the availability of rein-forcement contingent on behavior that is incompatible with substance abuse. However, unlike CM, CRA does not rely primarily on experimenter-arranged contingencies (e.g., vouchers contingent on abstinence). Rather, practitioners work together with patients to promote desirable behavior change in several key areas of the patient's life, including family relation-ships, recreational activities, social networks, and vocation (Budney & Higgins, 1998), thereby increasing alternative sources of reinforcement. In short, practitioners help patients find ways to make non-drug-related behavior more reinforcing than drug use (Meyers & Smith, 1995). Indeed, some research has shown that CRA not only works to promote abstinence from abused substances, but that it is more effective than standard care (Roozen et al., 2004).

Although no research to date has shown that adding CRA to a CM treatment protocol improves long-term abstinence rates relative to CM alone, Higgins et al. (2003) showed that CRA may enhance other treatment outcomes. For example, the researchers found that combining voucher-based CM with CRA improved treatment retention relative to CM alone. They also found that patients treated with CRA and CM reported fewer hospitalizations and legal problems during a 12-month follow-up assess-ment than patients treated with CM alone. Thus, integrating CRA into a CM intervention may have several advantages.

CBT has also been combined with CM in attempts to improve long-term treatment outcomes. For example, Rawson et al. (2006) divided stimulant-dependent participants into one of three 16-week treatment con-ditions: CM, CBT, or CM + CBT. CM + CBT did not significantly improve treatment retention relative to CM alone. Additionally, combining the two treatments did not produce an increase in the mean number of stimulant-free urine samples collected during treatment relative to CM alone. Fur-thermore, there were no differences in any outcome measures between any of the treatment conditions at 3-month follow-up assessments.

Motivational interviewing is another empirically supported psychoso-cial intervention (Hettema, Steele, & Miller, 2005) that has been combined with CM. Like CRA and CBT, the processes involved in behavior change in motivational interviewing can be framed in terms that are compatible with the theoretical foundations of CM (Christopher & Dougher, 2009). MET is a psychosocial intervention frequently used to treat alcohol dependence wherein counselors utilize motivational interviewing techniques. Research has shown that MET/CBT combined with CM increases abstinence rates among marijuana-dependent participants during treatment (Carroll et al., 2006) and posttreatment (Budney et al., 2006; Kadden et al., 2007) relative to either treatment alone.

Because group-based treatment modalities are common in substance abuse treatment clinics, researchers have recently combined CM with group therapy. For example, Petry, Weinstock, Alessi, Lewis, and Dieckhaus (2010) found that CM delivered in group settings is feasible and efficacious in increasing drug abstinence among HIV-positive substance abusers. The group CM intervention produced significantly greater consecutive drug-free samples (opiates, cocaine, alcohol) relative to a 12-step control group, although the overall proportions of negative samples did not differ between groups. Group CM also reduced viral loads during treatment, but this effect was not maintained at follow-up.

It is possible that arranging contingencies based on group performance (not just individual performance) may improve the compatibility of CM and group-therapy-based interventions. Kirby, Kerwin, Carpenedo, Rosenwasser, and Gardner (2008) found that delivering monetary consequences contingent on group performance (i.e., group contingencies) is a feasible treatment strategy for producing desirable behavior change among cocaine-dependent methadone-maintained patients. Similarly, Meredith, Grabinski, and Dallery (in press) employed group contingencies to promote abstinence from cigarette smoking. Vouchers were delivered via the Internet based on the Breath CO levels of individuals, and based on whether the entire group met the abstinence criterion. The study also integrated an online peer support forum. The forum allowed participants to provide social support for one another when they met their treatment goals. This forum could have implications for sustainability without increasing treatment costs. For example, access to the online peer support forum could continue after the monetary contingencies are removed from the intervention, which may help sustain treatment effects previously established by the monetary contingencies.

CM is often delivered in conjunction with psychosocial interventions. Although few studies to date have shown that integrating psychosocial therapy into a CM treatment program improves abstinence rates during treatment, some research shows that it can improve posttreatment outcomes. Thus, researchers should continue to investigate the short-term and long-term effects of combining psychosocial interventions with CM, and clinicians should be encouraged to include a psychosocial therapy component in their CM treatment protocols.

Dissemination of CM: Challenges and Opportunities

Evidence-based substance abuse treatments are slow to diffuse from research to practice (Lamb, Greenlick, & McCarty, 1998). CM is no exception to this rule. Despite overwhelming evidence supporting the efficacy of CM interventions, the treatment strategy is rarely used by community-based treatment providers (Herbeck, Hser, & Teruya, 2008; Lott & Jencius, 2009; McGovern, Fox, Xie, & Drake, 2004). Below we address some of the key challenges facing dissemination efforts, as well as some promising new directions in implementing CM on a broad scale.

Cost

Although some research suggests CM interventions are cost-effective (Olmstead, Sindelar, & Petry, 2007a; Olmstead, Sindelar, & Petry, 2007b; Sindelar, Elbel, & Petry, 2007), the cost of monetary incentives is often viewed as a significant barrier to dissemination (Petry & Simcic, 2002). A number of innovative strategies can be used to reduce costs without degrading treatment integrity or efficacy (Amass & Kamien, 2008; Petry et al., 2000). For example, treatment providers in the private sector can increase fees to recoup voucher costs. Increased fees could even be returned to patients as rebates when they meet treatment goals (i.e., utilize deposit contracts; Dallery et al., 2008). In the context of mental health clinics where the clinic acts as a representative payee of disability benefits, CM can be delivered based on a management of benefits without increasing costs (Ries et al., 2004). In the substance abuse clinic, clinic funds can be supplemented with donations from the community (Amass & Kamien, 2008).

Several studies have shown how low-cost CM interventions can result in clinically significant improvements in treatment outcomes. For example, a recent observational study suggests that low-cost, prize-based CM can be delivered in a community substance abuse treatment program for adolescents (Lott & Jencius, 2009). Expenses related to CM were minimal at $0.39 per patient per day, and the percentage of urine samples positive for multiple drugs decreased from 33.3 to 23.4%. The authors also noted that CM increased length of stay and that CM-based costs were likely offset due to the increased length of stay and associated increase in clinical charges.

Some authors have argued that the development of long-term sustainable interventions is one of the most important challenges in substance abuse treatment research (DeFulio et al., 2009; Silverman et al., 2002, 2007). Several promising models could be used to address this challenge, such as the use of contingent housing, or employment-based abstinence reinforcement (reviewed above). As noted by Defulio et al. (2009), employment-based CM may be an ideal long-term treatment for cocaine dependence. Many employment settings not only control powerful reinforcers, they can monitor drug status over long periods by virtue of the fact that drug testing is already used in many workplaces.

Another cost-saving strategy is to incorporate computerized therapies into community-based treatment clinics (Bickel, Marsch, Buchhalter, & Badger, 2008; Budney et al., 2011). Evidence-based, psychosocial interventions may be expensive to implement and require financial and staffing resources not available to the average treatment program. They can also be complex and require considerable staff training in order to be applied with fidelity. Computerized therapies could reduce staff burden and associated costs and deliver treatment with high fidelity. Moreover, a portion of the savings could be reallocated to administer CM programs.

Education and Training

In an effort to identify other variables that may inhibit dissemination, several studies have assessed clinicians' characteristics and practices, as well as their attitudes and beliefs regarding CM (Benishek, Kirby, Dugosh, & Padovano, 2010; Bride, Abraham, & Roman, 2010; McGovern et al., 2004). Results from these studies suggest that the most significant barrier to dissemination may be education and training. Nearly half of community-based treatment providers report being unfamiliar with CM (48%; McGovern et al., 2004) or not knowing if the treatment is effective (43%; Herbeck et al., 2008). Many, in fact, have unfavorable opinions about incentive-based strategies and believe them to be ineffective (McCarty et al., 2007). However, clinicians with more education and greater experience treating substance abuse report more favorable opinions of CM (Kirby, Benishek, Dugosh, & Kerwin, 2006; McCarty et al., 2007). Moreover, CM training and experience is associated with an increase in perceived effectiveness of the treatment (Bride et al., 2010; Kirby et al., 2006). Benishek et al. (2010) also found that treatment providers' opinions of CM improved and their willingness to implement the treatment increased after reading summaries of empirical findings related to CM.

Thus, one way to promote dissemination may be to educate and train community-based treatment providers. Researchers should publish in outlets other than academic journals and forge collaborative relationships with clinicians. Indeed, such collaboration was a major goal of the CTN. In one exemplary project, researchers and clinicians from the CTN collaborated with leaders from the New York City Health and Hospitals Corporation (HHC), the largest public hospital system in the United States, to integrate CM into the treatment protocols in five HHC clinics (Kellogg et al., 2005). One of the most notable findings to emerge from this collaborative effort was the reaction of clinicians to the new treatment approach. Kellogg et al. (2005) described how CM was initially met with resistance by many clinicians. After observing the effects of the treatment on patient behavior, however, attitudes began to change. When the staff observed improvements in patient behavior, including self-esteem, they stopped viewing the prize-based incentives as "bribes" and started viewing them as opportunities to praise patients for meeting treatment goals. Counselors and clinic staff not only developed more favorable opinions of CM, the overall mood and culture of the clinics changed. CM became the centerpiece of the psychosocial component of the HHC treatment programs. Rather than being critical of patients when they did not meet their treatment goals, counselors began to congratulate them when they did meet their goals.

Principles of Application and Recommendations

A wide variety of CM interventions can be found in a recently published text on this topic (Higgins et al., 2008). General overviews on the application of general behavior analytic principles can be found in a number of sources (Martin & Pear, 2010). Here we offer an abbreviated summary of these principles and examples of their application in a substance abuse setting.

The *delay to reinforcement* refers to the temporal relation between the target behavior and the delivery of the consequence. The efficacy of the contingency will generally increase as the temporal delay between the occurrence of the target behavior and delivery of the scheduled consequence decreases (Kirby, Petry, & Bickel, 1999; Petry et al., 1998; Roll et al., 2000). Thus, reinforcement or punishment should be applied as close in time to the detection of the target behavior as possible. For example, all else being equal, a clinic that provides positive reinforcement for cocaine abstinence 5 minutes after a client submits a cocaine-negative urine specimen would generate greater rates of cocaine abstinence than a clinic that waits 4 days after the submission of the specimen before reinforcement is delivered.

The *frequency of reinforcement* is another important variable. More frequent opportunities for reinforcement (e.g., three times per week) are preferable to less frequent (once per week) schedules in establishing an initial target behavior like drug abstinence or attendance at counseling sessions. Once a target behavior (e.g., abstinence) is established, a less frequent schedule of reinforcement that is delivered on a fixed or variable schedule may be used for maintenance purposes. Because different drugs may require different monitoring schedules (e.g., more frequent monitoring for smoking), consulting the literature is recommended to identify the proper frequency of and delay to reinforcement.

The *schedule of reinforcement* used in CM interventions is also a determinant of their effectiveness (Roll et al., 2000; Roll et al., 2006). Specifically, one study compared the effects of a constant, fixed monetary value to escalating values for each consecutive negative drug sample. The fixed value was always $9.80 for negative samples. One escalating schedule started at $3.00 and escalated by $0.50 for each consecutive negative sample, plus a $10.00 bonus for every third consecutive negative sample (Roll & Higgins, 2000). Another escalating schedule specified the same parameters, but with the addition of a *reset contingency* in which a positive or missing sample resulted in the monetary value for the next negative sample resetting to $3.00 (i.e., negative punishment). If participants remained abstinent the entire time, they could earn the same amount of money in all three conditions. The authors found a significant difference between the schedules in the percentage of smokers who initiated and sustained abstinence, with the fixed schedule resulting in 17% of participants, compared to 22% in the escalating schedule without a reset, and 50% in the escalating schedule with a reset contingency. The escalating schedule with a reset contingency is the most common voucher-based schedule of reinforcement.

One potential problem with an escalating schedule of reinforcement is the low initial value of the consequence for abstinence. Several researchers have noted that a number of participants in clinical trials evaluating CM do not contact the monetary reinforcers for abstinence (Correia, Sigmon, Silverman, Bigelow, & Stitzer, 2005; Petry, 2000). It is possible that the low initial value is not high enough to motivate initial abstinence. A study by Silverman and colleagues (1998), however, suggested that increasing the initial voucher earnings did not result in a higher rate of cocaine abstinence compared to the standard escalating schedule of reinforcement. Another possible reason why some participants do not achieve abstinence is that most CM interventions require an abrupt transition to abstinence. Gradual reductions in drug use may permit greater contact with monetary reinforcers for changing drug use. Several studies suggest that gradual reductions in drug use, or shaping procedures, can generate high initial rates of abstinence in cocaine- (Correia et al., 2005) and nicotine-dependent individuals (Lamb, Kirby, Morral, Galbicka, & Iguchi, 2010). In order to use shaping, it is necessary to employ a quantitative outcome measure of drug status (as opposed to a categorical drug present/absent outcome measure).

Reinforcer magnitude is another important variable (Businelle, Rash, Burke, & Parker, 2009; Carroll, Sinha, Nich, Babuscio, & Rounsaville, 2002; Dallery et al., 2001). For example, if a patient's goal is drug abstinence as indicated by a drug-negative urine test, the scheduled delivery of a voucher worth $10.00 for each negative specimen is more likely to motivate drug cessation than a voucher worth $2.50. Silverman, Chutuape, Bigelow, and Stitzer (1999) demonstrated the importance of magnitude with methadone maintenance patients showing that high-value vouchers produced more cocaine abstinence than low-value vouchers, which were superior to zero-value vouchers. Choice of what magnitude of reinforcement to use requires careful consideration of the severity of the behavior targeted for change and the difficulty patients experience trying to change such behavior. An effective reinforcer must compete with the reinforcement derived from the behavior targeted for change. Given the resilience of substance use habits typically developed over many years, and especially when treating individuals who use relatively large quantities of a drug, strong reinforcers are likely to be necessary. The importance of magnitude notwithstanding, creative use of relatively low magnitude reinforcers has been successful in modifying a wide variety of target behaviors among drug abusers, especially when used in combination with other treatment interventions (Lott & Jencius, 2009; Stitzer et al., 2010).

CM programs must also employ an effective *monitoring system* so that consequences can be applied accurately and systematically. Precise information on the occurrence of the therapeutic target response is necessary to implement a successful intervention. With drug abusers, this is usually whether they have used drugs recently and involves some form of biochemical verification of drug abstinence. Urinalysis testing is the most common verification procedure in CM treatments for drug abuse, and breath-based techniques for alcohol and cigarette smoking have also been employed. Such objective monitoring is necessary for fair and effective implementation of CM programs. When choosing other behavioral targets, such as medication compliance, attending counseling sessions, increasing social activities, and completion of skills-training homework, the treatment provider must always keep in mind the need to objectively verify whether the target behavior occurred.

For CM to be effective, it is critical to select parameters of reinforcement (delay, magnitude, etc.) that maximize the probability of successful outcomes. Knowledge of the basic principles outlined above will help increase the chance of choosing parameters that result in good outcomes. However, one must be aware that selection of "incorrect" parameters may render the intervention ineffective, which could lead to the conclusion that the principles underlying the intervention do not work. In practice, it is likely that the parameters of a specific CM program may need to be modified repeatedly prior to finding the optimal program for a specific population or treatment setting.

Conclusion

CM can help clients to engage in therapy and find alternative, nondrug sources of reinforcement. Nonetheless, CM, like many other effective drug abuse treatments, are not the models most commonly used in community clinics. Most of the work described in this chapter has been implemented only in research settings (Kellogg et al., 2005; Lott & Jencius, 2009; Stitzer et al., 2010). A number of philosophical and practical factors contribute to this situation. As one can imagine, the logistics of initiating such a program in a typical community clinic may appear daunting. The costs of incentives, regular drug testing, and the personnel to run the program may seem beyond reasonable expectations, particularly given today's tight market on health care spending. Moreover, asking experienced therapists with histories of providing treatments that are based on a very different understanding of substance dependence also may appear problematic. Yet the need for more effective interventions in the drug abuse community is so great and the CM approach has so much to offer that it seems imperative that the field turn its attention to the issue of dissemination of such programs.

This chapter has provided examples of how communities might be willing to fund voucher-based programs, how such programs have the potential to become self-sustaining while simultaneously enhancing the vocational skills of the substance abuser, and how creative, low-cost CM strategies can be developed by using existing clinic privileges to enhance therapeutic outcomes. The research suggests that investing in the development and dissemination of CM programs has the potential to produce a substantial, cost-effective payoff. The high cost of problems associated with drug dependence and its seemingly refractory course implore us to seek alternative strategies for intervening with this difficult treatment population. CM strategies certainly do not provide "the answer" that will eradicate this societal problem. They do, however, offer alternative and complementary strategies to effectively treat individuals suffering from substance use disorders.

References

Amass, L., & Kamien, J. B. (2008). Funding contingency management in community treatment clinics: Use of community donations and clinic rebates. In S. T. Higgins, K. Silverman, & S. H. Heil (Eds.), *Contingency management in substance abuse treatment* (pp. 280–297). New York: Guilford Press.

Azrin, N. H., Sisson, R. W., Meyers, R., & Godley, M. (1982). Alcoholism treatment by disulfiram and community reinforcement therapy. *Journal of Behavior Therapy and Experimental Psychiatry, 13*(2), 105–112.

Benishek, L. A., Kirby, K. C., Dugosh, K. L., & Padovano, A. (2010). Beliefs about the empirical support of drug abuse treatment interventions: A survey of outpatient treatment providers. *Drug and Alcohol Dependence, 107*(2–3), 202–208.

Bickel, W. K., Amass, L., Higgins, S. T., Badger, G. J., & Esch, R. A. (1997). Effects of adding behavioral treatment to opioid detoxification with buprenorphine. *Journal of Consulting and Clinical Psychology, 65*(5), 803–810.

Bickel, W. K., Marsch, L. A., Buchhalter, A. R., & Badger, G. J. (2008). Computerized behavior therapy for opioid-dependent outpatients: A randomized controlled trial. *Experimental and Clinical Psychopharmacology, 16*(2), 132–143.

Boyer E. W., Smelson, D., Fletcher, R., Ziedonis, D., & Picard, R. W. (2010). Wireless technologies, ubiquitous computing and mobile health: Application to drug abuse treatment and compliance with HIV therapies. *Journal of Medical Toxicology, 6,* 212–216.

Bride, B. E., Abraham, A. J., & Roman, P. M. (2010). Diffusion of contingency management and attitudes regarding its effectiveness and acceptability.

Substance Abuse: Official Publication of the Association for Medical Education and Research in Substance Abuse, 31(3), 127–135.

Budney, A. J., Fearer, S., Walker, D. D., Stanger, C., Thostenson, J., Grabinski, M., & Bickel, W. K. (2011). An initial trial of a computerized behavioral intervention for cannabis use disorder. *Drug and Alcohol Dependence, 115*(1–2), 74–79.

Budney, A. J., & Higgins, S. T. (1998). *A community reinforcement plus vouchers approach: Treating cocaine addiction.* Rockville, MD: U.S. Department of Health and Human Services.

Budney, A. J., Higgins, S. T., Delaney, D. D., & Kent, L. (1991). Contingent reinforcement of abstinence with individuals abusing cocaine and marijuana. *Journal of Applied Behavior Analysis, 24*(4), 657–665.

Budney, A. J., Higgins, S. T., Radonovich, K. J., & Novy, P. L. (2000). Adding voucher-based incentives to coping skills and motivational enhancement improves outcomes during treatment for marijuana dependence. *Journal of Consulting and Clinical Psychology, 68*(6), 1051–1061.

Budney, A. J., Moore, B. A., Rocha, H. L., & Higgins, S. T. (2006). Clinical trial of abstinence-based vouchers and cognitive-behavioral therapy for cannabis dependence. *Journal of Consulting and Clinical Psychology, 74*(2), 307–316.

Businelle, M. S., Rash, C. J., Burke, R. S., & Parker, J. D. (2009). Using vouchers to increase continuing care participation in veterans: Does magnitude matter? *American Journal on Addictions/American Academy of Psychiatrists in Alcoholism and Addictions, 18*(2), 122–129.

Carroll, K. M., Easton, C. J., Nich, C., Hunkele, K. A., Neavins, T. M., Sinha, R., et al. (2006). The use of contingency management and motivational/skills-building therapy to treat young adults with marijuana dependence. *Journal of Consulting and Clinical Psychology, 74*(5), 955–966.

Carroll, K. M., & Rounsaville, B. J. (2007). A perfect platform: Combining contingency management with medications for drug abuse. *American Journal of Drug and Alcohol Abuse, 33*(3), 343–365.

Carroll, K. M., Sinha, R., Nich, C., Babuscio, T., & Rounsaville, B. J. (2002). Contingency management to enhance naltrexone treatment of opioid dependence: A randomized clinical trial of reinforcement magnitude. *Experimental and Clinical Psychopharmacology, 10*(1), 54–63.

Christopher, P. J., & Dougher, M. J. (2009). A behavior-analytic account of motivational interviewing. *The Behavior Analyst, 32*(1), 149–161.

Chutuape, M. A., Silverman, K., & Stitzer, M. (1999). Contingent reinforcement sustains postdetoxification abstinence from multiple drugs: A preliminary study with methadone patients. *Drug and Alcohol Dependence, 54*(1), 69–81.

Correia, C. J., Sigmon, S. C., Silverman, K., Bigelow, G., & Stitzer, M. L. (2005). A comparison of voucher-delivery schedules for the initiation of cocaine abstinence. *Experimental and Clinical Psychopharmacology, 13*(3), 253–258.

Dallery, J., & Glenn, I. M. (2005). Effects of an Internet-based voucher reinforcement program for smoking abstinence: A feasibility study. *Journal of Applied Behavior Analysis, 38*(3), 349–357.

Dallery, J., Glenn, I. M., & Raiff, B. R. (2007). An Internet-based abstinence reinforcement treatment for cigarette smoking. *Drug and Alcohol Dependence, 86*(2–3), 230–238.

Dallery, J., Meredith, S., & Glenn, I. M. (2008). A deposit contract method to deliver abstinence reinforcement for cigarette smoking. *Journal of Applied Behavior Analysis, 41*(4), 609–615.

Dallery, J., Silverman, K., Chutuape, M. A., Bigelow, G. E., & Stitzer, M. L. (2001). Voucher-based reinforcement of opiate plus cocaine abstinence in treatment-resistant methadone patients: Effects of reinforcer magnitude. *Experimental and Clinical Psychopharmacology, 9*(3), 317–325.

DeFulio, A., Donlin, W. D., Wong, C. J., & Silverman, K. (2009). Employment-based abstinence reinforcement as a maintenance intervention for the treatment of cocaine dependence: A randomized controlled trial. *Addiction, 104*(9), 1530–1538.

DeGrandpre, R. J. (2000). A science of meaning: Can behaviorism bring meaning to psychological science? *American Psychologist, 55*(7), 721–739.

Donatelle, R. J., Hudson, D., Dobie, S., Goodall, A., Hunsberger, M., & Oswald, K. (2004). Incentives in smoking cessation: Status of the field and implications for research and practice with pregnant smokers. *Nicotine and Tobacco Research, 6*(Suppl. 2), S163–S179.

Donatelle, R. J., Prows, S. L., Champeau, D., & Hudson, D. (2002). Randomized controlled trial using social support and financial incentives for high risk pregnant smokers: Significant other supporter (SOS) program. *Tobacco Control, 2*(3), 67–69.

Donlin, W. D., Knealing, T. W., Needham, M., Wong, C. J., & Silverman, K. (2008). Attendance rates in a workplace predict subsequent outcome of employment-based reinforcement of cocaine abstinence in methadone patients. *Journal of Applied Behavior Analysis, 41*(4), 499–516.

Downey, K. K., Helmus, T. C., & Schuster, C. R. (2000). Treatment of heroin-dependent polydrug abusers with contingency management and buprenorphine maintenance. *Experimental and Clinical Psychopharmacology, 8*(2), 176–184.

Dunn, K. E., Sigmon, S. C., Reimann, E., Heil, S. H., & Higgins, S. T. (2009). Effects of smoking cessation on illicit drug use among opioid maintenance patients: A pilot study. *Journal of Drug Issues, 39*(2), 313–328.

Festinger, D. S., Marlowe, D. B., Croft, J. R., Dugosh, K. L., Mastro, N. K., Lee, P. A., et al. (2005). Do research payments precipitate drug use or coerce participation? *Drug and Alcohol Dependence, 78*(3), 275–281.

Griffiths, R. R., Bigelow, G. E., & Henningfield, J. E. (1980). Similarities in animal and human drug-taking behavior. In N. K. Mello (Ed.), *Advances in substance abuse: Behavioral and biological research* (pp. 1–90). Greenwich, CT: JAI Press.

Heil, S. H., Higgins, S. T., Bernstein, I. M., Solomon, L. J., Rogers, R. E., Thomas, C. S., et al. (2008). Effects of voucher-based incentives on abstinence from cigarette smoking and fetal growth among pregnant women. *Addiction, 103*(6), 1009–1018.

Henggeler, S. W., Chapman, J. E., Rowland, M. D., Halliday-Boykins, C. A., Randall, J., Shackelford, J., et al. (2007). If you build it, they will come: Statewide practitioner interest in contingency management for youths. *Journal of Substance Abuse Treatment, 32*(2), 121–131.

Henggeler, S. W., Halliday-Boykins, C. A., Cunningham, P. B., Randall, J., Shapiro, S. B., & Chapman, J. E. (2006). Juvenile drug court: Enhancing outcomes by integrating evidence-based treatments. *Journal of Consulting and Clinical Psychology, 74*(1), 42–54.

Herbeck, D. M., Hser, Y., & Teruya, C. (2008). Empirically supported substance abuse treatment approaches: A survey of treatment providers' perspectives and practices. *Addictive Behaviors, 33*(5), 699–712.

Hettema, J., Steele, J., & Miller, W. R. (2005). Motivational interviewing. *Annual Review of Clinical Psychology, 1*(1), 91–111.

Higgins, S. T., Bernstein, I. M., Washio, Y., Heil, S. H., Badger, G. J., Skelly, J. M., et al. (2010). Effects of smoking cessation with voucher-based contingency management on birth outcomes. *Addiction, 105*(11), 2023–2030.

Higgins, S. T., Budney, A. J., Bickel, W. K., Foerg, F. E., Donham, R., & Badger, G. J. (1994). Incentives improve outcome in outpatient behavioral treatment of cocaine dependence. *Archives of General Psychiatry, 51*(7), 568–576.

Higgins, S. T., Budney, A. J., Bickel, W. K., Hughes, J. R., Foerg, F., & Badger, G. (1993). Achieving cocaine abstinence with a behavioral approach. *American Journal of Psychiatry, 150*(5), 763–769.

Higgins, S. T., Heil, S. H., Solomon, L. J., Bernstein, I. M., Lussier, J. P., Abel, R. L., et al. (2004). A pilot study on voucher-based incentives to promote abstinence from cigarette smoking during pregnancy and postpartum. *Nicotine and Tobacco Research, 6*(6), 1015–1020.

Higgins, S. T., Sigmon, S. C., Wong, C. J., Heil, S. H., Badger, G. J., Donham, R., et al. (2003). Community reinforcement therapy for cocaine-dependent outpatients. *Archives of General Psychiatry, 60*(10), 1043–1052.

Higgins, S. T., Silverman, K., & Heil, S. H. (2008). *Contingency management in substance abuse treatment.* New York, NY U.S.: Guilford Press.

Higgins, S. T., Wong, C. J., Badger, G. J., Ogden, D. E. H., & Dantona, R. L. (2000). Contingent reinforcement increases cocaine abstinence during outpatient treatment and 1 year of follow-up. *Journal of Consulting and Clinical Psychology, 68*(1), 64–72.

Iguchi, M. Y., Belding, M. A., Morral, A. R., Lamb, R. J., & Husband, S. D. (1997). Reinforcing operants other than abstinence in drug abuse treatment: An effective alternative for reducing drug use. *Journal of Consulting and Clinical Psychology, 65*(3), 421–428.

Iguchi, M. Y., Lamb, R. J., Belding, M. A., Platt, J. J., Husband, S. D., & Morral, A. R. (1996). Contingent reinforcement of group participation versus abstinence in a methadone maintenance program. *Experimental and Clinical Psychopharmacology, 4*(3), 315–321.

Jones, H. E., Haug, N., Silverman, K., Stitzer, M., & Svikis, D. (2001). The effectiveness of incentives in enhancing treatment attendance and drug abstinence in methadone-maintained pregnant women. *Drug and Alcohol Dependence, 61*(3), 297–306.

Kadden, R. M., Litt, M. D., Kabela-Cormier, E., & Petry, N. M. (2007). Abstinence rates following behavioral treatments for marijuana dependence. *Addictive Behaviors, 32*(6), 1220–1236.

Kellogg, S. H., Burns, M., Coleman, P., Stitzer, M., Wale, J. B., & Kreek, M. J. (2005). Something of value: The introduction of contingency management interventions into the New York City Health and Hospital Addiction Treatment Service. *Journal of Substance Abuse Treatment, 28*(1), 57–65.

Kidorf, M., Brooner, R. K., & King, V. L. (1997). Motivating methadone patients to include drug-free significant others in treatment: A behavioral intervention. *Journal of Substance Abuse Treatment, 14*(1), 23–28.

Kidorf, M., & Stitzer, M. L. (1999). Contingent access to clinic privileges reduces drug abuse in methadone maintenance patients. In K. Silverman (Ed.), *Motivating behavior change among illicit-drug abusers: Research on contingency management interventions* (pp. 221–241). Washington, DC: American Psychological Association.

Kinnaman, J. E. S., Slade, E., Bennett, M. E., & Bellack, A. S. (2007). Examination of contingency payments to dually-diagnosed patients in a multi-faceted behavioral treatment. *Addictive Behaviors, 32*(7), 1480–1485.

Kirby, K. C., Benishek, L. A., Dugosh, K. L., & Kerwin, M. E. (2006). Substance abuse treatment providers' beliefs and objections regarding contingency management: Implications for dissemination. *Drug and Alcohol Dependence, 85*(1), 19–27.

Kirby, K. C., Kerwin, M. E., Carpenedo, C. M., Rosenwasser, B. J., & Gardner, R. S. (2008). Interdependent group contingency management for cocaine-dependent methadone maintenance patients. *Journal of Applied Behavior Analysis, 41*(4), 579–595.

Kirby, K. N., Petry, N. M., & Bickel, W. K. (1999). Heroin addicts have higher discount rates for delayed rewards than non-drug-using controls. *Journal of Experimental Psychology: General, 128*(1), 78–87.

Knealing, T. W., Roebuck, M. C., Wong, C. J., & Silverman, K. (2008). Economic cost of the therapeutic workplace intervention added to methadone maintenance. *Journal of Substance Abuse Treatment, 34*(3), 326–332.

Lamb, R. J., Kirby, K. C., Morral, A. R., Galbicka, G., & Iguchi, M. Y. (2010). Shaping smoking cessation in hard-to-treat smokers. *Journal of Consulting and Clinical Psychology, 78*(1), 62–71.

Lamb, S., Greenlick, M. R., & McCarty, D. (Eds.). (1998). *Bridging the gap between practice and research: Forging partnerships with community-based drug and alcohol treatment*. Washington, DC: National Academy Press.

Liebson, I. A., Tommaselo, A., & Bigelow, G. E. (1978). A behavioral treatment of alcoholic methadone patients. *Annals of Internal Medicine, 89*, 342–344.

Lott, D. C., & Jencius, S. (2009). Effectiveness of very low-cost contingency management in a community adolescent treatment program. *Drug and Alcohol Dependence, 102*(1–3), 162–165.

Magura, S., Casriel, C., Goldsmith, D. S., & Lipton, D. S. (1987). Contracting with clients in methadone treatment. *Social Casework: The Journal of Contemporary Social Work, 68*, 485–494.

Martin, G. L., & Pear, J. J. (2010). *Behavior modification: What it is and how to do it* (9th ed.). New York: Prentice-Hall.

McCarty, D., Fuller, B. E., Arfken, C., Miller, M., Nunes, E. V., Edmundson,

E., et al. (2007). Direct care workers in the National Drug Abuse Treatment Clinical Trials Network: Characteristics, opinions, and beliefs. *Psychiatric Services, 58*(2), 181–190.

McCollister, K. E., French, M. T., Sheidow, A. J., Henggeler, S. W., & Halliday-Boykins, C. A. (2009). Estimating the differential costs of criminal activity for juvenile drug court participants: Challenges and recommendations. *Journal of Behavioral Health Services and Research, 36*(1), 111–126.

McGovern, M. P., Fox, T. S., Xie, H., & Drake, R. E. (2004). A survey of clinical practices and readiness to adopt evidence-based practices: Dissemination research in an addiction treatment system. *Journal of Substance Abuse Treatment, 26*(4), 305–312.

McLellan, A. T., O'Brien, C. P., Lewis, D., & Kleber, H. D. (2000). Drug addiction as a chronic medical illness: Implications for treatment, insurance, and evaluation. *Journal of the American Medical Association, 284,* 1689–1695.

Meredith, S., Grabinski, M. J., & Dallery, J. (2011). Internet-based group contingencies to promote abstinence from cigarette smoking. *Drug and Alcohol Dependence, 118,* 23–30.

Meyers, R. J., & Smith, J. E. (1995). *Clinical guide to alcohol treatment: The community reinforcement approach.* New York: Guilford Press.

Milby, J. B., Schumacher, J. E., McNamara, C., Wallace, D., Usdan, S., McGill, T., et al. (2000). Initiating abstinence in cocaine abusing dually diagnosed homeless persons. *Drug and Alcohol Dependence, 60*(1), 55–67.

Milby, J. B., Schumacher, J. E., Wallace, D., Frison, S., McNamara, C., Usdan, S., et al. (2003). Day treatment with contingency management for cocaine abuse in homeless persons: 12-month follow-up. *Journal of Consulting and Clinical Psychology, 71*(3), 619–621.

Miller, P. M. (1975). A behavioral intervention program for chronic public drunkenness offenders. *Archives of General Psychiatry, 32*(7), 915–918.

Olmstead, T. A., Sindelar, J. L., & Petry, N. M. (2007a). Clinic variation in the cost-effectiveness of contingency management. *American Journal on Addictions/American Academy of Psychiatrists in Alcoholism and Addictions, 16*(6), 457–460.

Olmstead, T. A., Sindelar, J. L., & Petry, N. M. (2007b). Cost-effectiveness of prize-based incentives for stimulant abusers in outpatient psychosocial treatment programs. *Drug and Alcohol Dependence, 87*(2–3), 175–182.

Paxton, R. (1983). Prolonging the effects of deposit contracts with smokers. *Behaviour Research and Therapy, 21*(4), 425–433.

Peirce, J. M., Petry, N. M., Stitzer, M. L., Blaine, J., Kellogg, S., Satterfield, F., et al. (2006). Effects of lower-cost incentives on stimulant abstinence in methadone maintenance treatment: A National Drug Abuse Treatment Clinical Trials Network study. *Archives of General Psychiatry, 63*(2), 201–208.

Petry, N. M. (2000). A comprehensive guide to the application of contingency management procedures in clinical settings. *Drug and Alcohol Dependence, 58*(1–2), 9–25.

Petry, N. M., & Alessi, S. M. (2010). Prize-based contingency management is efficacious in cocaine-abusing patients with and without recent gambling participation. *Journal of Substance Abuse Treatment, 39*(3), 282–288.

Petry, N. M., Bickel, W. K., & Arnett, M. (1998). Shortened time horizons and insensitivity to future consequences in heroin addicts. *Addiction* (Abingdon, UK), *93*(5), 729–738.

Petry, N. M., Martin, B., Cooney, J. L., & Kranzler, H. R. (2000). Give them prizes, and they will come: Contingency management for treatment of alcohol dependence. *Journal of Consulting and Clinical Psychology, 68*(2), 250–257.

Petry, N. M., Peirce, J. M., Stitzer, M. L., Blaine, J., Roll, J. M., Cohen, et al. (2005). Effect of prize-based incentives on outcomes in stimulant abusers in outpatient psychosocial treatment programs: A National Drug Abuse Treatment Clinical Trials Network study. *Archives of General Psychiatry, 62*(10), 1148–1156.

Petry, N. M., & Simcic, F. Jr. (2002). Recent advances in the dissemination of contingency management techniques: Clinical and research perspectives. *Journal of Substance Abuse Treatment, 23*(2), 81–86.

Petry, N. M., Tedford, J., Austin, M., Nich, C., Carroll, K. M., & Rounsaville, B. J. (2004). Prize reinforcement contingency management for treating cocaine users: How low can we go, and with whom? *Addiction, 99*(3), 349–360.

Petry, N. M., Weinstock, J., Alessi, S. M., Lewis, M. W., & Dieckhaus, K. (2010). Group-based randomized trial of contingencies for health and abstinence in HIV patients. *Journal of Consulting and Clinical Psychology, 78*(1), 89–97.

Piotrowski, N. A., & Hall, S. M. (1999). Treatment of multiple drug abuse in the methadone clinic. In K. Silverman (Ed.), *Motivating behavior change among illicit-drug abusers: Research on contingency management interventions* (pp. 183–202). Washington, DC: American Psychological Association.

Prendergast, M., Podus, D., Finney, J., Greenwell, L., & Roll, J. (2006). Contingency management for treatment of substance use disorders: A meta-analysis. *Addiction* (Abingdon, UK), *101*(11), 1546–1560.

Preston, K. L., Umbricht, A., & Epstein, D. H. (2000). Methadone dose increase and abstinence reinforcement for treatment of continued heroin use during methadone maintenance. *Archives of General Psychiatry, 57*(4), 395–404.

Rawson, R. A., McCann, M. J., Flammino, F., Shoptaw, S., Miotto, K., Reiber, C., & et al. (2006). A comparison of contingency management and cognitive-behavioral approaches for stimulant-dependent individuals. *Addiction, 101*(2), 267–274.

Reilly, M. P., Roll, J. M., & Downey, K. K. (2000). Impulsivity and voucher versus money preference in polydrug-dependent participants enrolled in a contingency-management-based substance abuse treatment program. *Journal of Substance Abuse Treatment, 19*(3), 253–257.

Reynolds, B., Dallery, J., Shroff, P., Patak, M., & Leraas, K. (2008). A web-based contingency management program with adolescent smokers. *Journal of Applied Behavior Analysis, 41*(4), 597–601.

Ries, R. K., & Comtois, K. A. (1997). Managing disability benefits as part of treatment for persons with severe mental illness and comorbid drug/alcohol disorders: A comparative study of payee and non-payee participants. *American Journal on Addictions, 6*(4), 330–338.

Ries, R. K., & Dyck, D. G. (1997). Representative payee practices of community mental health centers in Washington State. *Psychiatric Services, 48*(6), 811–814.

Ries, R. K., Dyck, D. G., Short, R., Srebnik, D., Fisher, A., & Comtois, K. A. (2004). Outcomes of managing disability benefits among patients with substance dependence and severe mental illness. *Psychiatric Services, 55*(4), 445–447.

Rigsby, M. O., Rosen, M. I., Beauvais, J. E., Cramer, J. A., Rainey, P. M., O'Malley, S. S., et al. (2000). Cue-dose training with monetary reinforcement: Pilot study of an antiretroviral adherence intervention. *Journal of General Internal Medicine, 15*(12), 841–847.

Roll, J. M. (2005). Assessing the feasibility of using contingency management to modify cigarette smoking by adolescents. *Journal of Applied Behavior Analysis, 38*(4), 463–467.

Roll, J. M., & Higgins, S. T. (2000). A within-subject comparison of three different schedules of reinforcement of drug abstinence using cigarette smoking as an exemplar. *Drug and Alcohol Dependence, 58*(1–2), 103–109.

Roll, J. M., Higgins, S. T., Steingard, S., & McGinley, M. (1998). Use of monetary reinforcement to reduce the cigarette smoking of persons with schizophrenia: A feasibility study. *Experimental and Clinical Psychopharmacology, 6*(2), 157–161.

Roll, J. M., Huber, A., Sodano, R., Chudzynski, J. E., Moynier, E., & Shoptaw, S. (2006). A comparison of five reinforcement schedules for use in contingency management-based treatment of methamphetamine abuse. *Psychological Record, 56*(1), 67–81.

Roll, J. M., Reilly, M. P., & Johanson, C. (2000). The influence of exchange delays on cigarette versus money choice: A laboratory analog of voucher-based reinforcement therapy. *Experimental and Clinical Psychopharmacology, 8*(3), 366–370.

Roozen, H. G., Boulogne, J. J., van Tulder, M. W., van de Brink, W., de Jong, C. A., & Kerkhof, A. J. (2004). A systematic review of the effectiveness of the community reinforcement approach in alcohol, cocaine and opioid addiction. *Drug and Alcohol Dependence, 74*(1), 1–13.

Rosado, J., Sigmon, S. C., Jones, H. E., & Stitzer, M. L. (2005). Cash value of voucher reinforcers in pregnant drug-dependent women. *Experimental and Clinical Psychopharmacology, 13*(1), 41–47.

Rosen, M. I., Dieckhaus, K., McMahon, T. J., Valdes, B., Petry, N. M., Cramer, J., et al. (2007). Improved adherence with contingency management. *AIDS Patient Care and STDs, 21*(1), 30–40.

Schumacher, J. E., Milby, J. B., Wallace, D., Meehan, D. C., Kertesz, S., Vuchinich, R., et al. (2007). Meta-analysis of day treatment and contingency-management dismantling research: Birmingham homeless cocaine studies (1990–2006). *Journal of Consulting and Clinical Psychology, 75*(5), 823–828.

Shaner, A., Eckman, T. A., Roberts, L. J., & Wilkins, J. N. (1995). Disability income, cocaine use, and repeated hospitalization among schizophrenic cocaine abusers: A government-sponsored revolving door. *New England Journal of Medicine, 333*(12), 777–783.

Shaner, A., Roberts, L. J., Eckman, T. A., & Tucker, D. E. (1997). Monetary reinforcement of abstinence from cocaine among mentally ill patients with cocaine dependence. *Psychiatric Services, 48*(6), 807–810.

Sigmon, S. C., & Higgins, S. T. (2006). Voucher-based contingent reinforcement of marijuana abstinence among individuals with serious mental illness. *Journal of Substance Abuse Treatment, 30*(4), 291–295.

Sigmon, S. C., Lamb, R. J., & Dallery, J. (2008). Tobacco. In S. T. Higgins, K. Silverman, & S. H. Heil (Eds.), *Contingency management in substance abuse treatment* (pp. 99–119). New York: Guilford Press.

Silverman, K., Chutuape, M. A., Bigelow, G. E., & Stitzer, M. L. (1999). Voucher-based reinforcement of cocaine abstinence in treatment-resistant methadone patients: Effects of reinforcement magnitude. *Psychopharmacology, 146*(2), 128–138.

Silverman, K., Higgins, S. T., Brooner, R. K., Montoya, I. D., Cone, E. J., Schuster, C. R., et al. (1996). Sustained cocaine abstinence in methadone maintenance patients through voucher-based reinforcement therapy. *Archives of General Psychiatry, 53*(5), 409–415.

Silverman, K., Robles, E., Mudric, T., Bigelow, G. E., & Stitzer, M. L. (2004). A randomized trial of long-term reinforcement of cocaine abstinence in methadone-maintained patients who inject drugs. *Journal of Consulting and Clinical Psychology, 72*(5), 839–854.

Silverman, K., Svikis, D., Robles, E., Stitzer, M. L., & Bigelow, G. E. (2001). A reinforcement-based therapeutic workplace for the treatment of drug abuse: Six-month abstinence outcomes. *Experimental and Clinical Psychopharmacology, 9*(1), 14–23.

Silverman, K., Svikis, D., Wong, C. J., Hampton, J., Stitzer, M. L., & Bigelow, G. E. (2002). A reinforcement-based therapeutic workplace for the treatment of drug abuse: Three-year abstinence outcomes. *Experimental and Clinical Psychopharmacology, 10*(3), 228–240.

Silverman, K., Wong, C. J., Needham, M., Diemer, K. N., Knealing, T., Crone-Todd, D., et al. (2007). A randomized trial of employment-based reinforcement of cocaine abstinence in injection drug users. *Journal of Applied Behavior Analysis, 40*(3), 387–410.

Silverman, K., Wong, C. J., Umbricht-Schneiter, A., Montoya, I. D., Schuster, C. R., & Preston, K. L. (1998). Broad beneficial effects of cocaine abstinence reinforcement among methadone patients. *Journal of Consulting and Clinical Psychology, 66*(5), 811–824.

Sindelar, J., Elbel, B., & Petry, N. M. (2007). What do we get for our money?: Cost-effectiveness of adding contingency management. *Addiction, 102*(2), 309–316.

Sorensen, J. L., Haug, N. A., Delucchi, K. L., Gruber, V., Kletter, E., Batki, S. L., et al. (2007). Voucher reinforcement improves medication adherence in HIV-positive methadone patients: A randomized trial. *Drug and Alcohol Dependence, 88*(1), 54–63.

Stanger, C., & Budney, A. J. (2010). Contingency management approaches for adolescent substance use disorders. *Child and Adolescent Psychiatric Clinics of North America, 19*(3), 547–562.

Stanger, C., Budney, A. J., Kamon, J. L., & Thostensen, J. (2009). A randomized trial of contingency management for adolescent marijuana abuse and dependence. *Drug and Alcohol Dependence, 105*(3), 240–247.

Stitzer, M. L., Bickel, W. K., Bigelow, G. E., & Liebson, I. A. (1986). Effect of methadone dose contingencies on urinalysis test results of polydrug-abusing methadone-maintenance patients. *Drug and Alcohol Dependence, 18*(4), 341–348.

Stitzer, M. L., & Bigelow, G. (1978). Contingency management in a methadone maintenance program: Availability of reinforcers. *International Journal of the Addictions, 13*(5), 737–746.

Stitzer, M. L., Bigelow, G., Lawrence, C., Cohen, J., D'Lugoff, B., & Hawthorne, J. (1977). Medication take-home as a reinforcer in a methadone maintenance program. *Addictive Behaviors, 2*(1), 9–14.

Stitzer, M. L., & Bigelow, G. E. (1984). Contingent methadone take-home privileges: Effects on compliance with fee payment schedules. *Drug and Alcohol Dependence, 13*(4), 395–399.

Stitzer, M. L., Iguchi, M. Y., & Felch, L. J. (1992). Contingent take-home incentive: Effects on drug use of methadone maintenance patients. *Journal of Consulting and Clinical Psychology, 60*(6), 927–934.

Stitzer, M. L., Petry, N. M., & Peirce, J. (2010). Motivational incentives research in the National Drug Abuse Treatment Clinical Trials Network. *Journal of Substance Abuse Treatment, 38*(Suppl. 1), S61–S69.

Stoops, W. W., Dallery, J., Fields, N. M., Nuzzo, P. A., Schoenberg, N. E., Martin, C. A., et al. (2009). An Internet-based abstinence reinforcement smoking cessation intervention in rural smokers. *Drug and Alcohol Dependence, 105*(1–2), 56–62.

Tidey, J. W., O'Neill, S. C., & Higgins, S. T. (1999). Effects of abstinence on cigarette smoking among outpatients with schizophrenia. *Experimental and Clinical Psychopharmacology, 7*(4), 347–353.

Vandrey, R., Bigelow, G. E., & Stitzer, M. L. (2007). Contingency management in cocaine abusers: A dose–effect comparison of goods-based versus cash-based incentives. *Experimental and Clinical Psychopharmacology, 15*(4), 338–343.

Weiser, M. (1991, September). The computer for the 21st century. *Scientific American*, pp. 94–104.

Wilson, K. G., & Hayes, S. C. (2000). Why it is crucial to understand thinking and feeling: An analysis and application to drug abuse. *Behavior Analyst, 23*(1), 25–43.

Winett, R. A. (1973). Parameters of deposit contracts in the modification of smoking. *Psychological Record, 23*(1), 49–60.

Chapter 5

Cognitive-Behavioral Theories of Substance Abuse

Frederick Rotgers

Cognitive-behavioral (CB) theories of treatment for psychoactive substance use disorders (PSUDs) are based on principles of learning and behavior change (Eysenck, 1982). CB strategies are part of the larger group of techniques that fall under the rubric of "behavior therapy." The last decade has been a period of "normal science" (Kuhn, 1970) for CB theory. Recent advances have included increased attention to the importance of the therapeutic relationship in CB theory (Evans-Jones, Peters, & Barker, 2009) and on the use of CB approaches in combination with other approaches, such as motivational interviewing (Moyers & Houck, 2011), pharmacotherapy (Willenbring, 2010), mindfulness (Witkiewicz & Bowen, 2010), and contingency management (Lee & Rawson, 2008). This chapter begins by discussing basic assumptions of CB theory, followed by a brief outline of the processes presumed to operate in treatment of PSUDs. This review is followed by a consideration of the etiology, maintenance, and client characteristics that inform treatment from a CB perspective. Discussion then proceeds to the tasks that CB-oriented clinicians attempt to accomplish in treatment. The chapter concludes with a review of the advantages and disadvantages of CB theories of PSUDs.

Basic Assumptions

CB theories are based on psychological learning principles as delineated in animal and human experiments during the course of the last 75 years. The advent of the "cognitive revolution" in psychology in the 1970s (Baars, 1986) led to the addition of a number of components to theories of the development and treatment of PSUDs. The microtheories of behavior change that can be included under the rubric of CB differ from each other somewhat in the aspects of the person–environment interactions on which they focus. Nonetheless, regardless of the particular microtheory of behavior on which a set of CB techniques is based, all share basic assumptions that characterize a CB approach to therapeutic change (see Table 5.1).

First and most fundamental to these assumptions is the conviction that despite some evidence for biological or genetic components to human behavior, human behavior, especially at a macrolevel, is largely learned. Many behavioral theorists (Bandura, 1977; Eysenck, 1982) assume that biological factors form a substrate on which a person's experiences build in producing individual patterns of behavior. Learning is thus the result of interactions between the person and the environment. While the process of learning may vary depending on the particular behavior at issue, biological and genetic factors are presumed by most CB theorists to take a back seat in the formation and change of behavior (although in recent years, theorists have increasingly recognized that a combination of CB approaches with medications can increase the effectiveness of both; see Moyers & Houck, 2011, and Tooley & Moyers, Chapter 2, this volume). CB theorists tend to believe that biological and genetic factors are largely immutable given our current level of knowledge, and that change efforts are better focused on a higher order level: that of behavior itself. For instance, a CB clinician might target a behavior that would help the person cope with biological factors that may be maintaining substance use (e.g., withdrawal symptoms).

TABLE 5.1. Basic Assumptions of Cognitive-Behavioral Theories of Psychoactive Substance Use Disorders

1. Human behavior is largely learned rather than being determined by genetic factors.
2. The same learning processes that create problem behaviors can be used to change them.
3. Behavior is largely determined by contextual and environmental factors.
4. Covert behaviors such as thoughts and feelings are subject to change through the application of learning principles.
5. Practicing new behaviors in the contexts in which they are to be performed is a critical part of behavior change.
6. Each client is unique and must be assessed as an individual in a particular context.
7. The cornerstone of adequate treatment is a thorough CB assessment.

A corollary to the first assumption is that the same processes by which behavior develops can be harnessed to help a person to change behavior (Krasner, 1982). This technology is described in more detail in the companion chapter to this one (see Marinchok & Morgan, Chapter 6, this volume), based on the notion that any behavior shaped by learning can be reshaped, reduced, or even eliminated by the same process.

A third assumption is that contextual and environmental factors are significant in the initiation, maintenance, and change of behavior. Consistent with the focus of CB theories on person–environment interactions, many CB techniques focus explicitly on altering aspects of this interaction as a means of changing behavior. The degree to which importance is placed on changing environment versus individual reactions to the environment varies from microtheory to microtheory. Techniques such as the community reinforcement approach of Azrin and Sisson (Azrin, Sisson, Meyers, & Godley, 1982), based explicitly on operant learning theory, rely heavily on *environmental* changes to promote changes in behavior (see Murphy, MacKillop, Vuchinich, & Tucker, Chapter 3, and Dallery, Meredith, & Budney, Chapter 4, this volume). In contrast, cognitive theories, such as those of Ellis (Ellis, McInerney, DiGiuseppe, & Yeager, 1988), Beck (Beck, Wright, Newman, & Liese, 1993), and Ball (2004; Ball & Young, 2000) place a greater emphasis on changing individual *reactions* to the environment. Both approaches, however, recognize the importance of context *and* environment in the origins and treatment of PSUDs.

The fourth assumption common to CB approaches is that all internal behaviors (e.g., thoughts, feelings, and physiological changes) are changeable through the application of learning theory principles. This assumption has been borne out in numerous studies; changes in internal processes occur in response to treatment of a variety of disorders other than PSUDs. For instance, there is substantial evidence from research on anxiety disorders and depression that learning theory-based approaches can produce changes in internal processes as well as changes in overt observable behavior.

The fifth basic assumption is that techniques should emphasize practicing new behaviors in the contexts that are problematic for clients. Whereas the practice of new skills in the office setting is helpful as a first step, confrontation of problem situations in the real world is considered to be a more effective way of ensuring long-term behavior change.

Sixth, CB therapists assume that each client presents a unique case that requires a thorough understanding within a CB framework in order for treatment to be successful. Approaching each client uniquely means that CB therapists attempt to identify the particular configuration of forces that produce and maintain the target behavior. Thus, while a cognitive-behaviorist may believe that there are certain common errors in thinking and reasoning that produce or maintain substance use, each individual is still presumed to suffer from a unique combination of errors.

The previous assumption leads logically into the seventh assumption: treatment within a CB context must be preceded by a thorough and rigorous assessment of the client's behavior (Donovan, 1988). Without a thorough initial assessment focusing on how specific learning processes operate in a particular client's case, therapy and consequent behavior change are bound to fail.

The eighth and final assumption is one that has developed more significantly in the years since the publication of the second edition of this book: a strong working alliance is crucial to effective behavior change, regardless of therapy technique (Norcross, 2002). This additional assumption is also reflected in the increasingly frequent combination of CB with other approaches, such as motivational interviewing (see Rose & Walters, Chapter 1, and Tooley & Moyers, Chapter 2, this volume) and contingency management (see Murphy, MacKillop, Vuchinich, & Tucker, Chapter 3, and Dallery, Meredith, & Budney, Chapter 4, this volume). These two approaches in particular focus on retaining and engaging users in treatment. Thus, these strategies may be highly complementary with CB approaches, and thereby improve overall outcome.

CB theorists and practitioners have increasingly recognized that clients are not always receptive to or ready to implement the techniques that CB therapists have to offer. In the language of Prochaska, DiClemente, and Norcross (1992), many clients enter treatment in one of the three stages of change that precede actual taking action to effect change. In fact, in some settings, up to two-thirds of clients entering treatment are still in the precontemplation, contemplation, or preparation stages of change. For those clients, action-focused approaches such as CB theory may have little impact until the client has undergone the cognitive and emotional shifts from early stages of change to action.

In addition to adherence to these basic assumptions about the nature of PSUDs and the process of treatment and behavior change, CB theorists also place a heavy emphasis on empirical validation of the efficacy of their techniques. Although behavior therapy has often been equated with a rigid, mechanistic, and authoritarian approach, nothing could be further from the truth in practice. Those who adhere to a CB theory of substance abuse treatment tend to adopt an approach to the therapeutic enterprise that insists on rigorous, but humanistically based, application of well-validated principles to help people change unwanted behavior that is standing in the way of a more fulfilling life.

With the basic assumptions of CB theory as background, let us now turn to a consideration of the processes CB theorists view as central to the initiation, maintenance, and change of PSUDs. The discussion that follows presents only a bare outline of each process. (For more information about how these processes are applied to form a detailed theory of the development of PSUDs, see Abrams & Niaura, 1987.) Although focused on alcohol use disorders, this chapter provides a CB framework that is also applicable to other PSUDs.

Basic CB Processes and Models of PSUDs

Three basic learning processes contribute to the initiation, maintenance, and change of behavior: classical conditioning, operant conditioning, and psychological modeling. These three processes form the core of most behavioral theories of substance abuse treatment. In addition, since the cognitive revolution in psychology, increasing emphasis has been placed by some theorists (notably those who adopt Bandura's [1977] social learning models and followers of Ellis et al.'s [1988], Beck et al.'s [1993], and Ball & Young's [2005] cognitive approaches) on the role of cognitive processes in the initiation and maintenance of behavior. In the sections that follow, I outline classical conditioning and modeling formulations of various aspects of PSUDs (leaving out operant conditioning, which is addressed in Dallery, Meredith, & Budney, Chapter 4, this volume). I then discuss cognitive factors in substance abuse and treatment as presented in social learning theory (SLT) and CB theories. The focus in the final sections is on how basic learning and cognitive processes can be used to change substance use behavior.

Classical Conditioning

Classical conditioning is a basic learning process that was first intensively studied by the Russian physiologist Ivan Pavlov (1927) and the American psychologist J. B. Watson (1919). As one example of a classical conditioning paradigm, consider a person who drinks in a bar. The conditioned stimulus (CS), alcohol, is paired with the unconditioned stimulus (UCS), social interaction, until the alcohol itself elicits what the UCS formerly produced: feelings of warmth, satisfaction, and companionship. Of course, being with others might normally produce such feelings, but over time the alcohol on its own produces this conditioned response (CR). Whether a cue will elicit a CR depends, among other factors, on the frequency with which the UCS and the CS have been paired, the intensity of the CS when it is presented, and the physiological and psychological state of the organism at the time the CS is presented. Thus, for a hungry person, the mere sight of a picture of a Big Mac, without any of the associated cues of smell and taste, may elicit a salivation response or a subjective feeling of desire or craving to buy lunch.

Classical conditioning has been most often invoked as the primary process by which environmental cues come to elicit urges or cravings to use psychoactive substances. While working at the U.S. Public Health Service Hospital in Lexington, Kentucky, in the 1960s, Wikler discovered that some of the chronic heroin users being treated there experienced what appeared to be withdrawal symptoms from the mere sight of the paraphernalia associated with heroin use. In a series of studies, Wikler and others (outlined in Wikler, 1965, 1973) provided addicts with paraphernalia and an opportunity to engage in the ritual of preparing and injecting what they thought to be heroin, but what was in reality an inert substance. In many of the subjects, the sight of the paraphernalia elicited physiological and subjective signs of withdrawal, which Wikler began to view as conditioned withdrawal phenomena. Moreover, when presented with the opportunity to "use" what they thought was heroin, these individuals often experienced a "high" even when the substance they injected was merely an inert solution that looked like heroin.

According to a classical conditioning model, in Wikler's studies the UCS was heroin and the UCR was the withdrawal symptoms and subsequent high that the users experienced after injecting heroin. The CS was the paraphernalia associated with heroin preparation and use and the CR was the pseudowithdrawal and pseudohigh experienced by the experimental subjects when preparing and injecting an inert solution. Based on findings such as these, classical conditioning theorists postulate that substance users actually condition many stimuli in the environment to the rituals, paraphernalia, and use of their drug of choice by repeatedly using the drug in specific settings, with specific people, and according to a specific ritual. Each user may then have a vast number of CS cues based on his or her own experience and substance use pattern.

Classical conditioning theory has formed the basis for at least four prominent procedures in the treatment of PSUDs: cue exposure treatments (e.g., Childress et al., 1993; McLellan, Childress, Ehrman, & O'Brien, 1986), stimulus control techniques (e.g., Bickel & Kelly, 1988), relaxation training (e.g., Monti, Kadden, Rohsenow, Cooney, & Abrams, 2002), and covert sensitization and other aversion therapy techniques (Rimmele, Miller, & Dougher, 1989). In addition, they form part of the theoretical basis for teaching drinking refusal skills (Monti et al., 2002). Other than aversion therapy, all these procedures attempt, at least in part, to break the conditioned connection between particular aspects of the client's environment and the conditioned withdrawal or cravings presumed to form the motivational basis for substance use. Aversion therapy and its variant covert sensitization apply classical conditioning theory in a different fashion by attempting to condition a new, aversive response to substance use and the cues associated with it.

Modeling

Modeling (Bandura, 1977) is a second basic learning process that has been used to develop CB theories of substance abuse treatment. Of the three basic learning processes (the others being classical conditioning and operant conditioning), modeling appears to be most efficient and most rapid in producing new learning. Modeling involves, as its name implies, observation of another's behavior and then performance of that behavior given appropriate reinforcement contingencies. Modeling is an efficient way to learn new behaviors because humans can learn many complex behaviors with very few observations. In fact, many complicated behaviors can be learned and accurately performed after only a single observation.

The modern theory of modeling began with the work of Albert Bandura (1977). He and his coworkers mapped out the parameters of modeling as a learning process. Modeling involves two subprocesses: observational learning and performance. Learning can occur by observation, and the newly learned behavior can be reproduced quite accurately without any prior practice. Bandura postulates that a process of "cognitive mapping" occurs at this stage in which the individual stores aspects of the behavior that are later reproduced from this cognitive map. The adequacy with which this cognitive representation of the modeled behavior occurs depends on, among other factors, how well the observer attended to the model's behavior and how the behavior was encoded (e.g., verbal, visual, tactile). The more modalities the learner uses to encode the behavior, the more efficiently the behavior is learned. Thus, when sensory, emotional, cognitive, and motor modalities are all engaged in encoding newly modeled behavior, that behavior is most efficiently stored and retrieved. Whether behavior learned by observation will actually be performed depends on factors other than the cognitive map. The actual performance of the behavior depends on characteristics of the model (e.g., the degree to which the observer holds the model in esteem and as a person to be imitated), whether the model is seen as being reinforced or punished for engaging in the behavior, whether the observer has an incentive to perform the modeled behavior, and whether the observer expects to be reinforced if the behavior is performed.

Modeling processes have been strongly implicated in the development of PSUDs in adolescence. Adolescents who observe substance-using peers with whom they wish to relate, or the behavior of persons whom they view as powerful or popular and who use alcohol or drugs, may both learn and perform those behaviors quite rapidly. Modeling also influences the maintenance of PSUDs in that people will often engage in behaviors that members of their peer group engage in as a means of ensuring inclusion in the group.

The efficiency of modeling as a learning process (it can occur in only a few trials, without the necessity of repeated experiences, as is the case in both classical and operant learning) has led to its utilization as a major process in CB treatment of PSUDs. Persons with PSUDs often lack skills that would enable them to cope with situations that evoke substance use. Persons who lack assertiveness or refusal skills or who are prone to inappropriate thought processes that lead to substance use can be taught new skills and thought processes by observing skilled others modeling those processes and behaviors. Thus, modeling theory provides the theoretical basis for social skills approaches to the treatment of PSUDs, as well as forming a component of the teaching of other intrapersonal skills such as relaxation, coping self-statements, and anger management. Almost any new behavior that does not rely directly on repeated pairings of environmental stimuli with client responses can be taught or enhanced through modeling processes.

Cognitive Mediation of Behavior

Cognitive mediation of behavior is another basic process that has been integrated into CB theory. Several theoretical accounts of PSUDs heavily emphasize the roles of cognitive processes in the initiation, maintenance, and change of substance use behavior (e.g., Abrams & Niaura, 1987; Goldman, Brown, & Christiansen, 1987; Sher, 1987). These cognitive theories vary in the amount of emphasis they place on cognitive mediators, but all rely heavily on the three basic learning processes to promote behavior change.

SLT represents an extension of the theories of classical conditioning, operant conditioning, and modeling as previously discussed. SLT assumes that certain cognitive factors mediate these basic learning processes. Primarily associated with the work of Bandura (1977), SLT is a comprehensive theory of the development, maintenance, and change of learned behavior. In a nutshell, SLT postulates that human behavior develops by a combination of classical conditioning, operant conditioning, and modeling, which not only produce overt behaviors but lead to the development of patterns of thought and emotion that themselves guide and shape behavior.

A central concept in SLT is *reciprocal determinism*, the belief that people both influence and are influenced by their environments. This two-way interaction implies that behavior change can be brought about by changing a person's environment, but it also implies that behavior change can be engineered by the person him- or herself through a planned process of self-control or self-initiated changes in his or her environment. This "self" control is a central feature of SLT-based approaches to treatment of PSUDs.

In addition to postulating a reciprocally determined relationship between environment and behavior, SLT emphasizes the role of cognition in the control and performance of behavior. A person's expectations about whether a particular behavior will be reinforced, confidence about the adequacy with which the behavior can be performed, and the level of skill that person can bring to bear to cope with problematic situations—all these influence the coping strategies and behaviors he or she will use in navigating through life. The interaction of expectations and skill levels is encapsulated in the notion of self-efficacy, a central concept of SLT. *Self-efficacy* refers to a person's expectations that he or she will be able to perform a coping response in a given situation, coupled with the expectation that performance of that response will be reinforced. The extent to which a person lacks requisite coping skills, or views his or her ability to execute those skills as being deficient, contributes to the person's self-efficacy expectations for coping in a given situation. According to SLT, self-efficacy expectations are primary cognitive mediators that determine whether or not a person will engage in a particular coping response. When self-efficacy is high, a person will be more likely to enact that skill in an attempt to cope with life. If, on the other hand, self-efficacy is low, the person will likely choose some other skill or coping strategy with which he or she feels more comfortable.

SLT views PSUDs as basically a failure of coping (Abrams & Niaura, 1987). This failure may be due to any combination of inappropriate conditioning, reinforcement contingencies, modeling of inappropriate behaviors, failure to model appropriate coping skills, and reduced self-efficacy with regard to behaviors that not only enhance coping but are also widely reinforced. Failure to perform skills one already knows may also be the result of reduced self-efficacy or outcome expectations or may be due to physiological, emotional, or other cognitive factors that interfere with effective skill performance.

Following logically from this view of PSUDs, SLT-based treatment approaches emphasize skills training and practice. In addition, SLT approaches seek not only to teach skills for coping with known problems but also to help the client anticipate situations in which he or she either lacks appropriate coping skills or has low self-efficacy with regard to performance of those skills. This process, coupled with teaching clients to address the cognitive aspects of relapse (e.g., how to cope with the abstinence violation effect from a "slip" to returning to use after a period of abstinence) forms the core of relapse prevention approaches to PSUDs (Marlatt & Gordon, 1985). Treatments within this framework are initiated following a thorough functional analysis of substance use behavior to determine whether substance use is maintained because the person lacks other coping skills, because the person has adequate coping skills but low self-efficacy expectations toward using those skills, or because the person expects that using the available coping skills will be ineffective. The client is also assessed with regard to physiological or emotional factors that may be interfering with skill performance (e.g., high levels of anxiety, depression, or anger) or which may themselves drive substance use. Assessment of skills and expectations continues throughout treatment in order to measure progress toward adequate, substance-free coping.

Treatments that have been developed within an SLT framework include social and communication skills training, assertiveness training, anger and stress management training, self-control training, and relapse prevention training (Marlatt & Gordon, 1985; Marlatt & Donovan, 2008). Marital and family approaches to treatment have also been developed from an SLT perspective (see Lam, O'Farrell, & Birchler, Chapter 10, this volume).

Three other cognitive theories of treatment bear mention. These have grown primarily out of the work of two theorists: Ellis, the founder of rational–emotive therapy (RET), and Beck, the founder of cognitive therapy (CT). Although differing somewhat in their details, all three of these theories view thought (cognition) as a primary causal factor in emotion and substance use, and regard abuse primarily as an effort to cope with negative emotional states that arise as a result of illogical or distorted thinking.

Ellis et al.'s (1988) RET approach is one example of how a cognitive framework addresses the role of cognition (thoughts) in the development of emotional disturbance and the consequent development of PSUDs in some people as a means of coping with negative emotions. Ellis has developed what he calls the A–B–C model of emotion. According to the A–B–C model of emotion, the events or situations a person encounters (A) do not, in and of themselves, create negative emotions. Rather the person's interpretation (B) of the meaning of events based on his or her beliefs is what creates the negative emotion (C). In order for change in emotions to occur, the client must identify and challenge the thoughts occurring at B through a process of rational disputation. Ellis has identified a variety of irrational beliefs that, coupled with what he views as the addict's inability to tolerate frustration or other negative emotions, are believed to set the stage for substance use as a means of coping with negative emotions. According to Ellis, a further factor that triggers alcohol or drug use to cope with emotions is poor ability to tolerate negative affect. This results in a belief that Ellis calls "I-can't-stand-it-itis." This belief prompts people suffering from PSUDs to react impulsively in order to alleviate negative emotions immediately. Ellis refers to this tendency as low frustration tolerance and believes that this additional set of beliefs must be addressed for substance abuse to be successfully treated.

Beck (Beck, Rush, Shaw, & Emery, 1979; Beck et al., 1993) has articulated a second theory of negative emotion based on an inventory of illogical or irrational reasoning processes that he terms "core beliefs." These beliefs are commonly held but irrational ideas about the nature of the world or what a person needs in order to lead a contented life. When the person faces a problematic situation, these core beliefs are activated as a way of construing the meaning of the experience and of generating coping responses. Because these core beliefs are maladaptive, the coping responses they trigger are often maladaptive. Coupled with these core beliefs are highly stereotyped "automatic" thoughts, which are similar to the "B" component of Ellis's A–B–C model of emotion. The occurrence of these automatic thoughts is presumed to activate urges or cravings to use drugs or alcohol to alleviate negative emotions produced by the automatic thoughts. Action on urges or cravings in substance abusers is presumably triggered by additional thoughts or beliefs, which Beck terms "facilitating beliefs." Facilitating beliefs are, in Beck's model, the proximate cause of drug- and alcohol-seeking behavior in an addicted person faced with problematic situations or emotions.

Finally, Ball, Cobb-Richardson, Connolly, Bujosa, and O'Neil (2005) have recently published preliminary data on an approach with clients suffering from co-occurring substance use disorders and personality disorders based on schema therapy (Young, Klosko, & Weishaar, 2003). Schema therapy combines behavioral and cognitive techniques to challenge maladaptive or unstable behavior patterns. Though it assumes a more complex cognitive schema, this approach nonetheless relies on a similar theoretical basis as Beck's and Ellis's approaches.

Despite their emphasis on cognitive processes, cognitive therapies rely heavily on techniques based on SLT to facilitate the changes in cognition that are viewed as being crucial to the treatment of PSUDs. Cognitive theorists do, however, believe that lasting behavior change is difficult to achieve without changing the underlying faulty patterns of thinking that lie at the root of most emotional upsets.

Techniques for treating PSUDs that derive wholly or in part from cognitive theories include anger management training, rational disputation of positive thoughts about alcohol/drug use, and rational disputation of thoughts linking substance use to alleviation of negative emotional states. Techniques based on cognitive theory tend to blend quite nicely with SLT-based techniques. Current research aimed at enhancing aspects of techniques based on other behavioral theories (e.g., cue–exposure based on classical conditioning theory) is beginning to incorporate explicit cognitive strategies into treatment. With its flexibility and inclusiveness, SLT has emerged in the last two decades as the predominant CB theory of addictions origin and treatment.

With this brief overview of CB theories of substance abuse treatment in mind, let us now turn to a discussion of critical issues in treating substance abusers as viewed through the lens of CB theory. These issues are discussed from the perspective of SLT because that theory provides the most comprehensive behavior theoretical framework currently available.

Critical Issues in Substance Abuse Treatment

Etiology and Maintenance of Substance Use

CB theories view PSUDs as resulting from a combination of factors presumed to interact in different ways to produce PSUDs depending on each individual's unique characteristics and environment. Although explicitly endorsing a "biopsychosocial" perspective from which to view the origins of PSUDs, CB theories tend to minimize the causal role of genetic factors while placing a heavier emphasis on the interacting influences of an individual's environment, innate biological makeup or temperament, and learning processes.

CB theories view the initiation of substance use as primarily due to a combination of environmental factors (particularly substance availability and peer group norms) and individual physiological responses to initial use, resulting in substance use being either reinforcing or punishing for the individual. Whether substance use will be initiated and continued depends on factors such as the availability of substances in a person's environment, peer group behavior and norms with respect to substance use, the degree of importance of the peer group in the individual's life, and whether or not initial use of the substance is pleasurable. Parental attitudes and behaviors also play a role, with parental behavior being more likely to be modeled than parental dictates, especially if other factors (e.g., substance availability or peer group norms) favor substance use. The combined effect of these factors is the development of drinking and drug use outcome expectancies that appear to play an important role in the initiation and maintenance of early drinking (Christiansen, Smith, Roehling, & Goldman, 1989).

For persons who develop PSUDs, CB theories postulate that the pharmacological and social reinforcements attendant on initial use increase the probability of substance use behavior. With increased use, the person begins to recognize the role that drugs or alcohol can play in reducing negative emotions and may fail to learn alternative coping responses. In a somewhat different fashion, persons who have failed to learn adequate coping skills prior to the onset of substance use may begin to use drugs or alcohol as a means of compensating for the lack of those skills. Finally, some substance users may, by virtue of temperamental factors such as sensation seeking and impulsivity, use alcohol or drugs initially for their excitement-producing properties rather than as a means of coping.

The processes presumed to operate in the development of PSUDs at the earliest, or less severe, stages are largely modeling, operant conditioning (reinforcement of substance use), and cognitive mediators such as expectancies that substance use will result in positive outcomes. With repeated substance use and at more severe stages of dependence, classical conditioning factors begin to play a more prominent role in the development of PSUDs, with both conditioned craving and withdrawal playing an important part in producing severe dependence in some individuals. There is also evidence that tolerance is, at least to some extent, a learned phenomenon (Vogel-Sprott, 1992). At severe levels of dependence, use is often driven by the reinforcing value of avoiding withdrawal (negative reinforcement) rather than the pleasurable effects of use. It is clear that at more severe levels of dependence, the person's body has adapted to the continuing presence of alcohol or drugs, and that these physiological changes play an important role in shifting the reinforcing contingencies of substance use. At this latter stage, CB theories of treatment shift the focus of treatment somewhat toward coping with the effects of these physiological changes, particularly withdrawal symptoms that may trigger a return to use following brief abstinence. Nonetheless, the basic processes by which treatment proceeds remain the same and involve implementation of learning strategies to cope with the long-term effects of substance use.

As substance use begins to assume a greater role in the individual's life, the negative consequences of use may also increase. These consequences are unique to the individual and may require active coping responses. Coping skill deficits become important again as the individual may be unable to cope with the problems associated with substance use itself (e.g., family, work, or legal problems) and increase their use in an effort to cope with increasingly frequent negative emotions. The immediate reinforcing value of substance use assumes a prominent role in maintaining the habit, despite the negative consequences, because substance use produces immediate reinforcement whereas the punishment of negative consequences might be greatly delayed.

As the severity of an individual's PSUD increases, several things may happen. Often substance use itself becomes stereotyped and limited to certain situations. These settings and the associated stimuli may become conditioned to substance use and come to elicit physiological or psychological responses that further prompt it. With increasingly complex problems to face, the individual's coping skills may be overwhelmed and his or her substance use increased as a means of alleviating the negative emotions that stem from failure to cope adequately.

Associations with peer groups whose members are themselves substance users may exert pressure on the individual to maintain substance use as a means of interaction with peers or of retaining the reinforcement of group membership. Peers may also reinforce unrealistically positive expectancies for drug or alcohol by their own behavior under the influence.

Consistent with natural history studies of the development of PSUDs, CB theories suggest that although the nature and quality of reinforcement for substance use may change over the course of a individual's substance use history, principles of classical conditioning, operant conditioning, modeling, and cognitive mediation of behavior still operate in maintaining substance use behavior. In the many cases now being documented in which persons suffering from PSUDs stop using drugs or alcohol on their own without any treatment, a combination of shifting reinforcement contingencies and cognitive changes appears to explain the change in behavior (Sobell, Sobell, Toneatto, & Leo, 1993).

Homogeneity/Heterogeneity of Persons with PSUDs

CB theories are entirely consistent with current views of substance use as falling along a continuum ranging from no use at all to severely dependent use (Institute of Medicine, 1990). CB theories view each individual as forming a unique constellation of biological bases, learning history, and current environment. In spite of the uniqueness of every individual's substance use history, CB theories believe that there are also commonalities among substance users and abusers. Nonetheless, CB theories tend to minimize the importance of global subtyping or labeling of individuals in treatment. Although guided by empirical evidence that suggests differences in treatment outcomes and the advisability of various treatment goals among persons with PSUDs who have particular genetic backgrounds, personality makeups, and environments, CB theorists tend to use these data as guidelines rather than as strict determinants of treatment.

In essence, although CB theorists recognize groups of PSUDs that result from personality disorders, depression, or anxiety, a thorough assessment and treatment must still be based on an individualized CB analysis rather than on assumptions about group membership. CB theories of treatment emphasize the matching of treatment procedures and goals to patient needs to a greater extent than do other theories of treatment. Although the therapist's armamentarium of techniques is relatively constant, the application of those techniques is based on analyses of a particular client's skill assets and deficits.

Role of Genetics/Biological Factors in PSUDs

It would be foolish to deny that human beings are to some extent the product of their biology. All behavior at the levels at which therapy takes place (e.g., the overtly or subjectively observable) ultimately has a biological substrate. All learning, at bottom, involves changes at the neuronal level, if not change at the molecular level. The role of genetics in human behavior is not clearly specified, and at the present time the genetic substrate of human behavior is immutable by available methods. Thus, while biological and genetic factors are viewed as risk factors that must be taken into account in one's analysis of a particular individual's substance use patterns and addressed in the selection of treatment goals, they do not play a significant role in treatment itself.

CB theorists believe that changes in behavior require something more than changes in a person's biological or neurochemical functioning. This belief rests on the assumption that environmental contingencies play a key role in the cause and control of behavior, as well as on the notion that skill assets and deficits are important contributors to the development, maintenance, and change of PSUDs.

CB theories of change emphasize helping the client to learn coping skills that will be more effective in managing day-to-day life without using drugs or alcohol. While not rejecting the potential role of pharmacotherapeutic interventions (see Chung, Ross, Wakhlu, & Adinoff, Chapter 11, and Carroll & Kulik, Chapter 12, this volume), CB theorists point out that these approaches are still underused in the treatment of PSUDs. The reason for this relatively minimal impact to date is most likely due to difficulties in persuading persons with PSUDs to take these medications reliably, and to a lack of knowledge as to which clients will best respond to what forms of pharmacological interventions. This sort of client–treatment matching is an issue that CB treatment techniques are uniquely equipped to address.

Tasks of Treatment

Consistent with the increasing emphasis on the therapeutic relationship noted at the beginning of this chapter, CB therapists have recognized the importance of establishing a strong working alliance with clients at the beginning of treatment. This realization has led to efforts to combine motivational interviewing (which is focused on increasing motivation for change among clients who are in the earliest stages of change) and CB-based approaches (which are inherently action-focused). In one major research study (Project COMBINE; Moyers & Houck, 2011) motivational interviewing was implemented alongside a variety of CB techniques in a study of the use of medications conjointly with CB approaches. The assumption behind this aspect of development in CB approaches is that without a strong working alliance leading to high motivation for change, most, if not all, CB approaches will be ineffective.

CB theories typically view treatment as needing to accomplish several tasks in order to be successful. As with all psychosocial treatment approaches, the first task in treatment, if necessary, is to detoxify the client from hazardous or potentially life-threatening levels of substance use, preferably to a level of temporary abstinence, although CB theories do not usually make total abstinence a precondition for treatment or even a necessary treatment goal for some clients.

Once detoxification has been accomplished, the therapist must conduct a thorough functional analysis of substance use behavior. This analysis should focus on both skill deficits and on the client's environment, with a particular emphasis on identifying those person-specific (e.g., emotional states and thoughts) and environmental factors that are associated with, or perhaps trigger, substance use. These high-risk situations, which may be both internal and external, need to be addressed in order for treatment to succeed and treatment gains to be maintained. Without this thorough assessment, treatment cannot proceed and is likely to fail.

Following a functional analysis, work then proceeds on teaching the client a specifically tailored menu of techniques and strategies aimed at intervening in the problems identified in the assessment. In CB treatments, assessment and treatment are closely linked, and assessment is reiterated throughout the process of treatment to gauge progress and identify continuing problem areas and behaviors. The fact that problems may continue to emerge during treatment reinforces the importance of ongoing assessment.

The final task of CB treatments is to assist the client in identifying and planning strategies for coping with high-risk situations that may occur in the future. This task is designed to provide the client with the tools necessary to prevent relapse to substance use—the core of CB notions of relapse prevention. Clients are also taught how to cope with slips or relapses, should they occur, in ways that will shorten the length and intensity of any future return to substance use.

The three core tasks of treatment from a CB perspective—functional analysis, skills training, and relapse prevention—are accomplished both by individual work with the client and by helping the client make active attempts to change environmental factors that may be triggering or maintaining substance use. Thus, clients may be encouraged to make significant lifestyle changes or changes in their daily routine or interactions with family and friends, which the functional analysis suggests might enhance the client's ability to cope without the use of drugs or alcohol. Although not always explicitly addressed, the key role of the environment in PSUDs is always a factor in guiding treatment.

Treatment Goals

Because they place heavy emphasis on matching treatments to specific client characteristics and needs, CB approaches imply flexibility in the selection of treatment goals. Unlike other theoretical positions that insist on abstinence as the only legitimate goal of treatment and that often make abstinence a prerequisite for treatment entry, CB theories allow for a more flexible and incremental approach to substance use reduction that is often more attractive to clients who might otherwise avoid treatment.

Although individual therapists may vary in the degree to which they insist on an abstinence goal for their clients, there is a substantial body of literature suggesting that many persons with PSUDs, particularly those with less severe dependence, can and do become moderate users, often without any treatment at all (Booth, Dale, Slade, & Dewey, 1992; Duckert, Amundsen, & Johnsen, 1992; Sobell et al., 1993). In fact, many who have been treated for PSUDs in abstinence-oriented programs become moderate users, and many who set out to achieve only a reduction in substance use ultimately become abstinent. There appear to be cognitive variables that have an impact on the decision to change substance use behavior. There are also data to suggest that an individual's stage of readiness to change (Prochaska et al., 1992) strongly influences the process of treatment participation and commitment.

CB-oriented therapists will typically work with a client incrementally toward client-selected goals (either moderation or abstinence), although clinicians will provide evidence-based counterarguments to a client goal of moderation if the client's level of substance use at treatment entry carries with it the risk of immediate catastrophic consequences (e.g., liver failure, legal contingencies) if some level of use continues. The process of goal determination is one of negotiation rather than therapist insistence, consistent with the notion that the more committed the client is to the particular treatment goal, the greater the likelihood of reaching it.

Recently, another approach to treatment goals that has been termed "harm reduction" has emerged (Marlatt & Tapert, 1993; Dayton & Rotgers, 2002). The harm reduction approach attempts to reflect the realities of treating persons with PSUDs in recognizing that complete lifelong abstinence is often extremely difficult to accomplish, even though that may be the healthiest goal for a particular client, even when a client is committed to abstinence. When immediate cessation of substance use is not likely to or does not occur (due, perhaps, to the severity of the individual's PSUD), taking a harm reduction approach leads to working in an incremental fashion, in smaller steps, toward an ultimate goal of safer substance use (which in many cases may equate to permanent abstinence). The ultimate aim of harm reduction is to enhance health by minimizing or reducing the impact of behaviors or other factors that threaten health. From this perspective, any change in the environment or client behavior that leads to reduced substance use is one that should be promoted.

Empirical Research and CB Theory

Of all the approaches presented in this book, with the exception of motivational and pharmacotherapeutic approaches, cognitive-behaviorally-based approaches are the most closely linked with existing scientific knowledge of PSUDs. Empirical validation of treatment techniques has been an integral part of the CB theory of treatment from the beginnings of the behavior therapy movement in the early 1950s. CB therapists view each treatment case as, in a sense, a minilaboratory within which the therapist and the client collaborate to assess client needs and apply and evaluate the effect of various treatment technologies.

Not only are CB treatments open to scientific scrutiny, they insist on it. Without well-designed experimental studies of treatment outcomes, CB theorists believe that no progress can be made toward resolving the most difficult issue when treating PSUDs: what treatments work best under what conditions with what clients. This is the crux of the patient–treatment matching research that has been conducted under the auspices of the National Institute of Alcohol Abuse and Alcoholism (Donovan & Mattson, 1994). The behavior therapy movement, from which CB theories of treating PSUDs are derived, insists on empirical validation of the techniques used to treat clients as a cornerstone of ethical professional practice. To apply scientifically untested or untestable techniques routinely, solely on the basis of single case histories or client testimonials, is considered by most CB therapists to be unethical practice, especially when empirically validated techniques exist and could be more widely used were practitioners aware of them.

Advantages and Disadvantages of CB Approaches

Advantages of CB Approaches

Approaches to treating PSUDs based on CB theory have a number of advantages over other currently available approaches to treatment. This can be seen by the extent to which concepts that were originally developed by CB theorists (e.g., Marlatt's [Marlatt & Donovan, 2005; Marlatt & Gordon, 1985; Marlatt & Tapert, 1993] relapse prevention concept) have begun to be incorporated, although often in altered form, into the practice of therapists trained in other approaches (Morgenstern & McCrady, 1992; Rotgers & Morgenstern, 1994). There are seven clear advantages to adopting a CB view of PSUDs and their treatment. These are outlined briefly in Table 5.2.

Flexibility in Tailoring Treatment to Client Needs

Because CB approaches eschew global labeling and place a heavy emphasis on individualized assessment, they are ideally suited to matching treatments

---

TABLE 5.2. Advantages of Cognitive-Behavioral Theories of Psychoactive Substance Use Disorders

1. Flexibility in meeting specific client needs.
2. Readily accepted by clients due to high level of client involvement in treatment planning and goal selection.
3. Soundly grounded in psychological theory.
4. Emphasis on linking scientific knowledge to treatment practice.
5. Clear guidelines for assessing treatment progress.
6. Empowerment of clients in making their own behavior change.
7. Strong empirical and scientific evidence of efficacy.

to client needs. This flexibility extends to treatment goal selection as well as to selection of the particular interventions to be used with a given client. CB theory allows for specific matching of client problems, goals, and readiness for change, as well as selection of treatment interventions.

Avoidance of Labeling and Goal Imposition

CB treatments for PSUDs are readily accepted by clients. This is because therapists operating within this perspective adopt a collaborative rather than a confrontational stance with clients and avoid labeling clients with terms that in our society carry pejorative connotations. Likewise, CB approaches are explicitly carried out in a collaborative fashion in which client input is given a high level of attention and consideration. Clients are not forced to accept a unitary explanation of their behavior as a precondition for behavior change efforts. CB theory allows for a high degree of individualization of treatment, in contrast to other approaches that apply a similar formula for recovery to all clients.

Sound Basis in Psychological Theory

Unlike other widely used approaches, CB approaches have a clear, coherent, well-tested theoretical basis that is rooted in scientific psychology. Having a clear, coherent theory of behavior change has been cited as a factor in treatment success in substance abuse treatment (Onken, 1991).

Emphasis on Linking Science to Treatment

A corollary to this sound basis in psychological science is a strong emphasis on linking science to treatment. Scientific evaluation and knowledge are important both at the individual client–therapist level and at the systemic or treatment system level. In the client–therapist relationship, the emphasis on continuous testing of assessment hypotheses and technique success is integral to the achievement of behavior change. At the systemic level, scientific evaluation of techniques derived from CB theory plays an integral role in ensuring that consumers of CB treatments get the best available treatment and in providing the scientific knowledge that can lead to development of more efficient and more effective treatments in the future.

Clear Guidelines for Assessing Treatment Progress

By focusing on continued assessment of the factors contributing to a particular client's substance use, as well as the degree to which clients are learning and implementing new coping skills and lifestyle changes, CB approaches provide clear milestones for evaluating individual treatment progress or the lack thereof. Knowing whether and how well a client is progressing is essential both to altering treatment strategies that may be ineffective and to determining when it is appropriate to terminate treatment with a particular client. Because client and therapist mutually agree upon treatment goals at the beginning of treatment, progress toward termination is more easily assessed. This allows the length of treatment to be tailored explicitly to client needs on the basis of definable criteria.

Empowerment of Clients as Effective Agents in Changing Their Own Behavior

In contrast to traditional approaches that emphasize, in somewhat paradoxical (and often puzzling-to-clients) fashion, clients' powerlessness over their own addiction, CB approaches explicitly attempt to enhance clients' sense of personal efficacy. By teaching clients not only that they can be effective problem solvers without using alcohol or drugs, but that they can learn new skills necessary to solve new, unforeseen problems in the future, CB techniques accomplish two major tasks: they destigmatize addiction and help enhance self-efficacy and self-esteem. In a related way, they may also reduce the need for future treatment by teaching clients the requisite skills to analyze and solve problems themselves. In this, CB approaches are consistent with the adage, "When you give a man a fish, you feed him for a day, but when you teach him to fish, you feed him for a lifetime."

Empirical Evidence of Efficacy

Approaches based on CB theory have garnered substantial scientific evidence of efficacy in controlled clinical trials (Holder, Longabaugh, Miller, & Rubonis, 1991). In addition, there is evidence that CB approaches may be more effective than other approaches with a group of clients that have generally poor prognosis: those that suffer from antisocial personality disorder (Kadden, Cooney, Getter, & Litt, 1989). Given evidence that a very high percentage of clients with PSUDs also suffer from antisocial personality disorder (Regier et al., 1990; Ross, Glaser, & Germanson, 1988), the finding of relative efficacy of CB techniques with this group is a strong reason to consider them.

Disadvantages of CB Approaches

Despite the numerous advantages just presented, CB approaches also have disadvantages. These disadvantages have more to do with the current state of scientific knowledge than with any inherent difficulties with CB approaches. As scientific knowledge accumulates, it is likely that these disadvantages will disappear. As it now stands, these disadvantages could more reasonably be termed "limitations" of the approach.

First, while there is evidence of differential effectiveness for CB approaches, the exact reason for this is unclear. For example, the extent to which clients actually use the skills they are taught in treatment and the relationship of skill use to relapse or maintenance of change is unclear.

Second, there is a distinct, and surprising lack of empirical support for the advantage of adding relapse prevention procedures to treatment as a means of enhancing long-term outcomes. Although some data suggest that those who learn relapse prevention techniques are able to curtail the length and severity of their relapses, the overall advantage predicted to accrue to clients as a result of the introduction of relapse prevention technologies has not been strongly validated empirically (Wilson, 1992).

Third, and unrelated to the scientific basis of CB techniques, is the fact that few treatment providers are well trained in these techniques, and that some aspects of CB practice are rejected out of hand by some therapists working from a more traditional perspective. Specifically, some who hold a more traditional perspective reject the possibility of moderated use as a treatment goal, in spite of evidence that moderated use can be achieved by many clients (Miller, Walters, & Bennett, 2001).

The lack of emphasis on a spiritual aspect to PSUDs is also disturbing to some practitioners, particularly ones who have themselves benefited from more traditional, 12-step-based approaches to treatment, predominantly a reflection of the Alcoholics Anonymous philosophy. Although a CB approach is not inherently antithetical to a spiritual notion of PSUDs, the notion of powerlessness often associated with spirituality in addictions treatment is. For those who rely more strongly on personal belief rather than on scientific evidence to guide their practice, this may be an unbreachable barrier to the use of CB techniques in practice. For patients who reject the spiritual aspects of Alcoholics Anonymous, there are a number of alternative self-help approaches, such as S.M.A.R.T. Recovery (*www.smartrecovery.org*) and Moderation Management (*www.moderation.org*), that are more directly based on CB approaches to recovery (McCrady & Delaney, 1995; Rotgers, Kern & Hoeltzel, 2002; Steinberger, 2004).

Conclusion

In the last quarter century, CB theories have been among the most productive in advancing empirically validated knowledge of the origins and treatment of PSUDs. The notion of basing treatment on knowledge of the psychological processes of human behavior has led to the development of new and effective treatment technologies. Marital/family and motivational approaches (discussed elsewhere in this volume) are based largely on the work of CB theorists, although substantial progress beyond basic CB theory characterizes those approaches as well.

Although CB-based treatments still do not reliably and predictably produce the sorts of treatment outcomes all therapists desire (i.e., long-lasting, positive behavior change), they do offer some of the most promising approaches currently available to therapists treating patients with PSUDs. They also hold the promise, based on the strong emphasis by CB-oriented therapists on scientific study of both the efficacy and process of behavior change in addictions, of advancing our knowledge of how best to treat these difficult and costly problems.

References

Abrams, D. B., & Niaura, R. S. (1987). Social learning theory. In H. T. Blane & K. E. Leonard (Eds.), *Psychological theories of drinking and alcoholism* (pp. 131–178). New York: Guilford Press.

Azrin, N. H., Sisson, R. W., Meyers, R., & Godley, M. (1982). Alcoholism treatment by disulfiram and community reinforcement therapy. *Journal of Behavior Therapy and Experimental Psychiatry, 13*, 105–112.

Baars, B. J. (1986). *The cognitive revolution in psychology.* New York: Guilford Press.

Ball, S. A. (2004). Treatment of personality disorders with co-occurring substance dependence: Dual-focus schema therapy. In J. J. Magnavita (Ed.), *Handbook of personality disorders: Theory and practice* (pp. 398–425). Hoboken, NJ: Wiley.

Ball, S. A., Cobb-Richardson, P., Connolly, A. J., Bujosa, C. T., & O'Neil, T. W. (2005). Substance abuse and personality disorders in homeless drop-in center clients: Symptom severity and psychotherapy retention in a randomized clinical trial. *Comprehensive Psychiatry, 46,* 317–379.

Ball, S. A., & Young, J. E. (2000). Dual focus schema therapy for personality disorders and substance dependence: Case study results. *Cognitive and Behavioral Practice, 7,* 270–281.

Bandura, A. (1977). *Social learning theory.* Englewood Cliffs, NJ: Prentice-Hall.

Beck, A. T., Rush, A. J., Shaw, B. F., & Emery, G. (1979). *Cognitive therapy of depression.* New York: Guilford Press.

Beck, A. T., Wright, E. D., Newman, C. F., & Liese, B. S. (1993). *Cognitive therapy of substance abuse.* New York: Guilford Press.

Bickel, W. K., & Kelly, T. H. (1988). The relationship of stimulus control to the treatment of substance abuse. In B. A. Ray (Ed.), *Learning factors in substance abuse* (NIDA Research Monograph 84, pp. 122–140). Washington, DC: U.S. Government Printing Office.

Booth, P. B., Dale, B., Slade, P. D., & Dewey, M. E. (1992). A follow-up study of problem drinkers offered a goal choice option. *Journal of Studies on Alcohol, 53,* 594–600.

Childress, A. R., Hole, A. V., Ehrman, R. N., Robbins, S. J., McLellan, A. T., & O'Brien, C. P. (1993). Cue reactivity and cue reactivity interventions in drug dependence. In L. S. Onken, J. D. Blame, & J. J. Boren (Eds.), *Behavioral treatments for drug abuse and dependence* (NIDA Research Monograph 137, pp. 73–96). Washington, DC: U.S. Government Printing Office.

Christiansen, B. A., Smith, G. T., Roehling, P. V., & Goldman, M. S. (1989). Using alcohol expectancies to predict adolescent drinking behavior after one year. *Journal of Consulting and Clinical Psychology, 57*, 93–99.

Dayton, G., & Rotgers, F. (2002). The value of cognitive-behavioral strategies. In A. Tatarsky (Ed.), *Harm reduction psychotherapy: A new treatment for drug and alcohol problems* (pp. 72–105). Northvale, NJ: Jason Aronson.

Donovan, D. M. (1988). Assessment of addictive behaviors: Implications of an emerging biopsychosocial model. In D. M. Donovan & G. A. Marlatt (Eds.), *Assessment of addictive behaviors* (pp. 5–14). New York: Guilford Press.

Donovan, D. M., & Mattson, M. E. (Eds.). (1994). Alcoholism treatment matching research: Methodological and clinical approaches. *Journal of Studies on Alcohol*, Suppl. 12, 5–14.

Duckert, E., Amundsen, A., & Johnsen, J. (1992). What happens to drinking after therapeutic intervention? *British Journal of Addiction, 87*, 1457–1467.

Ellis, A., McInerney, J. F., DiGiuseppe, R., & Yeager, R. J. (1988). *Rational–emotive therapy with alcoholics and substance abusers.* New York: Pergamon Press.

Evans-Jones, C., Peters, E., & Barker, C. (2009). The therapeutic relationship in CBT for psychosis: Client, therapist and therapy factors. *Behavioural and Cognitive Psychotherapy, 37*(5), 527–540.

Eysenck, H. J. (1982). Neobehavioristic (S–R) theory. In G. T. Wilson & C. M. Franks (Eds.), *Contemporary behavior therapy: Conceptual and empirical foundations* (pp. 205–276). New York: Guilford Press.

Goldman, M. S., Brown, S. A., & Christiansen, B. A. (1987). Expectancy theory: Thinking about drinking. In H. T. Blane & K. E. Leonard (Eds.), *Psychological theories of drinking and alcoholism* (pp. 181–226). New York: Guilford Press.

Holder, H. D., Longabaugh, R., Miller, W. R., & Rubonis, A. V. (1991). The cost effectiveness of treatment for alcoholism: A first approximation. *Journal of Studies on Alcohol, 52*, 517–540.

Institute of Medicine. (1990). *Broadening the base of treatment for alcohol problems: Report of a study by a committee of the Institute of Medicine, Division of Health and Behavioral Medicine.* Washington, DC: National Academy Press.

Kadden, R. M., Cooney, N. L., Getter, H., & Litt, M. D. (1989). Matching alcoholics to coping skills or interactive therapies: Posttreatment results. *Journal of Consulting and Clinical Psychology, 57*, 698–704.

Krasner, L. (1982). Behavior therapy: On roots, contexts and growth. In G. T. Wilson & C. M. Franks (Eds.), *Contemporary behavior therapy: Conceptual and empirical foundations* (pp. 11–64). New York: Guilford Press.

Kuhn, T. S. (1970). *The structure of scientific revolutions* (2nd ed.). Chicago: University of Chicago Press.

Lee, N. K., & Rawson, R. A. (2008). A systematic review of cognitive and behavioural therapies for methamphetamine dependence. *Drug and Alcohol Dependence, 27*(3), 309–317.

Marlatt, G. A., & Donovan, D. M. (Eds.). (2008). *Relapse prevention: Maintenance strategies in the treatment of addictive behaviors, 2nd edition* New York: Guilford Press.

Marlatt, G. A., & Gordon, J. R. (Eds.). (1985). *Relapse prevention: Maintenance strategies in the treatment of addictive behaviors.* New York: Guilford Press.

Marlatt, G. A., & Tapert, S. F. (1993). Harm reduction: Reducing the risks of addictive behaviors. In J. S. Baer, G. A. Marlatt, & R. J. McMahon (Eds.), *Addictive behaviors across the life span: Prevention, treatment and policy issues.* Newbury Park, CA: Sage.

McCrady, B. S., & Delaney, S. I. (1995). Self-help groups. In R. K. Hester & W. R. Miller (Eds.), *Handbook of alcoholism treatment approaches: Effective alternatives* (2nd ed., pp. 160–175). Needham Heights, MA: Allyn & Bacon.

McLellan, A. T., Childress, A. R., Ehrman, R. N., & O'Brien, C. P. (1986). Extinguishing conditioned responses during treatment for opiate dependence: Turning laboratory findings into clinical procedure. *Journal of Substance Abuse Treatment, 3,* 33–40.

Miller, W. R., & Rollnick S. (2002). *Motivational interviewing: Preparing people to change* (2nd ed.). New York: Guilford Press.

Miller, W. R., Walters, S. T., & Bennett, M. E. (2001). How effective is alcohol treatment in the United States? *Journal of Studies on Alcohol, 62,* 211–220.

Monti, P. M., Kadden, R. M., Rohsenow, D. J., Cooney, N. L., & Abrams, D. B. (2002). *Treating alcohol dependence: A coping skills training guide* (2nd ed.). New York: Guilford Press.

Morgenstern, J., & McCrady, B. S. (1992). Curative factors in alcohol and drug treatment: Behavioral and disease model perspectives. *British Journal of Addiction, 87,* 901–912.

Moyers, T. B., & Houck, J. (2011). Combining motivational interviewing with cognitive-behavioral treatments for substance abuse: Lessons from the COMBINE Research Project. *Cognitive and Behavioral Practice, 18(1),* 38–45.

Norcross, J. C. (2002). *Psychotherapy relationships that work: Therapist contributions and responsiveness to patients.* New York: Oxford University Press.

Onken, L. S. (1991). Using psychotherapy effectively in drug abuse treatment. In R. W. Pickens, C. G. Leukefeld, & C. R. Schuster (Eds.), *Improving drug abuse treatment* (pp. 267–278). Washington, DC: U.S. Government Printing Office.

Pavlov, I. P. (1927). *Lectures on conditioned reflexes.* New York: International Publishers.

Prochaska, J. O., DiClemente, C. C., & Norcross, J. C. (1992). In search of how people change: Applications to addictive behaviors. *American Psychologist, 47,* 1102–1114.

Regier, D. A., Farmer, M. E., Rae, D. S., Locke, B. Z., Keith, S. J., Judd, L. L., et al. (1990). Comorbidity of mental disorders with alcohol and other drug abuse: Results from the Epidemiologic Catchment Area (ECA) study. *Journal of the American Medical Association, 264,* 2511–2518.

Rimmele, C. T., Miller, W. R., & Dougher, M. J. (1989). Aversion therapies. In R. K. Hester & W. R. Miller (Eds.), *Handbook of alcoholism treatment approaches: Effective alternatives* (pp. 134–147). New York: Pergamon Press.

Ross, H. E., Glaser, F. B., & Germanson, T. (1988). The prevalence of psychiatric disorders in patients with alcohol and other drug problems. *Archives of General Psychiatry, 45,* 1023–1031.

Rotgers, F., Kern, M.F., & Hoeltzel, R. (2002). *Responsible drinking: A moderation management approach for problem drinkers.* Oakland, CA: New Harbinger.

Rotgers, F., & Morgenstern, J. (1994). *Processes comprising successful substance abuse treatment: A survey of counselors.* Unpublished manuscript, Rutgers University, Center of Alcohol Studies, Piscataway, NJ.

Sher, K. J. (1987). Stress response dampening. In H. T. Blane & K. E. Leonard (Eds.), *Psychological theories of drinking and alcoholism* (pp. 227–271). New York: Guilford Press.

Sobell, L. C., Sobell, M. B., Toneatto, T., & Leo, G. I. (1993). What triggers the resolution of alcohol problems without treatment? *Alcoholism: Clinical and Experimental Research, 17,* 217–224.

Steinberger, H. (2004). *SMART recovery handbook.* Mentor, OH: Alcohol and Drug Abuse Self-Help Network, Inc.

Vogel-Sprott, M. (1992). *Alcohol tolerance and social drinking: Learning the consequences.* New York: Guilford Press.

Watson, J. B. (1919). *Psychology from the standpoint of a behaviorist.* Philadelphia: Lippincott.

Wikler, A. (1965). Conditioning factors in opiate addiction and relapse. In D. L. Wilner & G. G. Kassenbaum (Eds.), *Narcotics* (pp. 85–100). New York: McGraw-Hill

Wikler, A. (1973). Dynamics of drug dependence: Implications of a conditioning theory for research and treatment. *Archives of General Psychiatry, 28,* 611–616.

Willenbring, M. (2010). The future of research on the treatment of alcohol dependence. *Alcohol Research and Health, 33,* 55–63.

Wilson, P. H. (1992). Relapse prevention: Conceptual and methodological issues. In P. H. Wilson (Ed.), *Principles and practice of relapse prevention* (pp. 1–22). New York: Guilford Press.

Witkiewicz, K., & Bowen, S. (2010). Depression, craving and substance use following a randomized trial of mindfulness-based relapse prevention. *Journal of Consulting and Clinical Psychology, 78*(3), 362–374.

Young, J. E., Klosko, J. S., & Weishaar, M. E. (2003). *Schema therapy: A practitioner's guide.* New York: Guilford Press.

Chapter 6

Behavioral Treatment Techniques for Psychoactive Substance Use Disorders

James S. Marinchak
Thomas J. Morgan

Basic Tasks of All Behavioral Interventions

Whether working with substance abuse patients or with a general psychiatric population, there are several essential tasks that the behaviorally oriented clinician must accomplish during treatment. These tasks include (1) developing a collaborative working relationship, (2) enhancing patient motivation to engage in treatment exercises both within and outside therapy, (3) using a functional analysis to make a thorough individualized assessment of the patient's presenting problem/s, (4) developing the patient's treatment goals and assisting in their implementation, (5) evaluating treatment progress, and (6) providing information for long-term recovery strategies, including the warning signs of relapse.

Developing a Therapeutic Relationship

The importance of a positive relationship between therapists and patients in treatment has long been emphasized. Since Rogers (1957) first defined unconditional positive regard, accurate empathy, genuineness, and therapist congruence as necessary conditions for positive change, the scientific and treatment communities have been interested in understanding the contribution of the therapeutic relationship to treatment. Valle (1981) has shown that the level of a counselor's empathy and general interpersonal skills predicts long-term outcomes for alcoholics. Additionally, there is evidence that alcoholic patients have poorer treatment outcomes when clinicians use a confrontational style (Lieberman, Yalom, & Miles, 1973; MacDonough, 1976; Miller, Benefield, & Tonigan, 1993). In Project MATCH, higher therapeutic alliance ratings predicted increased treatment participation and improved drinking outcomes among outpatient clients (Connors, Carroll, DiClemente, Longabaugh, & Donovan, 1997). Finally, a recent review found that the formation of a positive working alliance in the initial sessions of substance abuse treatment was associated with increased patient engagement, treatment retention, and treatment improvement (Meier, Barrowclough, & Donmall, 2005).

In developing a positive collaborative relationship with a patient, the clinician should spend time focusing on key aspects of the therapeutic relationship. One aspect includes exploring patient expectations about treatment. It may be the case that patients have undergone previous treatments for their alcohol or drug use. Because of past difficulties in treatment or the experience of a relapse, patients may begin a new treatment episode with low expectations. Thus, it is important for clinicians to inquire about any expectations at the outset of treatment and discuss any factors that the client believes contributed to the lack of success with the previous treatment. Furthermore, the clinician should address the logistics of treatment, such as how long it might last, how sessions are structured, issues concerning confidentiality, and ways in which the current treatment will address factors associated with past failures.

Another important aspect of the collaborative relationship is a sense of empathy for the patient's experience. McCrady (2008) has suggested several actions therapists can take to enhance empathy for their substance–abusing patients. These actions include attempting to change an addictive behavior or deeply held habit of one's own, attending self-help meetings, and listening carefully to the client. Also, in developing a good therapeutic alliance, a clinician can ask questions that reflect an interest in the patient and his or her life outside of substance use. For example, one way to enhance rapport is to ask about a patient's family, work, hobbies, or family pet in addition to substance abuse history. This line of inquiry has the additional benefit of identifying potential therapeutic strengths, such as the presence of supportive individuals in the patient's social network who can be utilized during treatment.

Enhancing Motivation to Change

For more than 20 years motivational aspects of substance abuse treatment have been the subject of much discussion and research. The development of motivational interviewing (MI; Miller & Rollnick, 2002) and subsequently motivational enhancement therapy (MET; Miller, Zweben, DiClemente,

& Rychtarik, 1992) brought attention to the importance of addressing patient motivation throughout behavioral treatment. Today, MI is viewed as an effective add-on component to standard treatment; MET has been shown to be an effective stand-alone treatment in itself (Hettema, Steele, & Miller, 2005; Lundahl & Burke, 2009). Recent findings also suggest that the simple use of motivational-enhancement techniques during substance treatment, regardless if used specifically in a MET protocol, influenced the development of a positive therapeutic alliance (Crits-Cristoph et al., 2009). (See Rose & Walters, Chapter 1, and Tooley & Moyers, Chapter 2, this volume, for a more detailed discussion of motivation within the addictions field.) For purposes of this chapter, it is sufficient to say that motivation is a key part of engaging clients in behavioral therapy.

Assessment via Functional Analysis and Self-Monitoring

The prelude to good behavioral treatment is a thorough assessment and development of an individualized conceptualization of the patient's substance use. In a behavioral assessment, a patient's substance use is examined collaboratively to determine factors that precipitate and maintain his or her use of substances.

One area to assess is the unique precursors or triggers to a patient's substance use. This assessment includes evaluating interpersonal situations and relationships, internal emotional and somatic states, and environmental situations that are uniquely associated with a patient's drinking or drug use. Each patient is different, so it is important to identify the individualized "triggers" of substance use, as this information will be invaluable in identifying and coping with later high-risk situations. This type of assessment is often conducted by the therapist and patient in-session through the creation of a functional analysis (sometimes referred to as "behavioral analysis" or "behavior chain") and outside of session through the assignment of substance-use monitoring homework.

The clinician also needs to assess the consequences of the patient's substance use, both in the immediate and long term, as well as the positive and negative reinforcing consequences associated with the substance use. In identifying consequences, it is important to inquire about different areas of a patient's life that are often affected by substance use:

• *Relationship problems.* Arguments with family and/or friends about substance use; separations, breakups, or divorce due to substance use; family and/or friends becoming annoyed with or criticizing the patient's alcohol/drug use.

• *Work problems.* Coming in late or missing work due to intoxication or hangover; being intoxicated or high while at work; being warned and/or being fired due to substance use.

• *Legal problems.* Being arrested, placed on probation, and/or incarcerated for alcohol- or drug-related offenses such as driving while intoxicated (DWI); being disorderly; possessing controlled dangerous substances (CDS); possessing with intent to distribute. Additionally, dependence on alcohol and/or drugs may lead to other illegal activities such as burglary, larceny, or prostitution, and resultant criminal charges.

• *Medical/physical problems.* Having a history of alcohol-related traumas and liver or pancreatic problems, being hospitalized for alcohol- or drug-related illnesses, or having been advised by a physician to cut down on or quit drinking or drug use; having blackouts, hangovers, or withdrawal symptoms such as nausea, shakes, convulsions, or seizures after using substances.

• *Financial problems.* Experiencing heavy debt due to substance use; not paying bills in order to have money to buy alcohol and/or drugs.

• *Intrapersonal problems.* Experiencing feelings of guilt, shame, and regret about substance use; feeling depressed, paranoic, and/or anxious as a result of using substances; using substances to cope with depression or anxiety; deteriorating cognitive functioning as a result of long-term substance use. Whenever possible, it is important to gather collateral information from outside sources about the patient's substance use and its effects on other people. Gaining a perspective on the patient's substance use from his or her spouse/partner, an employer, a probation officer, and/ or physician can be extremely helpful during assessment. Before talking to collateral sources, however, the clinician must discuss with the patient the importance of getting collateral information and obtain appropriate releases. Finally, a clinician should assess a patient's beliefs and awareness regarding the antecedents or triggers to his or her substance use, as well as the patient's expectancies about the effects the substance use will have for him or her. For example, a patient who thinks "I deserve to have a beer and relax" after a particularly long and stressful day at work may have an interpretation of personal stress and discomfort as intolerable and hold a sense of entitlement to a stress-free life. Furthermore, this thought may reflect the patient's expectation that alcohol and only alcohol will have a soothing, calming effect during times of stress. (For those readers interested in more detailed accounts of substance abuse assessment, see Donovan, 1999; McCrady, 2008; or Miller, Westerberg, & Waldron, 1995.)

Developing and Implementing Treatment Goals

Developing individualized treatment plans has been one hallmark of behavioral treatment. However, within addictions treatment, the traditional disease model has historically prescribed a generic treatment plan for all. From this traditional perspective, treatment typically includes confrontation of patient denial, education about the disease concept of addiction, and facilitation of the patient into a 12-step-oriented program such as Alcoholics Anonymous (AA) or Narcotics Anonymous (NA). The goal for all patients has been acceptance of their powerlessness to control their substance use and lifetime abstinence from alcohol and drugs.

While this approach has traditionally been the norm in the substance treatment field, behavioral treatment plans are increasingly emphasizing the importance of providing multiple use options, particularly for alcohol abusers, in order to facilitate long-term treatment gains. The possibility of moderated drinking by alcoholic patients was first reported by Davies (1962) and later suggested by Sobell and Sobell (1976), Miller and Caddy (1977), and Polich, Armor, and Braiker (1981). Since that time, there has been a consistent and growing literature that supports moderated drinking for *some* problem drinkers. For instance, in their review of multisite treatment trials, Miller, Walters, and Bennett (2001) found that 10% of alcohol-dependent patients who underwent treatment were able to sustain moderate, asymptomatic drinking for at least 1 year. However, despite this evidence, it still is clear that most alcohol-dependent individuals are not appropriate candidates for moderation-based drinking goals. A more recent trend in the field has been to adopt a harm reduction approach (Tatarsky & Marlatt, 2010) in which treatment seeks to reduce harmful consequences associated with the substance use rather than the quantity of use itself.

From the behavioral perspective, it is important that treatment goals are determined collaboratively. Regardless of the preferences of treatment providers, studies have shown that patients will ultimately decide on substance use goals that suit them. This includes alcohol-dependent patients who moderate their drinking when treated in an abstinence-based program (McCabe, 1986; Nordstrom & Berglund, 1987; Sanchez-Craig, Annis, Bornet, & MacDonald, 1984; Vaillant & Milkofsky, 1982), as well as patients who abstain from drinking even after they have been treated in a moderation-based program (Miller, Leckman, Delaney, & Tinkcom, 1992; Rychtarik, Foy, Scott, Lokey, & Prue, 1987). Also, allowing patients to self-select their own goal is an important way to increase motivation, commitment, and engagement in treatment (Marlatt, Larimar, Baer, & Quigley, 1993; Ogborne, 1987; Sobell, Toneatto, & Sobell, 1992). Goal choice has become more popular as studies have suggested that successful outcomes are more likely if the treatment goals are consistent with the patient's goal preference (Booth, Dale, & Ansari, 1984; Orford & Keddie, 1986). (For further information on goal setting, see Kadden & Skerker, 1999.)

Evaluating Treatment Progress, Preparing a Relapse Prevention Plan, and Terminating Treatment

As treatment progresses, the therapist and patient must continually evaluate the progress of the work, or, if there is a lack of progress, immediately address this issue. By regularly assessing progress, both therapist and patient can see concrete evidence of positive change and the patient's sense of self-efficacy can be strengthened. When progress is not being made, the therapist and patient can identify and discuss obstacles to reaching treatment goals and possible solutions to overcome them. It may be true that the goals of treatment are unrealistic, that the patient has become ambivalent toward them, or that the assessment of the patient's circumstances was not accurate. Additionally, these continued progress evaluations allow the therapist to provide realistic feedback regarding the normative "ups and downs" of treatment progress and combat any unhelpful expectations the patient may hold.

Ideally, termination of treatment is mutually determined. Treatment ends when goals have been reached or there is an acknowledgment that treatment has not been effective and a different approach is warranted (e.g., referral to another practitioner or to a higher level of care). In terminating treatment, the clinician should review the course of treatment and acknowledge and reinforce behavior changes. At this time, there should also be a focus on relapse prevention, including discussion of "warning signs," the differences between a "slip" and a "relapse" (Marlatt & Gordon, 1985), and plans the patient can enact if he or she falls back into old patterns. Finally, the clinician and patient should agree upon a specific signal that would indicate the patient needs to come back into treatment.

Specific Behavioral Treatment Techniques and Interventions

It should be noted that the following description of behavioral treatment techniques is relevant for both alcohol- and drug-abusing patients. Due to space constraints, I will primarily describe the use of behavioral techniques with alcohol-abusing patients. (For a detailed description of behavioral treatment with drug abuse populations, see Higgins, Sigmon, & Heil, 2008; Onken, Blaine, & Boren, 1993; and Sobell et al., 1992.)

Classical conditioning theory assumes that substance users become conditioned to certain stimuli in the environment through the repeated pairing of substances with specific settings, people, and rituals. These cues, or "triggers" (conditioned stimuli), are quite diverse and unique to each individual. Conditioning research shows that if certain conditioned stimuli have come to be associated with substance use, then these cues can be unlearned through inhibitory responses (Bouton, 2000) created through repeated pairing of the conditioned stimulus (trigger) without the conditioned response (substance use). The following section provides a summary of the most well-known treatments for substance abuse disorders following the classical conditioning paradigm.

Aversion Treatments

One of the first behavioral treatments for alcohol dependence was aversion therapy. This treatment paired an aversive experience with the stimuli ("triggers") of drinking so that the patient would develop a negative reaction to alcohol, and thus lose the urge to drink. Over the years, electrical aversion, chemical aversion (e.g., disulfiram), and covert sensitization have been used in an attempt to condition an aversive response to the sensory cues of alcohol. Since electrical and chemical aversion have shown inconsistent empirical support and are no longer considered serious treatments for alcohol disorders, the discussion here is limited to covert sensitization techniques.

Covert Sensitization

In covert sensitization, the aversive conditioning to alcohol or drugs occurs through the patient's verbal and imaginal modalities. This treatment protocol continues to follow the learning principles of counterconditioning, but is not as invasive or painful as electrical or chemical aversion treatments. In addition, medical supervision and special equipment are not needed, so the protocol can be carried out on an outpatient basis.

In covert sensitization, specific information is gathered regarding the usual antecedents or cues to the patient's alcohol and/or drug use, as well as information regarding negative or feared consequences. This information is then incorporated into the conditioning scene or script. Patients are instructed to relax and imagine as vividly as possible a typical situation in which they are about to use alcohol or drugs. In the imaginal scene, immediately after the patient has used alcohol or drugs, he or she is provided with a specific and disgusting description of the aversive consequences of the substance use. Such scenarios might include graphic descriptions of nausea, vomiting, hangovers, heart racing, the hurt or frightened look from their children, or other feared results of use. The imaginal scene may also include the suggestion that the patient will have relief from these symptoms by leaving the situation and avoiding using alcohol or drugs in the future. Such scenes are paired repeatedly until the unpleasant images become associated with alcohol and drug use, and the urge for using the substances has been extinguished.

Data on the long-term efficacy of covert sensitization has been mixed (Institute of Medicine, 1990; Lawson & Boudin, 1992; Nathan & Niaura, 1985; O'Leary & Wilson, 1987; Rimmele, Howard, & Hilfrink, 1995). Rimmele et al. (1995) noted that the most encouraging results are found in those studies that have specific sensitization procedures and have verified the presence of conditioned aversion. Although the efficacy results are mixed, there continues to be optimism about the viability of covert sensitization as an outpatient treatment option. Especially when compared to electrical and chemical aversion treatments, it has the advantages of being less intrusive and physically stressful, and can be administered by an individual clinician on an outpatient basis. It may not be useful for all patients, especially those who have difficulty with visualizations. (For more specific information about a covert sensitization treatment protocol, see Rimmele et al., 1995.)

Cue Exposure

The intent of cue exposure is to extinguish conditioned behavioral responses to internal and external triggers. Internal triggers or cues can be physiological symptoms associated with craving and withdrawal, such as increased heart rate and sweating, and negative affective states such as feelings of anxiety or depression. External triggers are more likely to be the people, places, and things the patient associates with their use. As one would expect from the classical conditioning paradigm, extinction occurs through repeated *in-vivo* and interoceptive exposures to the patient's conditioned stimuli (e.g., affective distress, somatic symptoms, sight of drug, smell of alcohol) without the patient being able to execute the conditioned response (i.e., drinking or drug use). Thus, the patient's urges and cravings for substances become less frequent and intense over time as their ability to experience internal and external triggers without using substances increases. However, it appears that exposure alone does not produce significant long-term effects (Childress, Ehrman, Rohsenow, Robbins, & O'Brien, 1992; Monti et al., 1993). Other elements that must be addressed include self-efficacy, personally relevant cues for substance use, and coping skills training. Despite these caveats, empirical support for cue exposure treatments in the areas of phobia and obsessive–compulsive disorders (Foa, Huppert, & Cahill, 2006; Foa & Kozak, 1986) and bulimia (Wilson, Rossiter, Kleinfield, & Lindholm, 1986) offer some optimism for the use of exposure treatment with substance abuse disorders. In this vein, Otto, Safren, and Pollack (2004) recently adapted a protocol for the treatment of patients with panic disorder and benzodiazepine use to create a specific treatment design using interoceptive cue exposures for problematic drug use.

In providing cue exposure treatment, patients are given a rationale about the importance of reducing craving so that they are better able to cope with high-risk triggers. Patients are also given a simple description of the classical conditioning paradigm. In order to individualize treatment, a detailed description is needed of the patient's preferred drinks and drugs of abuse as well as details about internal and external situations that precipitate their use. Treatment typically consists of six to eight sessions, provided in an inpatient or outpatient facility. Each session begins and ends with an assessment of the patient's subjective and physiological responses to the alcohol cues. Patients receive a series of brief exposures to an alcoholic beverage. Patients can also be exposed to alcohol cues after they have been induced into a negative mood state. (For those readers interested in a more detailed cue exposure protocol, see Monti, Kadden, Roshenhow, Cooney, & Abbrams, 2002.)

The literature on efficacy of cue exposure is relatively small. Uncontrolled studies have provided promising results (Institute of Medicine, 1990; Pollack et al., 2002), although one review suggests that there is little consistent evidence for the efficacy of cue exposure as currently delivered (Conklin & Tiffany, 2002).

Behavioral Self-Control Training

Behavioral self-control training (BSCT) has been one of the most widely studied treatments in the alcohol field (Institute of Medicine, 1990; Miller & Wilbourne, 2002). BSCT is a brief, educationally oriented approach in which patients can achieve either a goal of nonproblematic drinking or abstinence. BSCT can be implemented either by a therapist (therapist-directed) or by a patient in the form of a guided self-help manual (self-directed). There are several advantages to BSCT over traditional treatment with alcohol-abusing patients. One advantage is that some patients will refuse to accept an abstinence goal without first attempting to drink moderately. A second rationale is that BSCT has the potential to reach a larger population of individuals who are having problems with drinking. It has been suggested that there are many more problem drinkers than those who are diagnosably dependent on alcohol (Cahalan, 1987; Institute of Medicine, 1990). In fact, a majority of those with alcohol problems never have any treatment contact with self-help groups or professional services (Cunningham, 1999; Institute of Medicine, 1990). Thus, a treatment approach that offers a choice of goals may be more attractive for those who are not yet ready for abstinence and who might not otherwise consider treatment. Third, treatments such as BSCT that show positive results using minimal resources may be viewed more favorably by reimbursing agencies and thus require less financial strain for patients and therapists.

The active ingredients of BSCT are believed to be self-efficacy and self-control. The patient maintains the primary responsibility for making decisions throughout treatment. BSCT is brief—usually consisting of between six and twelve 90-minute sessions. Follow-up "booster" sessions are scheduled to solidify gains and to assess whether patients need additional intervention. As described by Hester (1995), BSCT is made up of the following steps: (1) setting limits on the number of drinks per day and on peak blood alcohol concentrations (BACs), (2) self-monitoring of drinking behaviors, (3) changing the rate of drinking, (4) practicing assertiveness in refusing drinks, (5) setting up a reward system for achievement of goals, (6) learning which antecedents result in excessive drinking, and (7) learning other coping skills instead of drinking. Homework, role playing, and practice are emphasized in BSCT.

Although a great deal of research has been generated on BSCT over the past 25 years, results have been mixed. Studies have considered different populations (e.g., DWI offenders; chronic, alcohol-dependent veterans; early stage problem drinkers), settings (inpatient vs. outpatient), and treatment goals (abstinence vs. moderation), and varied treatment delivery (self-directed vs. therapist-directed). Many controlled studies suggest that BSCT fares no worse than abstinence-oriented treatments in terms of drinking outcomes and that patients have shown significant improvement when compared to control groups (Walters, 2000). One study by Foy, Nunn, and Rychtarik (1984) reported that BSCT patients had worse short-term outcomes when compared to an abstinence-oriented treatment, but also pointed out that at long-term follow-up there were no significant differences between groups. Several factors likely contribute to these mixed results. Treatment packages that are defined as BSCT can vary significantly. Also, BSCT has been used with heterogeneous populations and in a multitude of settings. It may therefore be the case that certain types of patients will respond better than others to BSCT.

Overall, results of empirical studies have suggested that BSCT is generally effective for treating those with alcohol problems. However, more information is needed to identify the active ingredients of BSCT and to determine which patients are most likely to benefit. (For those readers interested in a more detailed description of BSCT, see Hester, 1995.)

Social Skills Training

Social skills training addresses not only a patient's substance use, but also other problem areas that might be associated with excessive alcohol/drug use. The rationale for providing social skills training is the belief that the initiation and maintenance of addictive disorders is often related to problems with coping. That is, addictive behavior is seen as a habitual maladaptive way of coping with stressful life events that can be alleviated in part through training in alternative approaches.

In social skills treatment, patients identify situations that might place them at risk of substance use, such as negative emotional states, social pressure, and interpersonal conflicts. Patients are taught to use behavioral strategies to cope with these situations. Common strategies might include examining and challenging thoughts about substance use, developing drink/drug refusal skills, learning problem-solving skills, planning ahead for emergencies or anticipated high-risk situations, increasing pleasant activities not associated with substance use, developing a sober support network, and training in assertiveness, relaxation, and effective communication. As with other behavioral treatments, it is important to have the patient practice these coping skills *in vivo* with the therapist and with members of their social network in order to enhance self-efficacy and broaden generalization of the skills.

Results from Project MATCH suggest that treatment utilizing social skills training was a potent intervention for alcoholics in outpatient and aftercare environments. Overall, the literature has shown strong support for social skills training in a variety of settings (Carroll, 1996; Institute of Medicine, 1990; Irvin, Bowers, Dunn, & Wang, 1999; Miller & Wilbourne, 2002; Morgenstern, Blanchard, Morgan, Labouvie, & Hayaki, 2001; Project MATCH Research Group, 1998). (For detailed protocols for social skills training, see Kadden et al., 1992, or Monti, 2002.)

Contingency Management

Environmental contingencies have an extremely powerful effect on behavior. Substance abuse treatment that uses the operant conditioning paradigm emphasizes reinforcing desirable behavior (abstinence) while punishing undesirable behavior (substance use). Many patients enter treatment as part of an implicit contingency contract, such as a spouse who comes to treatment rather than face a divorce, or a motorist who enters treatment in order to get his or her driver's license back. However, at the same time it is ironic that in spite of strong contingencies, people often continue to use substances. Nathan and Niaura (1985) explain this paradox by noting that people are unique and that what is rewarding or punishing for one individual is not necessarily rewarding or punishing for another. Additionally, the authors emphasize the need for contingencies to be mutually agreed on, carefully observed, and consistently implemented. The consistent involvement of collaterals and institutions connected with the patient is essential for an effective contingency contract, but can be difficult to obtain. The effectiveness of contingency management programs will be mixed, depending on the type of contingency being used (e.g., revocation of professional licenses, increase in methadone dosages) and the consistency with which they are applied. Nonetheless, these approaches have begun to garner significant research support, particularly when combined with cognitive-behavioral approaches (see Murphy, MacKillop, Vuchinich, & Tucker, Chapter 3, and Dallery, Meredith, & Budney, Chapter 4, this volume).

Relapse Prevention

Recently, there has been an increase in interest in combining "third-wave" emotional acceptance techniques into existing relapse prevention protocols. For instance, Witkiewitz and Bowen (2010) argue that a patient's intolerance for negative mood states such as depression is highly associated with relapse. To address this issue, they have developed a relapse prevention protocol that incorporates mindfulness and acceptance techniques to help patients take a different approach to their experience of negative affect. Thus far, mindfulness-based techniques have been incorporated with a wide array of substance-using populations, including incarcerated individuals (Bowen et al., 2006), with notable success. Therefore, it is likely that the development and incorporation of mindfulness techniques into existing behavioral treatments will continue in the future. (For more information on mindfulness-based therapy for substance use disorders, see Zgierska & Marcus, 2010.)

Specific Issues in Implementing Substance Abuse Treatment from a Behavioral Perspective

Sequencing of Technique Use

Brownell, Marlatt, Lichtenstein, and Wilson (1986) conceptualize recovery in three phases in which specific techniques are more appropriate during certain phases. For a patient seeking to make any behavioral change, the first phase of treatment is becoming motivated and committed to making a change. This area of treatment has been described in detail earlier in the section "Enhancing Motivation to Change."

The second phase of treatment, lasting 3–6 months, is focused on initiating early changes. This phase is particularly crucial as roughly two-thirds of relapses occur within the first 3 months (Hunt, Barnett, & Branch, 1971). During this phase of treatment, several tasks and techniques are most appropriate. First, there is a strong emphasis on actions that facilitate substance use reduction or abstinence. These actions include setting up external supports, such as residential treatment, medication (to curb cravings or create aversion to use), and contingencies with spouses, friends, employers, or legal authorities. During this phase, the treatment techniques should be those that assist in initial reductions. The patient and clinician should identify high-risk situations for substance use and develop specific plans to deal with these situations. Such skills include drink/drug refusal skills, managing urges and cravings, understanding "seemingly irrelevant decisions," and managing negative thoughts.

The third phase of treatment is the maintenance of behavioral changes. Most patients can make short-term changes relatively easily. However, it is much more difficult to maintain new behaviors over time. Mark Twain, an inveterate smoker, was quoted as saying, "Quitting smoking is easy . . . I've done it a thousand times." The point is that the maintenance of change is a difficult task. Clinicians can facilitate this maintenance by encouraging the patient to self-monitor, remain aware of high-risk situations, and regularly weigh the advantages and disadvantages of both sobriety and returning to substance use. This is often difficult for the patient who has gone a length of time without using substances. The patient's level of confidence is often high immediately after treatment termination, but may begin to waver as time progresses.

Another area of focus is to help the patient develop and maintain a social network that is supportive of sobriety. For many this will include members of a 12-step program such as AA or NA. Other patients who do not utilize 12-step programs may also develop support networks through their church or synagogue, family members, or other recovery-based self-help groups (e.g., Women for Sobriety, Secular Organizations for Sobriety, and S.M.A.R.T. Recovery). The crucial factors in these support groups are that they are supportive of sobriety and that group members are not substance users themselves (Beattie & Longabaugh, 1999; Gordon & Zrull, 1991; Longabaugh, Beattie, Noel, Stout, & Malloy, 1993).

How (and in What Order) Problems Are Addressed

Substance abuse patients come into treatment with a variety of concomitant problems. Stress related to unemployment, financial problems, relationship difficulties, pending legal action, or severe psychiatric symptomatology is often found in those who present for substance abuse treatment. Individuals may feel depressed, guilty, and ashamed as they recount the toll their substance use has taken on themselves and others. In addition, some patients have preexisting psychiatric conditions that become more prominent as the patient begins abstaining from alcohol and/or drugs.

If at all possible, the initial focus of treatment should be on assisting the patient to make changes in substance use. Patients can rarely make headway with other problems while they continue to use alcohol and drugs. A slogan from the 12-step programs is relevant: the patient must remember to keep "first things first." However, it may be difficult for the clinician to focus only on substance use. Some patients come into sessions each week with a crisis that is begging for immediate attention. Other times, patients insist on dealing with relationship problems, depression, or anxiety rather than their substance use. For instance, it is understandably difficult for a caring clinician not to become engaged with a patient who begins to talk painfully about the abuse/trauma that he or she has suffered.

How can a clinician remain focused on substance abuse recovery while also tending to significant issues that the patient brings into treatment? There are several strategies one can employ:

1. Initially, when briefing the patient about what to expect in treatment, make it clear that the first order of business in treatment is to address

his or her substance use. Reminding the patient of the consequences of continued use will be useful in emphasizing the importance of dealing with the substance use first.

2. The clinician can structure the session into "minisessions" where the first third of the session is reserved for non-substance-abuse concerns, while the remaining two-thirds of the session is used to focus on initiating and maintaining changes in the patient's substance use. The advantage of this strategy is that the patient has time to vocalize problems that are important to him or her. Additionally, the clinician may have access to more material that can be used in the substance-focused part of the session. However, a disadvantage of breaking up the session in this way is that the transition between these parts can become incongruous. This also necessitates that the clinician have good assertiveness skills.

3. When the clinician finds him- or herself in sessions where the treatment is constantly focusing on non-substance-use material, this should be a signal to pause and reevaluate the goals of treatment. It may be that in avoiding discussions of substance use, the patient is expressing ambivalence about changing the behavior. It may also be that there are painful or pressing issues that were not initially assessed. In such cases, it may be useful to reevaluate the patient's treatment goals and modify them accordingly.

4. Finally, when a patient's psychiatric symptoms are interfering with the tasks of substance abuse treatment, it may indicate that a referral for a psychiatric consultation is in order. Based on the evaluation, it may be that medication, concurrent psychiatric therapy, or a higher level of care is indicated.

How Denial, Resistance, and Lack of Progress Are Addressed

The concept of denial has long been the cornerstone of traditional alcohol- and drug-dependency treatment. Denial has been said to be the "cardinal and integral feature of chemical dependency and the fatal aspect of alcoholism and other drug dependencies" (Hazelden, 1975, p. 9). Likewise, a substance abuse patient's lack of "motivation" or "resistance" has often been used to explain failure to enter, comply with, and succeed in treatment. Although confrontation of denial has been viewed historically as the first step in resolving substance abuse problems, this method has increasingly fallen out of favor in behavioral treatment approaches.

From a behavioral perspective, "denial" and "resistance" are not patient *traits* (Miller & Rollnick, 2002), but rather *states* in which the patient and therapist disagree on the definition of the problem. In this state, progress in treatment will inevitably stall. Thus, rather than defining "resistance" as a patient characteristic, it is more accurate (and helpful) to define it as a problem in the therapeutic *process*. Adapting a process perspective of treatment resistance makes it easier for both therapist and patient to distance themselves from their defensive stances and to reengage in the collaborative process of resolving differences in treatment goals. It is also important for clinicians to keep in mind that a patient's motivation is likely to fluctuate over the course of treatment.

In working with patients from the behavioral perspective, there are two things to keep in mind regarding patient–clinician agreement on treatment goals. First, it is important to routinely assess the patient's commitment to his or her original treatment goals. We cannot assume that an initial decision is etched in stone. Rather, a good therapeutic relationship allows the patient the ability to bring up changes he or she wants to make in his or her treatment goals. Thus, the clinician should routinely ask how the patient is feeling about the original goal choice and whether he or she has entertained thoughts about returning to limited alcohol or drug use. Also, when progress is not forthcoming, the clinician should initiate an honest discussion of the patient's treatment goals.

How Lapses/Relapses Are Viewed and Used in Treatment

Addiction is characterized by chronic episodes of relapse that Prochaska, DiClemente, and Norcross (1992, p. 1104) describe as being "the rule rather than the exception." According to Hunt et al. (1971), approximately two-thirds of patients who complete treatment for smoking, alcohol, and heroin addiction relapse within the first 90 days. The frequency of return to drinking (although not necessarily "full-blown" relapse) has been estimated to be between 70 and 74% within the first year (Hunt et al., 1971; Miller & Hester, 1980; Miller et al., 2001). In fact, because relapse is so prevalent, Prochaska et al. (1992) modified their stages-of-change model to include relapse as a stage of change.

From a behavioral perspective, clinicians should address the potential of relapse in the early stages of treatment. The clinician should initially discuss with the patient the distinction between a "lapse" and a "relapse." Marlatt and Gordon (1985) define a *relapse* as a return to a previous state, characterized by the perception of loss of control. However, a *lapse* is viewed as an event or situation in which one can take corrective action and not lose control. The cognitive and affective reactions to the first lapse after a period of abstinence exert a significant influence over whether or not the lapse is followed by a return to the former level of use. The clinician should emphasize that a relapse is not an inevitable result of a lapse. Rather, the clinician should advise the patient that lapses, or "slips," are part of the recovery process for many individuals. If one was to occur, the patient should have an "emergency plan" ready to implement that would keep the lapse from becoming a full-blown relapse. The clinician should convey to the patient the message that a lapse can be used as a learning experience by reviewing what happened, identifying where the patient may have been caught off-guard, and reexamining the patient's decision to change.

The advantage of this open discussion of lapses and relapses is that it provides an honest appraisal of what the patient might expect. For patients who slip, all is not lost. Rather, they can use the slip as a way of learning more about themselves and their plans to stay sober.

How to Integrate Other Treatment Supports Such as Self-Help Groups and Medication

Research in the areas of social support and recovery suggests that individuals have better treatment outcomes when they are involved with social networks supportive of abstinence (Beattie & Longabaugh, 1999; Gordon & Zrull, 1991; Longabaugh et al., 1993). Thus, support groups can be a valuable adjunct to behaviorally oriented substance abuse treatment.

Twelve-step-oriented groups such as AA and NA have been a prominent part of the treatment field for many years. In addition, the availability of alternative self-help groups has broadened in recent years with the emergence of Self-Management and Recovery Training (S.M.A.R.T.) and Rational Recovery groups to offer alternatives that are more theoretically compatible with the behavioral/social learning model. (See McCrady & Delaney, 1995, for a detailed description of alternative self-help groups.)

Medication has often been a part of treatment for patients with a concurrent psychiatric disorder. In fact, there is a large overlap between psychiatric and substance use disorders. The National Epidemiological Survey on Alcohol and Related Conditions (Grant et al., 2004) found that between 14 and 28% of individuals who had a current substance use disorder also met criteria for another DSM-IV diagnosis (American Psychiatric Association, 1994). In dually diagnosed patients, severe anxiety, depression, sociopathy, or psychotic symptomology may become a significant part of treatment.

The use of psychotropic medications will be appropriate in many cases in order to effectively treat the psychiatric disorder. Because symptoms resulting from the chronic use of substances often mimic psychiatric symptoms (such as depression, anxiety, and paranoia), it is important to conduct a thorough assessment of the patient's psychiatric history and allow for sufficient periods of abstinence to determine whether the psychiatric symptoms resolve with sobriety. There will be instances in which patients have a preexisting psychiatric condition that, during recovery from substance use, may increase in severity. Referral to a psychiatrist who has experience treating patients with addictions would be ideal. Those patients who participate in 12-step recovery meetings may feel uncomfortable in taking medication, as they might believe they are not totally drug-free. However, today, most 12-step groups accept the need for some individuals to be taking medications for psychiatric conditions. In fact, Alcoholics Anonymous

World Services has published a pamphlet specifically regarding the use of medications and recovery (Alcoholics Anonymous, 1984).

It should also be mentioned that medications are being used successfully to treat substance use disorders directly. Disulfiram (Antabuse) has long been used as a treatment for alcohol dependence, and other medications (e.g., acamprosate, naltrexone, buprenorphine) are currently being used as well in addictions treatment. (See Chung, Ross, Wakhlu, & Adinoff, Chapter 11, and Carroll & Kiluk, Chapter 12, this volume, for a more detailed presentation of the role of medications in addictions treatment.)

Case Example

Background and History

Teri is a 43-year-old married white female who self-referred to outpatient treatment because she felt her drinking had recently gotten "out of control." Teri had stopped drinking a week before the initial interview and hoped she could eventually learn how to drink moderately. Teri lives with her husband, Neil, in a house they have owned for 15 years. She and Neil have been married for 20 years and have no children. Teri is a college graduate and works as a loan processor for a large mortgage company. Neil dropped out of college after 2 years and currently works as a meter reader for the local gas and electric company.

Assessment

In addition to the clinical interview, Teri completed the Inventory of Drinking Situations (IDS; Annis, 1982) and the University of Rhode Island Change Assessment Scale (URICA; DiClemente & Hughes, 1990). The IDS is a 100-item questionnaire that asks about the likelihood a patient will drink heavily in a variety of drinking situations. The URICA (available at *casaa.unm.edu/inst.html*) is a 32-item questionnaire that asks about intentions to make changes regarding a problem behavior. A patient's score can be converted to a "readiness" indicator or to a change profile that shows an individual's score on each of the stages of change. The URICA stages include precontemplation, contemplation, action, and maintenance.

Alcohol and Drug Use History

Teri stated that she first used alcohol at age 15 when she drank some of her father's vodka with friends while her parents were out of the house. During high school, Teri reported that she would drink once or twice a month, typically at social events on weekends. She did not report any excessive drinking episodes or problems due to her drinking during high school. During college, Teri drank regularly on the weekends. She reported limiting herself to two or three glasses of wine or three to four beers over the course of a drinking day. When she started to date Neil, she continued to limit her drinking to the weekends. However, the amount she drank increased to five or six beers over the course of a drinking day. Since getting married and working full time, Teri's drinking has gradually increased in quantity and frequency. For the past 2 years, she has used alcohol nearly every day. During the week, she typically has three drinks of vodka (approximately 3 ounces per drink) after work. On the weekends, Teri will usually drink a bottle of wine plus four beers over the course of the weekend. In the past 6 months, Teri stated that she found herself drinking occasionally in the morning before work and having several drinks during lunch. Teri reported that her longest period of abstinence occurred 4 months ago. Her abstinence lasted 2 weeks and she felt pleased she could stop drinking on her own.

Teri also reported a history of marijuana and cocaine use. She stated that she had experimented with cocaine "a few times" during her freshman year in college. Teri described feeling jumpy and uncomfortable when she used cocaine and felt more attracted to the effects of marijuana. Teri described her use of marijuana as "infrequent," typically once a month, and generally at large social events. When she met Neil during her sophomore year, her use of marijuana became more regular. She described studying hard and abstaining from alcohol and marijuana during the week, but then "partying" all weekend long with Neil. Since her marriage, Teri stated that she and Neil smoked marijuana three to four times per month. Most often, they got high when going to concerts or when socializing with friends. Teri reported that she occasionally would smoke marijuana at home after a particularly stressful day at work.

Initial Phase of Treatment

During these sessions, the primary focus of treatment was to develop a therapeutic relationship, conduct a functional analysis of Teri's alcohol and drug use, and enhance her commitment to make changes in her use of substances.

Developing a Therapeutic Relationship

During the initial session, I explored Teri's expectations for treatment. She reported that this was her first treatment episode for drinking and drug use. She stated that she had several friends (one her mail carrier) whom she knew were recovering from addictions. She had attended an AA meeting with one of her friends but felt her drinking "wasn't that bad." As I discussed the expectations for our treatment, Teri seemed surprised. She feared I would tell her she had to stop drinking and dictate how to get and stay sober. I described how we would work together to understand her drinking and marijuana use from a variety of perspectives. We would talk also about possible treatment goals, but the ultimate decision about drinking and drug use would be up to her.

Functional Analysis

Over the first four sessions, using both the assessment questionnaires and information from our treatment sessions, Teri reported that the following situations were associated with heavier alcohol and marijuana use: (1) negative emotional states such as anxiety, depression, and anger; (2) pleasant times with others in social situations; and (3) free time spent with Neil. Table 6.1 shows three of Teri's self-monitoring exercises, which detail the functional analysis for high-risk situations during the initial phase of treatment.

Commitment and Motivation to Change

In listening to Teri's perceptions of her drinking and noting her responses on the URICA, I concluded that she was in the action stage of abstaining from marijuana and alcohol. She acknowledged that her alcohol and drug

TABLE 6.1. Examples of Teri's Functional Analysis Worksheets

Thoughts/feelings	Response	Positive consequence	Negative consequence
Trigger: End of work week			
Restless and bored. "A drink will help calm me down."	Started house projects. Read in a bubble bath.	Satisfied with accomplishments. Felt proud of self.	None
Trigger: Dinner with Neil and father-in-law			
Tense. "I want to loosen up and have fun." "A drink will help me socialize."	Drank two "Virgin Marys" and soda with dinner	Felt more awake. Felt "with it." Proud of myself. Neil was very happy.	Felt like I didn't belong. Felt like an outcast.
Trigger: Funeral			
Sad and helpless. "This is a heavy experience." "A drink will help me be less upset."	Drank two (3 oz.) glasses of vodka after the funeral.	Brief relief.	Felt more sad and helpless. Disappointed in self for "slipping."

use were problems, was committed to abstaining during treatment, and was faithful in completing practice assignments between sessions. However, there were times when her ambivalence toward abstinence from alcohol became evident, especially when considering the long term. During this time, Teri and I worked together to complete a decisional balance worksheet using a modified version of the Carlson model (Carlson, 1991). Table 6.2 shows Teri's decisional balance worksheet.

As noted in Table 6.2, Teri listed a number of drawbacks of continuing to drink. She was most concerned about the emotional consequences, such as feeling "out of control" when she drank. Additionally Teri was concerned about the strain on her marriage with Neil, her difficulty concentrating at

TABLE 6.2. Teri's Decisional Balance Worksheet

Disadvantages of using alcohol/drugs	Advantage of using alcohol/drugs	Achieving the same benefits without using alcohol/drugs
1. Emotional consequences: feeling guilty, depressed, and angry. 2. Failed obligations at home (laundry, care for the dog, bills). 3. Physical problems such as "fuzzy" thinking the next day. 4. Strained relationship with Neil. 5. Feeling "out of control."	1. Feels relaxed in social situations. 2. Escapes feelings such as anger, anxiety, boredom, and grief. 3. Helps to fall asleep. 4. Provides a break from responsibilities. 5. Feels "normal."	1. Think through situations where she has drank in the past. Link alcohol use to more stress in the long term. 2. Develop alternative activities to cope with negative feelings, such as reading, walking the dog, and talking with friends. 3. Relaxation exercises and meditation. 4. Use alternative activities (noted above) to take a break. Work toward more balance and guilt-free leisure time.

Advantages of abstinence	Drawbacks of abstinence	Coping with the difficulties of abstinence and early recovery
1. Feeling proud and having a sense of accomplishment. 2. Feeling better physically. 3. Losing weight. 4. Getting more accomplished at work and home. 5. Getting more involved with family and friends.	1. Belief that "I'm not normal." 2. Requires a lot of time and energy to recover. 3. Seeing Neil might have a problem with alcohol. 4. Uncomfortable to experience painful feelings like anger, grief, and frustration while sober.	1. Talk with others in recovery and challenge this belief. 2. Balance lifestyle with self-care activities. 3. Talk to Neil about her concerns and disengage from shared activities where he drinks heavily. 4. Examine thoughts that contribute to negative feelings. Talk to others about her feelings and utilize alternative coping strategies.

work, and her failure to accomplish tasks around the house. In discussing the advantages of drinking, Teri was quick to point out that she felt more comfortable in social situations when drinking. She also noted that drinking helped her escape uncomfortable feelings such as anger, tension, and grief, and helped her fall asleep after a stressful day. Finally, Teri noted that drinking made her feel "normal" when she was with her friends, and she didn't want to have to explain to them why she had quit.

Table 6.2 also shows Teri's list of advantages and disadvantages of sobriety. Teri had been sober for about 5 weeks and noted she felt better physically, had lost some weight, was accomplishing more at home and work, and felt her relationship with Neil had improved. Teri was able to list several drawbacks of her sobriety. She acknowledged that changing her thoughts and behavior was hard work, requiring a good deal of attention and energy. For Teri, additional drawbacks of sobriety included feeling more intensely her frustration with Neil's drinking, her grief around the death of family members, and her embarrassment that she was "abnormal" by being abstinent.

Initial Behavior Change

The next phase of treatment included making initial behavioral changes to support Teri's goal of abstinence. We used information from the functional analysis, decisional balance worksheet, and IDS to focus on "high-risk" situations. Of the two primary risk situations for Teri, one involved drinking in social situations with friends and Neil, and the other was drinking in response to negative emotional states, such as depression, anxiety, and boredom. Due to space limits, I will describe the strategies developed for only one of Teri's high-risk situations: social pressure to drink.

Teri described a social life that was active and highly involved with alcohol use. Teri and Neil had a regular restaurant they went to on Friday nights, where they would often have dinner at the bar. Additionally, at least two or three times a week Teri and Neil would socialize with friends or family where heavy drinking would be typical. There were three specific coping strategies we focused on in treatment to address these high-risk social situations: (1) drink refusal, (2) problem solving, and (3) challenging thoughts about the role of drinking. As one might expect, the discussion and development of these coping strategies were often closely related and overlapped during the treatment sessions.

Drink Refusal

Teri stated that she had only told a few of her friends about her decision to abstain from alcohol. She feared going out socially as she was unsure how people would respond to her choice. We used the example of her Friday night dinner to prepare her to have dinner but to drink a nonalcoholic beverage. We discussed a variety of options, beginning with making an intentional decision *not* to have dinner at the bar for the time being. Also, we rehearsed how Teri would respond to the server asking for her drink order. This would be somewhat challenging as Teri was a familiar face at the restaurant and servers would often assume she wanted "the usual," a bottle of imported beer. Teri agreed to decide before she entered the restaurant what nonalcoholic beverage she planned to drink. When they were seated, Teri would ask the server to bring her this beverage. Teri noted it would be more challenging for her to refuse alcoholic drinks when she and Neil were with friends. Several friends were quite heavy drinkers and Teri feared they would push her to drink if she declined. We role-played such a scenario and focused on how she could immediately and directly say "No," having an explanation prepared. Teri didn't feel comfortable telling these friends she had a drinking problem. She did, however, think it would be effective to explain that she wasn't drinking because she was trying to lose weight and was watching her diet. Teri also agreed that it would be helpful if she didn't make plans to socialize with these friends, at least for the next few months.

Problem Solving

Teri found that working through problem-solving exercises was particularly helpful in coping with social situations without drinking. As we examined specific problem areas, Teri was quite engaged in generating possible solutions and deciding on realistic applications. Teri acknowledged that one problem area was that her social network was made up mostly of heavy drinkers. We examined a variety of potential solutions. One solution was for Teri to develop new friendships with individuals who didn't drink. In the past year, Teri had attended some AA meetings but did not feel that they were helpful. I encouraged Teri to try a few more AA meetings as well as to attend a few local S.M.A.R.T. Recovery groups. Another solution we discussed was to renew old friendships with individuals who didn't drink. Eventually, Teri began to spend more time with a friend, Rebecca, who was also in recovery and regularly attending AA. In fact, Teri and Neil began to socialize more frequently with Rebecca and her husband.

Challenging Thoughts about the Role of Drinking

I encouraged Teri to use a daily monitoring form to assess urges and thoughts about drinking. This form helped us to discuss her beliefs about the role of drinking in her life. For example, she noted the following thoughts during the early part of our treatment: "I need a drink to relax" and "I deserve a drink to celebrate." I acknowledged Teri's need to relax and celebrate. However, I also asked her to identify other ways she might accomplish these goals. I challenged her belief that alcohol was the *only* way to achieve them. Through her initial period of abstinence, Teri had several experiences where she celebrated good times with friends and family without drinking. These experiences made it easier for her to challenge the old beliefs she had that linked alcohol with celebrating. Teri was quite successful at quickly finding and utilizing activities to help her relax. For example, she rediscovered her interest in reading novels and found it enjoyable to take the family dog out for long walks.

Maintenance and Termination Phase

The final stage of treatment focused on reestablishing sobriety after experiencing a slip. She had experienced the deaths of three close family members over the last 2 months of treatment. After the most recent funeral, she went home and drank 9 ounces of vodka. Teri was able to return to abstinence immediately after her lapse and we focused on how she might learn from this experience. What became apparent, particularly with her reactions to these deaths, was Teri's lack of support for her spiritual self. She began talking about how she might reconnect with her church or explore other places of worship. Teri felt she needed to address her spiritual needs in order to have a more balanced life and a stronger recovery.

During the termination phase of treatment, Teri and I discussed her progress and the specific skills she felt were most helpful. She reported regularly using the problem-solving method I had taught her with problems at home, with work, and with her parents. Teri also reported that she was consistently taking time for self-care activities and assertively communicating with Neil and colleagues at work. Finally, Teri stated she was spending a lot of time with her friend Rebecca and was socializing more with people who weren't drinkers.

Teri and I also discussed relapse warning signs and wrote out a detailed emergency plan she could follow in case she experienced another lapse. Teri identified specific relapse warning signs including (1) increases in arguments with Neil, (2) isolating herself from friends and family, and (3) reducing her self-care activities. Teri stated that if she experienced problems with sobriety, she would utilize her friend Rebecca as a support and/or reach out to me for a consultation. Toward the end of treatment Teri and I spoke more about her concern with Neil's drinking. We discussed how she could assertively communicate her concerns to him, as well as how couple treatment might be of some help.

Conclusion

Behaviorally based approaches are among the best supported models for addictions treatment (Miller & Wilbourne, 2002). The behavioral model, with its emphasis on assessment and evaluation, lends itself well to studies of effectiveness. In addition, the health care system continues to demand accountability and quality treatment, and behavioral treatments are a good match given this climate. The behavioral approach offers patients flexibility in treatment. However, in treating substance use disorders from a behavioral perspective, one of its strengths is also one of its biggest drawbacks. By individualizing treatment, it is difficult to study "treatment" because the "package" varies from individual to individual. There continues to be a need for research attention on the active elements in successful behavioral treatment (Finney, 2007; Litt, Kadden, Kabela-Cormier, & Petry, 2008; Morgenstern & Longabaugh, 2000). There also is a need for translation, dissemination, and training of these empirically supported behavioral approaches to frontline substance abuse counselors. Indeed, despite the existing support for behaviorally based treatment approaches, many treatment programs continue to operate according to a 12-step orientation that stresses the disease model of addiction and abstinence as the singular goal (Substance Abuse and Mental Health Services Administration, 1999). The future of behavioral addictions treatment is likely to include more focus on harm reduction (Marlatt et al., 1993; Tatarsky & Marlatt, 2010), augmenting existing treatments with distress-tolerance techniques, and increasing the availability of brief interventions to populations of people with less severe substance use problems.

References

Alcoholics Anonymous. (1984). *The A.A. member: Medications and other drugs.* New York: Alcoholics Anonymous World Services.

American Psychiatric Association (1994). *Diagnostic and statistical manual of mental disorders* (4th ed.). Washington, DC: Author.

Annis, H. M. (1982). *Inventory of drinking situations.* Toronto: Addiction Research Foundation of Ontario.

Beattie, M. C., & Longabaugh, R. (1999). General and alcohol-specific social support following treatment. *Addictive Behaviors, 24,* 593–606.

Booth, P. G., Dale, B., & Ansari, J. (1984). Problem drinker's goal choice and treatment outcome: A preliminary report. *Addictive Behaviors, 9,* 357–364.

Bouton, M. E. (2000). A learning theory perspective on lapse, relapse, and the maintenance of behavior change. *Health Psychology, 19,* 57–63.

Bowen, S., Witkiewitz, K., Dillworth, T. M., Chawla, N., Simpson, T. L., Ostafin, B. D., et al. (2006). Mindfulness meditation and substance use in an incarcerated population. *Psychology of Addictive Behaviors, 20,* 343–347.

Brownell, K. D., Marlatt, G. A., Lichtenstein, E., & Wilson, G. T. (1986). Understanding and preventing relapse. *American Psychologist, 41,* 765–782.

Cahalan, D. (1987). *Understanding America's drinking problem: How to combat the hazards of alcohol.* San Francisco: Jossey-Bass.

Carroll, K. M. (1996). Relapse prevention as a psychosocial treatment: A review of controlled clinical trials. *Experimental and Clinical Psychopharmacology,* *4,* 46–54.

Childress, A. R., Ehrman, R., Rohsenow, D. J., Robbins, S. J., & O'Brien, C. P. (1992). Classically conditioned factors in drug dependence. In J. H. Lowinsohn, P. Ruiz, & R. B. Millman (Eds.), *Comprehensive textbook of substance abuse* (2nd ed., pp. 56–69). New York: Williams & Wilkins.

Conklin, C. A., & Tiffany, S. T. (2002). Applying extinction research and theory to cue–exposure addiction treatments. *Addiction, 97,* 155–167.

Connors, G. J., Carroll, K. M., DiClemente, C. C., Longabaugh, R., & Donovan, D. M. (1997). The therapeutic alliance and its relationship to alcoholism treatment participation and outcome. *Journal of Consulting and Clinical Psychology, 65,* 588–598.

Crits-Cristoph, P., Temes, C. M., Woody, G., Gallop, R., Ball, S. A., Martino, S., et al. (2009). The alliance in motivational enhancement therapy and counseling as usual for substance use problems. *Journal of Consulting and Clinical Psychology, 77,* 1125–1135.

Cunningham, J. A. (1999). Resolving alcohol-related problems with and without treatment: The effects of different problem criteria. *Journal of Studies on Alcohol, 60,* 463–466.

Davies, D. L. (1962). Normal drinking by recovered alcoholics. *Quarterly Journal of Studies on Alcohol, 23,* 94–104.

DiClemente, C. C., & Hughes, S. O. (1990). Stages of change profiles in outpatient alcoholism treatment. *Journal of Substance Abuse, 2,* 217–235.

Donovan, D. M. (1999). Assessment strategies and measures in addictive behaviors. In E. E. Epstein & B. S. McCrady (Eds.), *Addictions: A comprehensive guidebook* (pp. 187–215). New York: Oxford University Press.

Finney, J. W. (2007). Treatment processes and mediators of substance use disorder treatment effects: The benefits of side road excursions. *Alcoholism: Clinical and Experimental Research, 31*(Suppl. 3), 80S–83S.

Foa, E. B., Huppert, J. D., & Cahill, S. P. (2006). Update on emotional processing theory. In B. O. Rothbaum (Ed.), *Pathological anxiety: Emotional processing in etiology and treatment* (pp.3–24). New York: Guilford Press.

Foa, E. B., & Kozak, M. S. (1986). Emotional processing of fear: Exposure to corrective information. *Psychological Bulletin, 99,* 20–35.

Foy, D. W., Nunn, B. L., & Rychtarik, R. G. (1984). Broad-spectrum behavioral treatment for chronic alcoholics: Effects of training in controlled drinking skills. *Journal of Consulting and Clinical Psychology, 52,* 218–230.

Gordon, A. J., & Zrull, M. (1991). Social networks and recovery: One year after inpatient treatment. *Journal of Substance Abuse Treatment, 8,* 143–152.

Grant, B. F., Stinson, F. S., Dawson, D. A., Chou, S. P., Dufour, M. C., Compton, W., et al. (2004). Prevalence and co-occurrence of substance use disorders and independent mood and anxiety disorders. *Archives of General Psychiatry, 61,* 807–816.

Hazelden. (1975). *Dealing with denial.* Center City, MN: Hazelden Caring Community Services.

Hester, R. K. (1995). Behavioral self-control training. In R. K. Hester & W. R. Miller (Eds.), *Handbook of alcoholism treatment approaches: Effective alternatives* (2nd ed., pp. 148–159). Needham Heights, MA: Allyn & Bacon.

Hettema, J., Steele, J., & Miller, W. R. (2005). Motivational interviewing. *Annual Reviews of Clinical Psychology, 1,* 91–111.

Higgins, S. T., Sigmon, S. C., & Heil, S. H. (2008). Drug abuse and dependence. In D. H. Barlow (Ed.), *Clinical handbook of psychological disorders: A step-by-step treatment manual* (4th ed., pp. 547–577). New York: Guilford Press.

Hunt, W. A., Barnett, L. W., & Branch, L. G. (1971). Relapse rates in addictions programs. *Journal of Clinical Psychology, 27,* 455–456.

Institute of Medicine. (1990). *Broadening the base of treatment for alcohol problems.* Washington, DC: National Academy Press.

Irvin, J. E., Bowers, C. A., Dunn, M. E., & Wang, M. C. (1999). Efficacy of relapse prevention: A meta-analytic review. *Journal of Consulting and Clinical Psychology, 67,* 563–570.

Kadden, R. M., Carroll, K., Donovan, D., Cooney, N., Monti, P., Abrams, D. et al. (1992). *Cognitive-behavioral coping skills therapy manual: A clinical research guide for therapists treating individuals with alcohol abuse and dependence.* (NIAAA Project MATCH Monograph Series, Vol. 3). Rockville, MD: National Institute on Alcohol Abuse and Alcoholism.

Kadden, R. M., & Skerker, P. M. (1999). Treatment decision making and goal setting. In E. E. Epstein & B. S. McCrady (Eds.), *Addictions: A comprehensive guidebook* (pp. 216–231). New York: Oxford University Press.

Lawson, D. M., & Boudin, H. M. (1992). Alcohol and drug abuse. In M. Hersen & A. S. Bellack (Eds.), *Handbook of clinical behavior therapy with adults* (pp. 293–318). New York: Plenum Press.

Lieberman, M. A., Yalom, I. D., & Miles, M. B. (1973). *Encounter groups: First facts.* New York: Basic Books.

Litt, M. D., Kadden, R. M., Kabela-Cormier, E., & Petry, N. M. (2008). Coping skills training and contingency management treatments for marijuana dependence: Exploring mechanisms of behavior change. *Addiction, 103,* 638–648.

Longabaugh, R., Beattie, M., Noel, N., Stout, R., & Malloy, R. (1993). The effect of social investment on treatment outcome. *Journal of Studies on Alcohol, 54,* 465–478.

Lundahl, B., & Burke, B. L. (2009). The effectiveness and applicability of motivational interviewing: A practice-friendly review of four meta-analyses. *Journal of Clinical Psychology, 65*(11), 1232–1245.

MacDonough, T. S. (1976). Evaluation of the effectiveness of intensive confrontation in changing the behavior of alcohol and drug abusers. *Behavior Therapy, 7,* 408–409.

Marlatt, G. A., & Gordon, J. R. (Eds.). (1985). *Relapse prevention: Maintenance strategies in the treatment of addictive behaviors.* New York: Guilford Press.

Marlatt, G. A., Larimar, M. E., Baer, J. S., & Quigley, L. A. (1993). Harm reduction for alcohol problems: Moving beyond the controlled drinking controversy. *Behavior Therapy, 24,* 461–504.

McCabe, R. J. R. (1986). Alcohol-dependent individuals sixteen years on. *Alcohol and Alcoholism, 21,* 165–171.

McCrady, B. S. (2008). Alcohol use disorders. In D. H. Barlow (Ed.), *Clinical handbook of psychological disorders: A step-by-step treatment manual* (4th ed., pp. 492–547). New York: Guilford Press.

McCrady, B. S., & Delaney, S. I. (1995). Self-help groups. In R. K. Hester & W. R.

Miller (Eds.), *Handbook of alcoholism treatment approaches: Effective alternatives* (2nd ed., pp. 160–175). Needham Heights, MA: Allyn & Bacon.

Meier, P. S., Barrowclough, C., & Donmall, M. C. (2005). The role of the therapeutic alliance in the treatment of substance misuse: A critical review of the literature. *Addiction, 100,* 304–316.

Miller, W. R., Benefield, R. G., & Tonigan, J. S. (1993). Enhancing motivation for change in problem drinking: A controlled comparison of two therapist styles. *Journal of Consulting and Clinical Psychology, 61,* 455–461.

Miller, W. R., & Caddy, G. R. (1977). Abstinence and controlled drinking in the treatment of problem drinkers. *Journal of Studies on Alcohol, 38,* 896–1003.

Miller, W. R., & Hester, R. K. (1980). Treating the problem drinker: Modern approaches. In W. R. Miller (Ed.), *The addictive behaviors: Treatment of alcoholism, drug abuse, smoking and obesity* (pp. 11–141). Elmsford, NY: Pergamon Press.

Miller, W. R., Leckman, A. L., Delaney, H. D., & Tinkcom, M. (1992). Long-term follow-up of behavioral self-control training. *Journal of Studies on Alcohol, 53,* 249–261.

Miller, W. R., & Rollnick, S. (2002). *Motivational interviewing: Preparing people for change* (2nd ed.). New York: Guilford Press.

Miller, W. R., Walters, S. T., & Bennett, M. E. (2001). How effective is alcohol treatment in the United States? *Journal of Studies on Alcohol, 62,* 211–220.

Miller, W. R., Westerberg, V. S., & Waldron, H. B. (1995). Evaluating alcohol problems in adults and adolescents. In R. K. Hester & W. R. Miller (Eds.), *Handbook of alcoholism treatment approaches: Effective alternatives* (2nd ed., pp. 61–88). Needham Heights, MA: Allyn & Bacon.

Miller, W. R., & Wilbourne, P. L. (2002). Mesa Grande: A methodological analysis of clinical trials of treatments for alcohol use disorders. *Addiction, 97,* 265–277.

Miller, W. R., Zweben, A., DiClemente, C. C., & Rychtarik, R. G. (1992). *Motivational enhancement therapy manual: A clinical research guide for therapists treating individuals with alcohol abuse and dependence.* (NIAAA Project MATCH Monograph Series, Vol. 2). Rockville, MD: National Institute on Alcohol Abuse and Alcoholism.

Monti, P. M., Kadden, R. M., Roshenow, D. J., Cooney, N. L., & Abrams, D. B. (2002). *Treating alcohol dependence: A coping skills training guide* (2nd ed.). New York: Guilford Press.

Monti, P. M., Rohsenow, D. J., Rubonis, A. V., Niaura, R. S., Sirota, A. D., Colby, S. M., et al. (1993). Cue exposure with coping skills treatment for male alcoholics: A preliminary investigation. *Journal of Consulting and Clinical Psychology, 61,* 1011–1019.

Morgenstern, J., Blanchard, K., Morgan, T. J., Labouvie, E., & Hayaki, J. (2001). Testing the effectiveness of cognitive behavioral treatment for substance abuse in a community setting: Within treatment outcomes. *Journal of Consulting and Clinical Psychology, 69,* 1007–1017.

Morgenstern, J., & Longabaugh, R. (2000). Cognitive-behavioral treatment for alcohol dependence: A review of evidence for its hypothesized mechanisms of action. *Addiction, 95,* 1475–1490.

Nathan, P. E., & Niaura, R. S. (1985). Behavioral assessment and treatment of alcoholism. In J. H. Mendelson & N. K. Mello (Eds.), *The diagnosis and treatment of alcoholism* (pp. 391–45). New York: McGraw-Hill.

Nordstrom, G., & Berglund, M. (1987). A prospective study of successful long-term adjustment in alcoholic dependence: Social drinking versus abstinence. *Journal of Studies on Alcohol, 48,* 95–103.

Ogborne, A. C. (1987). A note on the characteristics of alcohol abusers with controlled drinking aspirations. *Drug and Alcohol Dependence, 19,* 159–164.

O'Leary, K. D., & Wilson, G. T. (1987). Alcoholism and cigarette smoking. In K. D. O'Leary & G. T. Wilson (Eds.), *Behavior therapy: Application and outcome* (pp. 293–319). Englewood Cliffs, NJ: Prentice-Hall.

Onken, L. S., Blaine, J. D., & Boren, J. J. (Eds.). (1993). *Behavioral treatments for drug abuse and dependence* (NIDA Research Monograph Series No. 137). Rockville, MD: National Institute of Drug Abuse.

Orford, J., & Keddie, A. (1986). Abstinence or controlled drinking in clinical practice: A test of the dependence and persuasion hypothesis. *British Journal of Addictions, 81,* 495–504.

Otto, M. W., Safren, S. A., & Pollack, M. H. (2004). Internal cue exposure and the treatment of substance use disorders: Lessons from the treatment of panic disorder. *Anxiety Disorders, 18,* 69–87.

Polich, J. M., Armor, D. J., & Braiker, H. B. (1981). *The course of alcoholism: Four years after treatment* (National Institute on Alcohol Abuse and Alcoholism). Santa Monica, CA: Rand Corporation.

Pollack, M. H., Penava, S. A., Bolton, E., Worthington, J. J., Allen, G. L., Farach, F. J., et al. (2002). A novel cognitive-behavioral approach for treatment-resistant drug dependence. *Journal of Substance Abuse Treatment, 23,* 335–342.

Prochaska, J. O., DiClemente, C. C., & Norcross, J. C. (1992). In search of how people change: Applications to addictive behaviors. *American Psychologist, 47,* 1102–1114.

Project MATCH Research Group. (1998). Matching alcoholism treatments to client heterogeneity: Project MATCH three-year drinking outcomes. *Alcoholism: Clinical and Experimental Research, 22,* 1300–1311.

Rimmele, C. T., Howard, M. O., & Hilfrink, M. L. (1995). Aversion therapies. In R. K. Hester & W. R. Miller (Eds.), *Handbook of alcoholism treatment approaches: Effective alternatives* (2nd ed., pp. 134–147). Needham Heights, MA: Allyn & Bacon.

Rogers, C. R. (1957). The necessary and sufficient conditions for therapeutic personality change. *Journal of Consulting Psychology, 21,* 95–103.

Rychtarik, R. G., Foy, D. W., Scott, T., Lokey, L., & Prue, D. M. (1987). Five-six-year follow-up of broad-spectrum behavioral treatment for alcoholism: Effects of training controlled drinking skills. *Journal of Consulting and Clinical Psychology, 55,* 106–108.

Sanchez-Craig, M., Annis, H. M., Bornet, A. R., & MacDonald, K. R. (1984). Random assignment to abstinent and controlled drinking: Evaluation of a cognitive-behavioral program for problem drinkers. *Journal of Consulting and Clinical Psychology, 52,* 390–403.

Sobell, M. B., & Sobell, L. C. (1976). Second-year treatment outcome of alcoholics treated by individualized behavior therapy: Results. *Behavior, Research and Therapy, 14,* 195–215.

Sobell, L. C., Toneatto, A., & Sobell, M. B. (1992). Behavior therapy. In R. B. Millman & J. G. Langrod (Eds.), *Substance abuse: A comprehensive textbook* (pp. 479–505). Baltimore: Williams & Wilkins.

Substance Abuse and Mental Health Services Administration Office of Applied Sciences. (1997). *Uniform facility data set: Data on substance abuse treatment facilities.* Washington, DC: U.S. Government Printing Office.

Tatarsky, A. & Marlatt, G. A. (2010). State of the art in harm reduction psychotherapy: An emerging treatment for substance misuse. *Journal of Clinical Psychology: In Session, 66,* 117–122.

Vaillant, G. E., & Milkofsky, E. S. (1982). Natural history of male alcoholism: IV. Paths to recovery. *Archives of General Psychiatry, 39,* 127–133.

Valle, S. K. (1981). Interpersonal functioning of alcoholism counselors and treatment outcome. *Journal of Studies on Alcohol, 42,* 783–790.

Walters, G. D. (2000). Behavioral self-control training for problem drinkers: A meta-analysis of randomized control studies. *Behavior Therapy, 31,* 135–149.

Wilson, G. T., Rossiter, E., Kleinfield, E., & Lindholm, L. (1986). Cognitive-behavioral treatment of bulimia nervosa: A controlled evaluation. *Behaviour Research and Therapy, 24,* 277–288.

Witkiewitz, K., & Bowen, S. (2010). Depression, craving, and substance use following a randomized trial of mindfulness-based relapse prevention. *Journal of Consulting and Clinical Psychology, 78,* 362–374.

Zgierska, A., & Marcus, M. T. (2010). Mindfulness-based therapies for substance use disorders: Part 2. *Substance Abuse, 31,* 77–78.

Chapter 7

Theory of 12-Step-Oriented Treatment

John Wallace

D espite considerable variability among 12-step-oriented treatment programs, it is possible to discern some common characteristics. This chapter focuses on these common characteristics and the fundamental principles of 12-step-oriented treatment. In addition, the chapter presents evidence for the effectiveness of 12-step-oriented treatment and explores possible reasons for its effectiveness.

Concept of Addiction

The 12-step approach to the origins, maintenance, and modification of addictive behaviors has long constituted an informal bio–psycho–social–spiritual model of addiction (Wallace, 1989a). Although 12-step talk uses layman's terms and not technical psychology language, it is a rich language full of references to the physical, psychological, social, and spiritual aspects of human beings.

From its inception, Alcoholics Anonymous (AA; Alcoholics Anonymous, 1976) seemed to offer at least a two-dimensional concept of addiction. William Silkworth (1937) in the classic work *Alcoholics Anonymous* pointed to biological and psychological factors in alcoholism. For Silkworth, alcoholism was the result of an allergy to alcohol (physical) coupled with an obsession with the substance (psychological). Silkworth's allergy

hypothesis has never been shown to be correct, but it is historically important since it was an early attempt to identify a possible biological factor
in alcoholism, in addition to psychological factors. Likewise, Bill Wilson
(1953), the founder of AA, spoke of alcoholism as an "illness" but wrote
extensively on the psychodynamic aspects of drinking problems. In effect,
both history and modern thinking reveal implicit and explicit concerns
with multidimensional models of addiction.

Disease Models

In what sense are alcoholism and other drug addictions diseases? Perhaps
the simplest answer involves the many biomedical consequences of drinking and drug use; alcoholics and addicts are often seriously ill people as a
direct result of excessive drug consumption. Whether or not one believes
in biological etiological factors is simply irrelevant in many practical treatment contexts. Dangerous withdrawal symptoms, overdoses, cardiac conditions, liver and pancreatic disease, hypertension, and so forth must be
treated despite one's beliefs about the origins of addictive problems. This
first and probably least controversial of the disease models can be termed
the "medical consequences model."

A more complicated disease model can be termed the "bio–psycho–
social–spiritual consequences/maintenance model." This disease model is
much richer than the narrow medical consequences model, since biological,
psychological, social, and spiritual factors are at issue rather than medical problems. Furthermore, rather than focusing on the complex question
of etiology, this model permits both theorists and clinicians to attend to
the critical factors involved in changing addictive behaviors by addressing
the multiple factors that maintain these behaviors. This model asserts that
over time excessive alcohol and other drug use leads to profound biological, psychological, social, and spiritual negative consequences. The distress
associated with these consequences leads to further excessive drinking and/
or drug use, which, in turn, leads to more consequences and more distress.
Hence, a vicious cycle is established that maintains excessive drug and alcohol use. Each of the dimensions of the bio–psycho–social–spiritual model is
discussed separately in the following sections.

The Biological Dimension

The brain is an electrochemical information-processing system. Important neuromodulators, neurotransmitters, and neurohormones have been
identified, and the processes involved in presynaptic and postsynaptic neurotransmission of information have been studied extensively. In effect, the

brain is a sea of chemicals. Alcohol and other drugs enter this chemical environment of the brain and produce profound changes. These changes in the chemistry of the brain are associated with important positive and negative physical, cognitive, affective, and behavioral changes. It is most probable that the reinforcement values of various drugs lies in their capacities to effect acute changes in brain chemistry. For example, cocaine initially produces positive feelings of alertness, euphoria, and arousal because of its impact on synapses associated with dopamine, serotonin, and noradrenaline. But whereas the initial effects of cocaine enhance neurotransmission, the drug's longer term effect is to disrupt such neurotransmission (Dackis & Gold, 1985). As the levels of dopamine and other neurotransmitters fall as a result of continued cocaine use, this results in negative changes in mood, affect, cognition and behavior.

Despite these negative outcomes, the cocaine addict remains obsessed with the chemical in seeming defiance of all that is reasonable and rational. The paradox, however, is explained when we realize that the addict is caught in a vicious cycle: positive reinforcement occurs with initial drug use, which leads to abnormal changes in brain chemistry with chronic use, which, in turn, leads to negative mood, affect, and cognitive states. These negative psychological states motivate further drug-seeking behavior to attain the positive psychological states associated with initial use. Hence, the addict seeks relief from distress through use of the drug only to find him- or herself in even greater distress, which again can be temporarily alleviated through use. It is beyond the scope of this chapter to discuss the many recent studies of the neurobiology of addictions. However, the reader can find informative discussions in the following sources: the neurobiology of reward and stress in alcohol dependence (Gilpin & Koob, 2008); appetite regulatory peptides (Hillemacher et al., 2007); homocysteine levels and seizures (Bleich et al., 2004); drug-related genetic changes in the nucleus acumbens (Albertson, Schmidt, Kapatos, & Bannon, 2004; Albertson, Schmidt, Kapatos, & Bannon, 2006); the neurobiology of craving and relapse (Weiss, 2005). Comprehensive summaries of research and other matters can be found in *Neurobiology of Addiction* (Koob & Le Moal, 2005) and also in the National Institute on Alcohol Abuse and Alcoholism's (2004) *Alcohol Alert No. 61* which reviews the genetic basis of alcoholism.

The Psychological Dimension

Chronic use of psychoactive substances may produce profound changes in brain chemistry and these changes, in turn, may significantly alter mood and affect. Chronic consumption of large quantities of alcohol may, for example, lead to depression and anxiety. Patients admitted to alcoholism treatment facilities routinely show depressive and anxiety symptoms upon admission. By the third to fourth week of treatment, however, these symptoms disappear in the great majority of patients (Brown, Irwin, & Schuckit, 1991; Brown & Schuckit, 1988).

Although the often noted low self-esteem of some alcoholics and addicts may have preceded their addiction, it is also possible that negative self-esteem is an outcome of shame and embarrassment associated with drunken public comportment, arrests for drunken driving, relationship damage, or other personal consequences. Negative psychological consequences of alcoholism and drug addiction can include resentments toward others, denial and resistance to feedback, excessive self-pity and sensitivity, lack of self-confidence, low frustration tolerance, impaired ability to delay gratification, impulsiveness, and irrational fears. Of course, not all alcoholics and addicts have every one of these psychological issues, but they do occur with such frequency in addicted populations that clinicians should expect them and plan therapeutic activities to address them. The important point, however, is not that alcoholics and addicts show a universal set of negative psychological consequences of chemical use. Rather, negative consequences may enter into negative cycles that paradoxically maintain the patterns of heavy psychoactive substance use that gave rise to them. The stress associated with these psychological problems can lead to further drug-seeking behavior and consumption, which in turn leads to intensification of personal difficulties.

The Social Dimension

Alcoholics and other drug addicts must contend with mounting social problems as well as the intense discomfort and stress associated with the physical and psychological outcomes discussed above. The marriages of addicted people are often filled with frustration and anger turning into smoldering resentments, fear, and pervasive feelings of hopelessness and helplessness. In the face of this emotional stress, alcoholics and other addicts often feel that they have no other choice but to seek relief by continuing to use the substances that led to their marital problems in the first place. As a further consequence of their drinking and drug use, addicted persons do not develop skills for addressing relationship problems. In effect, their strategy of dealing with the pain of relationship problems is to drink or use drugs. Moreover, the partners of addicted people have often learned maladaptive strategies for coping with relationship problems. For instance, they may react to their addicted partners' intoxicated behaviors in ways that make matters worse. The wives, husbands, and lovers of addicted people are not the only intimates caught up in the stress and turmoil of addiction. The children of alcoholics and addicts also react to the stress, pain, conflict, and emotional upheaval of the alcoholic or drug-addicted marriage. These children may show emotional and social problems of their own including excessive fears, learning difficulties, delinquent behavior, or drug and alcohol problems of their own (Wallace, 1987). These problems in parenting and childrearing bring further stress and disorder into a family situation that is already overwhelmed. As a result, family treatment is frequently a part of primary treatment of addiction and occupies a central role in most modern treatment programs that utilize AA concepts.

Marital and family difficulties are not the only negative consequences of drinking and drug use that maintain addictive behavior. Alcoholics and addicts show a host of other difficulties that may involve one or more of the following: employment and career troubles, legal and financial problems, disturbed friendships, legal difficulties, community rejection and other forms of social stigma, and a decline in social status. The stress associated with these outcomes usually results in further deterioration of the alcoholic and addict and further drinking and drug use. Obviously, without vigorous intervention and treatment services, this downward spiral is not likely to be reversed.

The Spiritual Dimension

Spirituality is the fourth and final dimension in the bio–psycho–social–spiritual consequences/maintenance model. For many alcoholics and addicts, the consequences of heavy drinking and drug use culminate in intense feelings of alienation, emptiness, and meaninglessness. Moral values may have been compromised in the erratic acting out of intoxicated behaviors. As addiction develops, one's conviction about personal goals, objectives, and direction becomes less certain. In a very real sense, alcoholics and addicts seem to be ships without rudders cast adrift on turbulent seas. This may explain why a popular definition of "God" in the AA fellowship is simply "good orderly direction."

Nothing fills the inner void of alcoholics and addicts as do alcohol and other drugs. Never mind that alcohol and drugs caused the suffering in the first place. Alcohol and drugs can quickly "fix" these painful states of being. The fix, of course, is always temporary and usually followed by even greater spiritual distress, but alcoholics and addicts do not care about delayed punishments. The desire for immediate relief drives addicted people to make choices contrary to their best long-term interests.

The Predisposition Disease Models

In contrast to the consequences disease models discussed above, the "predisposition disease models" assume that alcoholics and other drug-addicted people were "set up" for addiction by biological differences that preceded the onset of drinking and/or drug use. In actuality, there are several types of predisposition models. The first type could be called the "genetic determination predisposition model." In this model, environment is irrelevant in determining alcoholism and addiction. All that is required in the genetic determination model is the gene for a specific disorder. Alcoholism, for example, is thought to be the result of an alcoholism "gene," cocaine dependence is associated with a cocaine "gene," and so on. Earlier research on the genetics of addiction is illustrative of this type of thinking (Goodwin et al., 1974; Blum et al., 1990).

A second genetic predisposition model is the "genetic influence model." This model assumes that multiple biological risk factors interact with psychosocial environmental factors to determine addiction. In effect, neither genetics nor environment alone are sufficient to produce alcoholism or drug addiction. Alcoholism and drug addiction require the joint presence of *both* biological and psychosocial environmental factors (Tarter & Edwards, 1986).

A third predisposition model is a "mixed genetic determination/ influence model." In this model, different types of etiological theories are needed to explain different types of addictions. Cloninger's (1983) distinction between Type I and Type II alcoholism is an example of this approach. According to Cloninger, Type I alcoholism (late onset, environmentally influenced) is explained by a genetic influence model since both genetic and environmental influences are necessary to produce illness. Type II alcoholism (early onset, heritable), however, is thought to be determined by genetic factors operating independently of the environment. Other mixed models include the fourfold typology proposed by Lesch and Walter (1996) and utilized in research by Hillemacher and Bleich (2008), and the subtypes identified by Babor and Caetano (2006) and Hesselbrock and Hesselbrock (2006). Studies have identified several possible predisposing biological risk factors such as defects in one or more neurotransmitter or neuromodulator systems, deficiencies in enzymes involved in neurotransmission, arousal system deregulation, irregularities in cell membrane processes and structures, and differences in brain reward pathways (Wallace, 1989b).

Theoretical Implications of Disease Models for 12-Step-Oriented Treatment

Regardless of the specific disease model, the contribution of biological factors has important implications for those who work with addicted persons.

The Admission of Powerlessness over Alcohol and Other Drugs

The first step of AA asserts that an admission of one's *powerlessness* over the substance must take place before progress can be expected. The individual does not need to accept a label of "alcoholic" or "addict" or to admit to being powerless in general. All that is required is an admission that one's use of the substance is no longer under one's personal control. That is, people who cannot *consistently* control when, where, and how much they drink and use drugs and/or cannot *guarantee* their actions once they start must recognize that they are powerless over this behavior.

Twelve-step theorists differ in how they approach the issues of loss of control and powerlessness. Some persons take an all-or-none position, which seems to imply that the individual is not only powerless over alcohol or some other chemical, but powerless over all aspects of his or her life. Other persons seem to take more balanced positions, and consider powerlessness in terms of degree rather than absolutes. Impaired control and unpredictability of one's behavior once alcohol or drug use has begun are seen as critical. This more moderate position recognizes that at various stages in the person's drinking history considerable control over alcohol may have been evident, and may in fact still be present. The key, however, is that the person cannot exercise consistent control over chemical use and cannot consistently predict and control his or her behavior once chemical use has begun on any given occasion. Moreover, the reason that the individual has impaired control and cannot guarantee his or her behavior once drinking or drug use has begun is because the individual is suffering from a disease not unlike other diseases in which choice, will, and moral conviction do not make much difference in the long run. Regardless of one's view, what is important is that the person becomes willing to admit that he or she has developed a serious problem with substances. Without such an admission, it is difficult to see how progress in treatment would be possible.

Recognition, Identification, and Acceptance

Many addicted people make tactical use of a variety of defenses to prevent them from seeing even the most devastating consequences of alcohol and drug use. Denial, rationalization, minimization, and other forms of repressive defenses make it difficult for the addicted person to see his or her life clearly and to take the steps necessary for change. Many of these defenses have their roots in shame, guilt, remorse, fear, and strong motivation to continue drinking and drug use. Whatever their origins, a person must overcome these defenses and become aware of the problems that the substance has caused. The person must come to recognize the bio–psycho–social–spiritual consequences that drinking and drug use have caused in his or her life. Recognition of consequences may take some time; as treatment progresses, the person is brought to see how many of his or her problems are directly attributable to the disease of alcoholism and/or other drug addiction. In the early stages of treatment and recovery, information about the disease concept may be helpful to the patient in managing otherwise overwhelming feelings of guilt, shame, anger, and remorse that may accompany the process of uncovering defenses.

Persons in recovery are encouraged to identify with others with similar problems of alcoholism and drug dependency. Identification with others can help to reduce guilt, shame, anger, anxiety, and remorse. Moreover, it eases entry into supportive fellowships such as AA, where the many benefits of community can be made available to recovering people. These benefits often include emotional support; a sense of belonging; a means to deal with loneliness, alienation, and isolation; shared problem solving; exposure to clean-and-sober social role models; and enhanced motivation to avoid alcohol and drug use.

Finally, acceptance of some disease model is critical. It is not enough to simply know the elements of a disease model. One must fully accept its implications. Perhaps the most significant outcome of acceptance of a disease model is the decision to remain abstinent from alcohol and other drugs.

The Central Role of Abstinence

All disease models stress the central role of abstinence in recovery. Controlled chemical use is not seen as feasible. Reviews of the more important studies of controlled drinking have generally failed to substantiate previous optimistic findings (Pendery, Maltzman, & West, 1982; Rychtarik, Foy, Scott, Lokey, & Prue, 1987; Wallace, 1978, 1979, 1990, 1993). Other research has demonstrated that stable moderate drinking is a relatively rare outcome among treated alcoholics (Helzer et al., 1985) and that the most stable outcome following treatment is abstinence (Pettinati, Sugarman, DiDonato, & Maurer, 1982).

The issue of controlled drinking and controlled drug use goals for alcoholics and addicts is not a trivial one. Alcoholics who continue to drink and addicts who continue to use drugs are at sharply increased risk for many bio–psycho–social–spiritual consequences including death, disease, traumatic injury, marital problems, legal and financial difficulties, and employment problems. For instance, using data from the U.S. Census Bureau, Bullock and Reed (1992) showed that abstinent alcoholics had a mortality rate that was indistinguishable from their matched peers. Alcoholics who continued to drink, however, died at a rate 4.96 times that of controls.

From a 12-step perspective, little progress can be expected in recovery if alcoholics and addicts continue to drink and/or use unauthorized drugs. One reason for this is that the pharmacological actions of drugs such as alcohol and cocaine increase the likelihood of compulsive use. In fact, changes in brain chemistry probably serve as important internal conditioned cues for compulsive use. In addition, alcoholics and other addicts often suffer from poor impulse control, low frustration tolerance, inability to delay gratification, anger management issues, and cognitive impairments. Because alcohol and certain other drugs appear to exacerbate these difficulties, it seems most appropriate for alcoholics and addicts to avoid these chemicals. Finally, the continued use of psychoactive chemicals keeps addicted people from practicing behavioral, emotional, cognitive, interpersonal, and spiritual strategies, which results in an overall poorer outcome.

Not only do attempts to drink and use drugs keep alcoholics and addicts caught up in chemical solutions to day-to-day problems, they also separate addicted people from sober friends and 12-step fellowship programs. It is difficult to be part of an AA group if one's brain is thoroughly soaked in alcohol. Historically, there have been no enduring support groups devoted to the pursuit of moderate intoxication for alcohol-dependent persons, moderate cocaine use for cocaine addicts, moderate cigarette smoking for nicotine addicts, and so forth. Although there have been attempts to establish groups such as these, none have stood the test of time as have AA, Narcotics Anonymous, and other abstinence-oriented programs.

It is sometimes argued that controlled drinking should be the treatment goal for alcohol abusers and abstinence should be reserved for alcohol-dependent persons. At first blush, this appears to be a simple and direct solution. However, the situation is complicated by several factors. First, it is not always easy in practice to differentiate alcohol abuse from alcohol dependence. Second, the argument ignores the fact that because of genetic and social learning factors, children of alcoholics are at increased risk for alcoholism themselves. Teenage and young adult children of alcoholics who may be abusing alcohol, but who have not yet reached the stage of alcohol dependence, could be mistreated with an inappropriate controlled drinking goal. Third, alcohol problems are often progressive, moving from abuse to dependence over time. At present, there are no reliable and valid means of predicting which cases of alcohol abuse will progress to alcohol dependence and which will not.

Spirituality and the Problem of Powerlessness

Once addicted people have admitted their powerlessness over alcohol and/or other drugs, they find themselves faced with a new dilemma. If they cannot personally control their behavior, who or what will do it for them? The 12-step answer to this dilemma appears disarmingly simple, but becomes far more complicated upon further analysis. According to the second and third steps of AA, addicted people are urged to believe in and to turn their will and their lives over to a power greater than themselves. This emphasis on spirituality in 12-step fellowship programs and in 12-step treatment has proven to be a boon to some, but a stumbling block to others. Some critics have seized upon the similarities between AA and religion and as a result have rejected the AA claim that it is a spiritual program and not a religious program. This criticism on similarities, however, ignores the many differences between AA and organized religions. Similarities do not prove identities. Of course, the literature of AA and the talk of some of its members contain double messages and ambiguities that encourage misunderstanding. Holding hands at the end of an AA meeting or after a group therapy session in a 12-step-oriented treatment program and chanting the Lord's Prayer or the "Serenity Prayer" does raise some serious issues for atheists and agnostics. The same is true of a number of the 12 steps in which God is given a central role in helping AA members deal with the dilemma posed by powerlessness. If Bill Wilson and others who had written the steps had consistently used the phrase "a power greater than self" or even "a power other than self," the issue of whether or not AA and 12-step-oriented treatment constitute "religious" rather than "spiritual" programs might never have arisen. But it is difficult to say whether or not the AA program would have held the same dynamic for change that it has obviously had for so many persons if the language of the program had been cast in terms of a psychosocial change program only.

In the final analysis, AA and other 12-step-oriented treatment programs do show important differences from organized religions. The steps of AA, for example, are not requirements but rather suggestions for recovery. In fact, strictly speaking the 12 steps are descriptions (e.g., "We admitted . . . " "We came to believe"), rather than prescriptions. Although AA does have a founder in the form of Bill Wilson (and Dr. Bob to a lesser extent), AA has no central religious figure who is worshiped and adored as do Christianity, Buddhism, Hinduism, and Judaism. In religions such as Christianity, a person must profess belief in a central figure before membership is bestowed. In AA, however, the only requirement for membership is a "desire to stop drinking."

In practice, many AA members and 12-step-oriented theorists manage to deal with the issue of religiosity versus spirituality by redefinition of a power greater than self in terms other than God. How does the concept of a higher power work out in the real-world contexts of the AA fellowship program and in 12-step treatment? Many 12-step fellowship groups and 12-step-oriented treatment programs encourage people to construe the power greater than self in terms of the group. There is a certain cunning in this position because the problem is not that addicted people need to find a conventional religion but that they need to become open to outside help. In AA terms, addicted people need to "get out of the driver's seat." By giving up their will concerning alcohol and other drugs to other persons at the beginning of their recoveries, addicted people become open to advice, new beliefs, and alternative strategies for dealing with problems.

While the group as a power greater than self can serve many addicted people well in the beginning stages of recovery, it is also useful to introduce patients to other ways of construing a "God of their understanding." Some people, of course, do enter recovery programs with well-developed religious convictions. Others, however, have virtually no understanding of how to proceed in these matters or are openly hostile to anything resembling religiosity. Resistance to religion and spirituality may constitute a reasoned intellectual position or may flow from negative childhood experiences with organized religions. In either case, addicted people may benefit from consideration of alternative ways of construing religious matters. As the theologian Paul Tillich (1952) asserted, God is a person's ultimate concern in life. From this perspective, almost anything can become a god or higher power. People have made gods of money, sexuality, fame, power over others, prestige, social status, and so forth.

In the case of addicted people, alcohol and drugs often achieve this power of ultimate concerns and, as such, take precedence over all other aspects of the addict's life. Family, friendships, careers, health, and well-being often take a backseat to the addict's drive to seek out his or her drug of choice. In effect, drugs and alcohol become powers greater than self (directing forces that drive all aspects of the addict's feelings, beliefs, and behaviors). In a very real sense, the goal is not to find a higher power, but rather to switch from a destructive higher power to a constructive and beneficial one.

As sobriety lengthens, the person may consider nondeistic directing forces for his or her life in addition to the recovery group. These might include love, truth, creativity, compassion, and justice. Ordering one's life in terms of abstract principles rather than concrete religious figures is one way nonreligious persons may be able to open the door to a nondeistic spirituality.

It is unfortunate that the emphasis on a "God of one's understanding" has driven some people away from 12-step programs. No one is required to believe in a conventional "God" in properly conceived 12-step fellowship programs. If introduced carefully to the concepts of such programs, atheists and agnostics as well as religious persons can benefit greatly from 12-step treatment and fellowship programs.

Awareness, Self-Examination, and Self-Criticism

Because of the alcoholic's and addict's use of repressive defenses and general mindlessness when drinking and using drugs, 12-step theory emphasizes the importance of self-knowledge. Many 12-step fellowship and treatment programs encourage people to share a personal inventory with at least one other person as a means of recognizing personal shortcomings and strengths. In 12-step-oriented treatment programs, group therapy and individual counseling can serve the same purpose.

Twelve-step-oriented treatment also stresses awareness of emotional states, attitudes, and actions that may signal the beginning of an active relapse process. Many 12-step theorists hold that alcoholics and addicts are never completely "fixed." They would encourage individuals to think of themselves as always "in recovery" and never as "recovered." Other theorists, however, argue that addicted people, although never "cured," can essentially recover from addictive disease. Whatever the theorist's position, virtually all agree that continued self-scrutiny and self-examination is critical to avoiding relapse.

Along with continued self-scrutiny, individuals are also encouraged to engage in self-criticism. Several steps of the AA fellowship program speak directly to these matters. For instance, members are encouraged to make a list of all the people they harmed during their period of active addiction, and wherever possible to make amends except where to do so would harm them or others. Making amends has several desirable outcomes. First, making amends for past wrongdoing enables alcoholics and addicts to deal with excessive remorse and fear over past actions. Second, it often results in mending relationships that were once broken by addiction. In many cases, these mended relationships are important to the addicted person's sense of community and self-esteem. Third, making amends permits the addicted person to see his or her past behaviors more clearly and reduces the need for continued use of repressive defenses.

In a very real sense, the Buddhist concept of *mindfulness* describes the passage of addicted people from states of blind acting out, lack of insight, and poor self-knowledge to the states of heightened awareness and joyful consciousness that are considered the hallmarks of ideal recoveries. Many persons committed to spiritual growth and development utilize the tools of meditation, prayer, and other rituals to achieve such mindfulness. In AA and in some other 12-step treatment programs, these tools are encouraged along with the writing of daily journals.

Personal Responsibility, Powerlessness, and Helplessness

It is sometimes argued that encouraging people to view their addictions as diseases takes away their sense of responsibility. From this point of view, alcoholics and addicts will simply continue to drink and use drugs because they believe they cannot help themselves. Twelve-step theory neither endorses shirking of personal responsibility for one's addiction nor sees such shirking of responsibility as a necessary part of the disease models of addiction. The usual position taken on this matter by 12-step theorists is that because of genetic and other biological factors, addicted people are not responsible for having developed an addictive disease, but they become responsible for doing something about it once they know they have it. Indeed, rather than encouraging people to disclaim responsibility, 12-step theory advocates a thoroughgoing sense of responsibility, not only for addictive behaviors but for all aspects of one's conduct. In 12-step approaches, people are not permitted to "cop out" by blaming their illness or, for that matter, anything else. Part of the misunderstanding here stems from confusion of the concepts of powerlessness and helplessness. In 12-step theory, addicted people are encouraged to view themselves as powerless over their drug of choice, but they are not encouraged to perceive themselves as powerless in general. Because addicted people are powerless over a chemical does not mean they are helpless; in fact, there may be many ways that addicted people can help themselves. The addicted person may not be able to choose to stop using cocaine in the middle of a cocaine run, but he or she is certainly able to choose to attend a treatment program or a Cocaine Anonymous group when not in the middle of a run. Addicted people can choose to become actively involved in their therapy groups or in their 12-step fellowship groups. Once clean and sober, addicted people can exercise choices about all aspects of their lives including jobs, relationships, marriages, parenting, investing, and so forth. In the beginning of recovery, such choices are better made in consultation with professionals and, when appropriate, with sponsors in fellowship programs. As recovery progresses, the ideal outcome is a self-governing person who has the ability to make choices that are in his or her best interests.

Mental Illness and 12-Step Theory

It is well accepted by the majority of 12-step theorists that addicted people may suffer from additional mental illnesses that need to be diagnosed and treated accordingly. In many cases, treatment will include use of antipsychotic and/or antidepressant medications. Twelve-step theorists, however, do object to the overprescribing of anti-anxiety medications that can accompany poorly informed psychiatric treatment in early stages of recovery. As research has shown (Brown et al., 1991; Brown & Schuckit, 1988), some of the symptoms seen in the first days and weeks of primary treatment can be a result of addictive use of chemicals and do not necessarily warrant a formal psychiatric diagnosis. In fact, symptoms of depression and anxiety commonly seen in alcoholics in the beginning of treatment usually resolve without medication within 3 weeks when the person is treated in a supportive and caring environment.

Priority Setting and Time Binding

Most 12-step theorists agree that therapeutic change should be orderly and consist of clear priority-setting activities. Newcomers to AA, for example, are often advised to deal with "first things first." This phrase is usually taken to mean that in the early stages of recovery, attempts to deal with issues other than those directly involved with drinking or drug use should be delayed until a stable base of sobriety has been achieved. It is not that other issues are unimportant, but rather it is an issue of timing. In the absence of sobriety, the vast majority of chemically dependent people do not improve their problems despite attempts at solving them. As we have already noted, drinking and drug use have important impacts including negative effects on the brain and cognitive processes involved with reasoning, judgment, problem solving, and decision making. Since these cognitive deficits tend to improve as sobriety lengthens, it may make sense to delay addressing other problems for a time. Of course, it may be impossible to delay some problems. A primary affective disorder, for example, must be dealt with early in recovery. In marital/family treatment, the same concern applies to priority setting. Clinicians working from a 12-step perspective generally endorse structured family approaches with more modest initial recovery goals and objectives in the beginning of treatment.

Throughout recovery, then, the phrase "first things first" serves as a reminder that problem solving should proceed in an orderly fashion from the primary concerns of addiction to more secondary matters as treatment proceeds. In a sense, this approach encourages people to approach problems in small, manageable units rather than flying off in all directions at once. The AA slogan "Easy does it" is intended to accomplish the same goal by slowing down the tempo of problem-solving attempts. "Easy does it" also cautions the addicted person to avoid a high-intensity, emotionally charged approach in which all problems must be solved immediately. Because problems in the real world often require a considerable amount of time and effort to solve, problem-solving styles characterized by impulsive actions and inability to delay gratification are not optimal for addicted people.

Perhaps one of the more ingenious ideas to come out of 12-step theory is the simple but important concept of "time binding." Newcomers to AA and 12-step-oriented treatment programs are urged to take life "24 hours at a time." This is because alcoholics and addicts may have difficulty maintaining a here-and-now perspective. Many chemically dependent persons make themselves miserable by living in the past or projecting into the future. On the one hand, an obsession with the past can keep alcoholics stuck in the painful stuff of regret, guilt, and resentments. On the other hand, a preoccupation with the future stirs anxiety, fear and dread over events that may or may not take place. By placing one's consciousness in the reality of each day as it unfolds, addicted people can learn to avoid the painful emotional triggers that often lead to relapse.

In effect, addicted people need to learn how to learn from their histories and not wallow in events they can no longer do anything about. Furthermore, they need to learn how to plan for the future without projecting themselves into a future that may or not unfold. In both cases, they need to live in the reality of the here-and-now.

Change, Acceptance, and Gratitude

The "Serenity Prayer" that is so popular in AA fellowships asks God to "grant the serenity to accept the things I cannot change, courage to change the things I can, and wisdom to know the difference." In 12-step treatment programs, both change and acceptance are viewed as important to a stable, enduring, and fulfilling recovery. In many cases, addicted people may make themselves miserable by trying to accept some situations or problems that are, in fact, not in their best interests. For instance, people may be unwilling to address difficult and destructive relationships. Recovering persons may also find themselves in difficult situations at work, such as performing demeaning, nonfulfilling, and boring jobs under the direction of impossible bosses. Unfortunately, many persons may choose relapse as a way of getting out of these difficult situations. In doing so, they allow alcohol and other drugs to make the decisions for them.

Treatment is all about change. Persons in recovery are encouraged to stay out of bars, keep away from heavy-drinking and/or drug-using friends, and to avoid relationships and situations that conflict with early recovery. Changes in decision making, problem solving, and skills for coping with emotions are priorities along with changes in beliefs and attitudes toward self and others.

In addition to change, acceptance is critical. While actively drinking and using drugs, addicted people as a rule did not learn the skills of acceptance. Disappointments were drowned in alcohol. Loss of a promotion or a job meant time to get drunk or high. Illness, death of a loved one, divorce, financial losses, or other life reversals were not accepted but were used as excuses for becoming intoxicated. Hence, 12-step theory stresses the need for recovering people to learn the skills that lead to acceptance. As the saying in AA goes, sometimes alcoholics in recovery need to learn to "sit still and hurt."

Perhaps the single most crucial attitude that addicted people can learn is "an attitude of gratitude." The pessimism and chronic dissatisfaction that seem to characterize the lives of many active alcoholics and addicts must yield to optimism, trust, and sense of fulfillment. By helping addicted people to appreciate what they have rather than complaining bitterly about what they do not have, 12-step-oriented therapists can encourage the development of cognitive structures that support decisions to remain abstinent.

Evaluation of 12-Step-Oriented Treatment

Research on 12-step-oriented treatment is complicated by a number of factors. Random assignment to treatment and nontreatment conditions, the "gold standard" of research, is not feasible in all real-world contexts. For instance, it is difficult to imagine how random assignment to treatment and nontreatment conditions could be accomplished in the private treatment system. As a consequence, research involving socially stable patients attending private system programs has lagged behind research involving socially unstable patients attending public programs. Moreover, socially unstable populations have been much more available to researchers than socially stable populations, an unfortunate situation since social stability is an important predictor of outcome (Baekeland, 1977). Since socially unstable persons typically present for treatment with many problems in addition to addiction, outcome research with socially unstable populations has led to a degree of pessimism about the effectiveness of addiction treatment in general that may be unwarranted (Miller & Hester, 1990; Peele, 1988, 1990). This writer, for example, worked in an outpatient addiction treatment program in Harlem, New York. Patients attending this program were extremely unstable socially and were characterized by lack of opportunity, discrimination, high unemployment rates, poverty, and other social disadvantages. In situations like this, it is unrealistic to expect outpatient addiction treatment alone to succeed without assistance in these other major life areas.

Fortunately, the studies involving more socially stable patients do demonstrate the effectiveness of 12-step-oriented treatment. In a study of socially stable patients attending a private treatment facility in Georgia, Cross, Morgan, Mooney, Martin, and Rafter (1990) reported on a 10-year follow-up of 200 randomly selected patients from a single inpatient facility. Treatment consisted of detoxification followed by daily meetings on the 12 steps of AA, counseling and didactic sessions, and family involvement. Aftercare was emphasized and all patients were given an AA contact in the local community. A 3-year follow-up showed that 60% were in remission and 84% were in a stable psychosocial condition.

Moos, Finney, Ouimette, and Suchinsky (1999) conducted a major treatment outcome study involving 3,000 Veterans Administration (VA) patients. The study was one of very few that involved a direct comparison of 12-step-oriented treatment and cognitive-behavioral therapy (CBT). The results demonstrated superior outcomes for 12-step-oriented treated patients over patients treated with cognitive behavioral therapy (CBT). At 1 year, 45% of 12-step-program patients were abstinent as compared to 36% for CBT patients. Additionally, Humphreys and Moos (2007) showed that 12-step-oriented treatment was more cost-effective than CBT. Finally, Stinchfield and Owen (1998) studied 1,083 patients who had attended treatment at the Hazelden 12-step-oriented treatment program. At a 12-month follow-up, 53% of the subjects reported complete abstinence from alcohol and other drugs. Although some follow-up bias was noted by the researchers, the results still suggested a lower bound estimate of approximately 45% remission. These results were consistent with an earlier study of Hazelden patients conducted by Laundergan (1982) and with results obtained by Harrison, Hoffman, and Streed (1991) on a more general population.

Several neglected studies by Smith (1985, 1986) of women ($N = 78$) and men ($N = 274$) showed very positive outcomes for 12-step-oriented treatment patients versus nontreatment patients who received detoxification. Of the treated women, 79% reported abstinence throughout the 15-month follow-up interval, while only 3% of the untreated women reported abstinence. Moreover, treated women had significantly more weeks of employment than did untreated women. Similar findings were reported for the treated men, who showed a 62% abstinence rate at 15-month follow-up while the untreated men had only a 5% abstinence rate. With regard to employment, treatment group men reported 51 weeks of employment in the follow-up period compared to 33 weeks of employment in the comparison group.

The relatively recent Project MATCH Research Group (1997) study involved comparisons among CBT, motivational enhancement therapy (MET), and 12-step facilitation (TSF). TSF consisted of individual counseling from a professional counselor intended to orient the person to the first three steps of AA and to encourage him or her to join a 12-step fellowship. As such, the TSF condition studied in Project MATCH lacked the important social processes and dynamics that characterize real-world 12-step engagement. Despite this incomplete version of 12-step-oriented treatment, TSF showed higher abstinence rates at all follow-up intervals. After 3 years, abstinence rates were 36%, 24%, and 27% for TSF, CBT, and MET, respectively.

McLellan et al. (1993) studied treatment outcomes for 198 alcohol-and/or cocaine-dependent men referred from employee assistance programs. The men were treated in two inpatient and two outpatient treatment programs that were 12-step-oriented programs. At 6-month follow-up, a 94% follow-up rate was achieved. For alcohol, there was a 59% abstinence rate, while for drugs there was a 78% abstinence rate.

McLellan et al's. (1993) results for an employed population at 6 months were similar to results obtained by Wallace, McNeill, Gilfillan, Maclean, and Fanella (1988) in a study of 181 socially stable patients treated in a private facility. Wallace et al. (1988) found that 66% of alcohol-only dependent patients and 52% of patients dependent on both drugs and alcohol were abstinent throughout an entire 6-month follow-up period. The follow-up rate was 94% and collateral verification of abstinence was obtained.

Slaymaker and Owen (2006) showed similar results to both McLellan et al. (1993) and Wallace et al. (1988). Slaymaker and Owen studied employed men and women. These investigators pointed out that 77% of the estimated 20 million substance-abusing or substance-dependent people in the United States are gainfully employed and do not fit the stereotype of the "skid row" alcoholic. Continuous abstinence was achieved by 65% at 6-month follow-up and 51% at 12-month follow-up. While follow-up rates were 82% and 75% at 6 and 12 months, respectively, followed and nonfollowed patients did not differ on baseline Addiction Severity Index scores.

Fiorentine and Hillhouse (2000) found that clients who stayed in treatment and attended AA meetings weekly had significantly higher rates of abstinence than those who did not. Moreover, the longer patients stayed in treatment, the more likely they were to contact their 12-step program sponsor at least once time per week. Fiorentine and Hillhouse concluded that when patients attended AA as well as treatment, they experienced a "powerful advantage" over either activity alone.

Kaskutas, Subbaraman, Wilbrodt, and Zemore (2009) studied the use of a manual-guided intervention to help patients to connect with other recovering people in AA. This procedure proved to be especially helpful for those patients with prior AA experience, pstients with severe psychiatric problems, and patients who were agnostic or atheists.

An important study conducted in the Federal Republic of Germany (Feuerlein & Kufner, 1989; Kufner & Feuerlein, 1989) involved 21 different inpatient treatment facilities and data were reported on 1,410 consecutively admitted patients. Although the programs studied by Kufner and Feuerlein were not literally 12-step-oriented treatment programs, an examination of the therapeutic principles employed were entirely consistent with 12-step-oriented treatment (Wallace, 2009). Moreover, patients in all programs were encouraged to attend AA meetings in aftercare and many patients did so with very good effect. At 18-month follow-up, 84% of the original 1,410 patients were interviewed. Fifty-three percent were abstinent for the entire 18-month interval. At 48-month follow-up, 81% of the original sample were interviewed and 46% were abstinent for the entire 4-year period since discharge. Utilizing a 6-month window prior to the 48-month interview, 66% were abstinent and 4% were improved.

Relationship of 12-Step-Oriented Treatment to Other Psychological Principles

While not every alcoholic or addict is helped by 12-step treatment or fellowship programs, the evidence points to substantial effectiveness of this body of principles and practices. Why is 12-step-oriented treatment effective? The answer to this question may very well involve important psychological principles that have long been recognized to have powerful influence over behavior. Critics of 12-step fellowship programs and of 12-step-oriented treatment programs (Marlatt, 1983; Peele, 1985) have tended to base their criticisms on assumptions about 12-step ideology and not on *substantial, direct, empirical* observations of the actual behaviors of persons in 12-step program settings.

This writer's observations of the behavior of persons in both AA fellowship programs and 12-step treatment programs indicate that both kinds of programs can be readily categorized as *social learning programs*. For instance, in both AA and Narcotics Anonymous (NA), newcomers are immediately exposed to models who display successful recovery-oriented beliefs, behaviors, attitudes, and emotions. In 12-step fellowship programs, models are those persons who have achieved substantial recovery and who openly describe their recovery experiences. Sponsors are members who have been clean and sober for substantial periods and who are willing to work directly with new members in a mentoring or "coaching" style. In 12-step-oriented treatment programs, mentoring and coaching functions are provided by professional counselors, many of whom are in recovery themselves and who also model the beliefs, behaviors, attitudes, and emotions that are appropriate to successful recovery. Sponsors and counselors not only model recovery-oriented beliefs, behaviors, attitudes, and emotions, they also serve as role models who exercise control over social reinforcements. As such, they have even greater social influence potential over newcomers to 12-step fellowship and 12-step-oriented treatment.

Group participation is critical to the effectiveness of 12-step fellowship and treatment programs. Participants have access to an ocean of talk and behaviors that pertain to both success and failure at recovery. Observational learning opportunities are abundant in social situations in which participants openly share about problem-solution attempts and outcomes, strategies for dealing with difficult persons and situations, coping with emotions, factors that may have led to relapses, and so on. Reinforcement of recovery-appropriate behaviors are present in both fellowship and treatment programs. In most AA and NA groups, achievement of each year of sobriety is rewarded by cakes, cookies, greeting cards, parties, and much social recognition and praise. In some fellowship groups and treatment centers, reinforcements may take the form of different colored chips signifying achievement of different periods of sobriety.

Identification with the group is encouraged in both AA/NA fellowship programs and 12-step-oriented treatment programs. When people begin to identify with the shared values, goals, and mores of a given group, the group becomes a *reference group*. The power of reference groups to influence the beliefs, behaviors, and attitudes of members is well known in the social sciences. In AA/NA and in many treatment programs, labeling oneself as an alcoholic and/or addict provides the means through which identification with the group and its members becomes possible. The slogans of AA and NA are important tools for achieving and maintaining sobriety and also for creating group identification through use of a common language. Adages like "First things first," "Easy does it," "A day at a time," "This too shall pass" not only help members to deal with life problems, they also provide the means through which members can communicate effectively with each other and identify further with the other members.

The cognitive-behavioral tool of *reframing* is clearly evidenced in the activities of fellowship and treatment programs. Persons entering recovery are asked to consider alternative explanations for their beliefs about addictions. Many persons entering fellowship or treatment programs are bewildered by their actions while intoxicated and by addiction in general. They can't understand why this is happening to them. The disease model "reframe" helps to free them from irrational guilt, self-hate, remorse, and punitive attitudes. It also helps them to begin to see themselves in a new light. An often heard remark in AA circles is "I'm not a bad person trying to be a good person, I'm a sick person trying to get well." This strong emphasis upon education is the means through which changes in the belief systems of alcoholics and addicts are encouraged.

Finally, the use of the common, unambiguous, shared goal of abstinence is a means through which members bond to each other and to the group as a whole. In AA/NA circles and in 12-step-oriented treatment programs, a member *is* clean and sober or is *not* clean and sober. There is no in between. Sobriety is the universally shared goal toward which all members are understood to be working. Clean-and-sober persons have access to group recognition and approval while those who continue to drink and use drugs do not.

Conclusion

This chapter has examined the basic concepts and principles that make up the theory of 12-step-oriented treatment. If one strips away the ambiguities and complexities of the 12 steps, a set of actions emerge that may be strongly related to the effectiveness of 12-step programs. In effect, the 12 steps suggest that the person undertake a set of actions as follows (1) *admit* to the problem of alcoholism or chemical dependency; (2) *accept* the fact that one's efforts alone will not solve the problem; (3) *seek help* from a source outside of self; (4) *gain self-understanding* including one's strengths and shortcomings; (5) *ask for help* in dealing with these shortcomings; (6) *make amends* for past destructive behaviors when appropriate; (7) *examine one's motives and behaviors* on a daily basis and promptly admit when wrong; (8) *find serenity* through meditation and other activities that increase spirituality; (9) *help other alcoholics and addicts* to achieve sobriety; and (10) *bond* with and continue to associate with other recovering people.

References

Alcoholics Anonymous. (1976). *Alcoholics Anonymous*. New York: Alcoholics Anonymous World Services.

Albertson, D. N., Schmidt, C. J., Kapatos, G., & Bannon, M. J. (2004). Gene expression in the human nucleus acumbens of human cocaine abusers: Evidence for dysregulation of myelin. *Journal of Neurochemistry, 88*, 1211–1219.

Albertson, D. N., Schmidt, C. J., Kapatos, G., & Bannon, M. J. (2006). Distinctive profiles of gene expression in the human nucleus acumbens associated with cocaine and heroin abuse. *Neuropsychopharmacology, 31*, 2304–2312.

Babor, T. F., & Caetano, R. (2006). Subtypes of substance dependence and abuse: Implications for diagnostic classification and empirical research. *Addiction, 101*(Suppl. 1), 104–110.

Baekeland, F. (1977). Evaluation of treatment methods in chronic alcoholism. In B. Kissin & H. Begleiter (Eds.), *The biology of alcoholism: 5. Treatment and rehabilitation of the chronic alcoholic* (pp. 385–440). New York: Plenum Press.

Bleich, S., Bayerlein, K., Reulbach, U., Hillemacher, T., Bonsch, D., Mugele, B., et al. (2004). Homocysteine levels in patients classified according to Lesch's typology. *Alcohol and Alcoholism, 39*(6), 493–498.

Blum, K., Noble, E. P., Sheridan, P. J., Montgomery, A., Ritchie, T., Jagadeeswaran, P., et al. (1990). Allelic association of human dopamine D2 receptor gene in alcoholism. *Journal of the American Medical Association, 263*, 2055–2060.

Brown, S. A., Irwin, M., & Schuckit, M. A. (1991). Changes in anxiety among abstinent male alcoholics. *Journal of Studies on Alcohol, 52*, 55–61.

Brown, S.A., & Schuckit, M. A. (1988). Changes in depression among abstinent alcoholics. *Journal of Studies on Alcohol, 49*, 412–417.

Bullock, K. D., & Reed, R. J. (1992). Reduced mortality risk in alcoholics who achieve long-term abstinence. *Journal of the American Medical Association, 5*, 668–672.

Cloninger, C. R. (1983). Genetic and environmental factors in the development of alcoholism. *Journal of Psychiatric Treatment and Evaluation, 5*, 487–496.

Cross, G. M., Morgan, C. W., Mooney, A. L., Martin, C. A., & Rafter, J. A. (1990). Alcoholism treatment: A ten-year follow-up study. *Alcoholism: Clinical and Experimental Research, 14*, 169–173.

Dackis, C. A., & Gold, M. S. (1985). Bromocriptine as a treatment of cocaine abuse. *Lancet, 1*, 1151–1152.

Feuerlein, W., & Kufner, H. (1989). A prospective multicenter study of inpatient treatment for alcoholics: 18 and 48–month follow-up (Munich Evaluation for Alcoholism Treatment, MEAT). *European Archives of Psychiatry and Neurological Science, 239*, 144–157.

Fiorentine, R., & Hillhouse, M. P. (2000). Drug treatment and 12-step participation: The additive effects of integrated recovery activities. *Journal of Substance Abuse Treatment, 18*, 65–74.

Gilpin, N. W., & Koob, G. F. (2008). Neurobiology of alcohol dependence: Focus on motivational mechanisms. *Neuroscience, 31*(3), 185–196.

Goodwin, F. D., Schulsinger, F., Moller, N., Hermansen, L., Winokur, G., & Guze, S. (1974). Drinking problems in adopted and nonadopted sons of alcoholics. *Archives of General Psychiatry, 31*, 164–169.

Harrison, A. H., Hoffmann, N. G., & Streed, S. G. (1991). Drug and alcohol addiction treatment outcome. In N. S. Miller (Ed.), *Comprehensive handbook of drug and alcohol addiction* (pp. 1163–1197). New York: Marcel Dekker.

Helzer, J. E., Robins, L. N., Taylor, J. R., Carey, K., Miller, R. H., Combs-Orne, T., et al. (1985). The extent of long-term moderate drinking among alcoholics discharged from medical and psychiatric treatment facilities. *New England Journal of Medicine, 312*, 1678–1682.

Hesselbrock, V. M., & Hesselbrock, M. N. (2006). Are there empirically supported and clinically useful subtypes of alcohol dependence? *Addiction, 101*(Suppl. 1), 97–103.

Hillemacher, T., & Bleich, S. (2008). Neurobiology and treatment in alcoholism—Recent findings regarding Lesch's typology of alcohol dependence. *Alcohol and Alcoholism, 43*(3), 341–346.

Hillemacher, T., Kraus, T., Rauh, J., Weifs, J., Schanze, A., Frieling, H., et al. (2007). Role of appetite-regulating peptides in alcohol craving: An analysis in respect to subtypes and different consumption patterns in alcoholism. *Alcoholism: Clinical and Experimental Research, 31*(6), 950–954.

Humphreys, K., & Moos, R.H. (2007). Encouraging post-treatment self-help group involvement to reduce demand for continuing care services: Two year clinical and utilization outcomes. *Alcoholism: Clinical and Experimental Research, 31*(1), 64–68.

Kaskutas, L. A., Subbaraman, M. S., Wilbrodt, J., & Zemore, S. E. (2009). Effectiveness of making Alcoholics Anonymous easier: A group format 12-step facilitation approach. *Journal of Substance Abuse Treatment, 37*, 228–239.

Koob, G. F., & Le Moal, M. (2005). *Neurobiology of addiction.* Maryland Heights, MO: Elsevier Science.

Kufner, H., & Feuerlein, W. (1989). *Inpatient treatment for alcoholism.* Berlin: Springer-Verlag.

Laundergan, J. C. (1982). *The outcome of treatment. A comparative study of patients 25 years old and older admitted to Hazelden in 1979.* Center City, MN: Hazelden Foundation.

Lesch, O. M., & Walter, H. (1996). Subtypes of alcoholism and their role in therapy. *Alcohol and Alcoholism, 31*(Suppl. 1), 63–67.

Marlatt, G. A. (1983). The controlled drinking controversy: A commentary. *American Psychologist, 38*(10), 1098–1110.

McLellan, A. T., Grisson, G. R., Brill, P., Durell, J., Metzger, D. S., & O'Brien, C. P. (1993). Private substance abuse treatments: Are some programs more effective than others? *Journal of Substance Abuse Treatment, 10*, 243–254.

Miller, W. R., & Hester, R. K. (1986). Inpatient alcoholism treatment: Who benefits? *American Psychologist, 41*(7), 794–805.

Moos, R. H., Finney, J. W., Ouimette, P. C., & Suchinsky, R. T. (1999). A comparative evaluation of substance abuse treatment: 1. Treatment orientation, amount of care and 1–year outcomes. *Alcoholism: Clinical and Experimental Research, 23*, 529–536.

National Institute on Alcoholism and Alcohol Abuse. (2004). *Genetic basis of alcoholism* (Alcohol Alert No. 61). Rockville, MD: Author.

Peele, S. (1985, January–February). Change without pain. *American Health*, pp. 36–39.

Peele, S. (1988). Can alcoholism and other drug addiction problems be treated away or is the current treatment binge doing more harm than good? *Journal of Psychoactive Drugs, 20*, 375–383.

Peele, S. (1990). Why and by whom the American alcoholism treatment industry is under siege. *Journal of Psychoactive Drugs, 22*, 1–13.

Pendery, M. L., Maltzman, I. M., & West, L. J. (1982). Controlled drinking by alcoholics?: New findings and a reevaluation of a major affirmative study. *Science, 217*, 169–175.

Pettinati, H., Sugerman, A., DiDonato, N., & Maurer, H. (1982). The natural history of alcoholism over four years after treatment. *Journal of Studies on Alcohol, 43*, 201–215.

Project MATCH Research Group. (1997). Matching alcoholism treatments to client heterogeneity: Project MATCH post-treatment drinking outcomes. *Journal of Studies on Alcohol, 58*, 7–29.

Rychtarik, R. G., Foy, D. W., Scott, T., Lokey, L., & Prue, D. M. (1987). Five-to-six year follow-up of broad-spectrum treatment for alcoholism: Effects of training controlled drinking skills. *Journal of Consulting and Clinical Psychology, 55*, 106–108.

Silkworth, W. (1937). The doctor's opinion. In *Alcoholics Anonymous*, xxiii–xxx. New York: Alcoholics Anonymous World Services.

Slaymaker, V. J., & Owen, P. (2006). Employed men and women substance abusers: Job troubles and treatment outcomes. *Journal of Substance Abuse Treatment, 31*, 347–354.

Smith, D. I. (1985). Evaluation of a residential AA programme for women. *Alcohol and Alcoholism, 20*, 315–327.

Smith, D. I. (1986). Evaluation of a residential AA programme. *International Journal of Addiction, 21*, 33–49.

Stinchfield, R., & Owen, P. (1998). Hazelden's model of treatment and its outcome. *Addictive Behavior, 23*, 669–683.

Tarter, R. E., & Edwards, K. L. (1986). Antecedents to alcoholism: Implications for prevention and treatment. *Behavior Therapy, 17*, 346–361.

Tillich, P. (1952) *The courage to be*. New Haven, CT: Yale University Press.

Wallace, J. (1978). Alcoholism and treatment: A critical analysis. *ALFAWAP Journal, 1*(2), 1–7.

Wallace, J. (1979). Alcoholism and treatment revisited: Further criticism of the Rand Report. *World Alcohol Project, 1*, 3–18.

Wallace, J. (1987). Children of alcoholics: A population at risk. *Alcoholism Treatment Quarterly, 43*, 13–30.

Wallace, J. (1989a). Ideology, belief, and behavior: Alcoholics Anonymous as a social movement. In *Writings: The alcoholism papers of John Wallace* (pp. 335–352). Newport, RI: Edgehill.

Wallace, J. (1989b). The relevance to clinical care of recent research in neurobiology. In *Writings: The alcoholism papers of John Wallace* (pp. 185–207). Newport, RI: Edgehill.

Wallace, J. (1990). Controlled drinking, treatment effectiveness, and the disease model of addiction: A commentary on the ideological wishes of Stanton Peele. *Journal of Psychoactive Drugs, 22,* 261–280.

Wallace, J. (1993). Fascism and the eye of the beholder: A reply to J. S. Searles on the controlled intoxication issue. *Addictive Behaviors, 18,* 239–251.

Wallace, J. (2009, April). *The two cultures of chemical dependence treatment: Time for reconciliation?* Plenary address to the annual leadership conference of the National Association of Addiction Treatment Programs, Miami Beach, FL.

Wallace, J., McNeill, D., Gilfillan, D., Maclean, K., & Fanella, F. (1988). Six month treatment outcomes in socially stable alcoholics: Abstinence rates. *Journal of Substance Abuse Treatment, 5,* 247–252.

Weiss, F. (2005). Neurobiology of craving, conditioned reward and relapse. *Current Opinion in Pharmacology, 5,* 9–19.

Wilson, B. (1953). *Twelve steps and twelve traditions.* New York: Alcoholics Anonymous World Services.

Chapter 8

Facilitating 12-Step Recovery from Substance Abuse

Joseph Nowinski

Twelve-step-facilitation (TSF) is an intervention for facilitating recovery from alcohol or drug abuse or addiction. TSF can be used by practitioners who do not necessarily have extensive knowledge of or experience with 12-step fellowships such as Alcoholics Anonymous (AA) or Narcotics Anonymous (NA) but who wish to actively encourage their patients' use of such programs. Research suggests that treatment, in tandem with AA or NA attendance, is a powerful intervention. Moos and Moos (2005) reported on a longitudinal study of 362 initially untreated individuals who were surveyed at baseline, 1 year, 3 years, 8 years, and 16 years later. They found that, compared to individuals who initially participated only in treatment but later entered AA, those who entered AA and treatment simultaneously participated in AA more frequently and were more likely to achieve abstinence.

Patients need not be dependent on alcohol or drugs in order to benefit from TSF; rather, they need merely to meet the primary criterion for becoming members of AA (or NA), namely, having "a desire to stop drinking" (Alcoholics Anonymous, 1952, p. 139) and/or using drugs. All 12-step fellowships share a common goal of abstinence from alcohol or drug use, as these fellowships were founded by and exist for the benefit of those who have failed to control their use of alcohol and/or drugs (Alcoholics Anonymous, 2001, pp. 21, 24, 30–31).

Evidence-Based Treatment

TSF (Nowinski, 2006; Nowinski & Baker, 2003) has been designated as an evidence-based treatment by the National Registry of Evidence-Based Programs and Practices. TSF was one of three manual-guided treatments evaluated as part of Project MATCH, a multisite study of alcohol interventions. TSF led to significant reductions in alcohol abuse at 12 months posttreatment (Project MATCH Research Group, 1997) as well as at 3 years posttreatment (Project MATCH Research Group, 1998). Among clients with alcohol-supportive social networks (family, friends), TSF was found to be more effective at reducing drinking than cognitive-behavioral treatment (CBT) and motivational enhancement therapy (MET; Longabaugh, Wirtz, Zweben, & Stout, 1998). TSF was equally effective for "problem drinkers" and severe alcoholics, and no gender differences in outcome were found. In a randomized clinical trial comparing TSF to MET those assigned to TSF were more active in AA and had a higher percentage of days abstinent (Walitzer, Dermen, & Barrick, 2009).

TSF has also been used in research involving subjects with concurrent mental illness and substance abuse disorders. In separate studies, TSF led to significant reductions in substance use and depression symptoms (Glassner-Edwards et al., 2007), as well as drinking and posttraumatic stress disorder symptoms (Triffleman, 2000). An adaptation of TSF targeted at the dually diagnosed client (TSFDD) is provided in Nowinski (2011b).

Compatibility with Other Treatment Models

Motivational Enhancement Therapy

MET is a treatment protocol originally developed for Project MATCH (Miller, Zweben, DiClemente, & Rychtarik, 1995) that involves a combination of motivational interviewing and personalized feedback (Miller & Rollnick, 2002). MET assumes that clients will pursue change once they have decided that a personal problem exists that requires action. As a template for client–therapist interaction, MET is fully compatible with TSF. One major difference between the two is that TSF advocates for involvement in 12-step fellowships as the preferred means of achieving long-term recovery, while MET does not advocate for any fixed solution.

Cognitive-Behavioral Therapy

CBT is a treatment model based on the assumption that substance abuse is a dysfunctional means of coping. It therefore aims to teach clients more functional ways of coping with stress (Kadden et al., 1992). CBT also teaches clients how to decline invitations to drink or use drugs. Many CBT interventions overlap the kind of practical advice that is routinely offered at 12 step meetings, and which also appear in the AA publication *Living Sober* (Alcoholics Anonymous, 1975).

Overview of TSF

TSF is organized into a set of interventions that include a "core" (basic) program, an "elective" (advanced) program, and a "conjoint" program. Usually, some combination of core, elective, and conjoint topics can be used to create individualized treatment plans; however, the primary focus of this chapter will be on the TSF core program.

Interventions in the core program are most appropriate for what could be termed the "early" or initial stage of recovery from alcohol or drug dependence. Early recovery is typically marked by ambivalence as the individual struggles with admitting "powerlessness" over substance abuse and commits to following the collective wisdom of a fellowship of men and women whose shared goal is to stay clean and sober. Within the recovery culture, these two steps are referred to as "acceptance" and "surrender," respectively.

TSF was intended to be a time-limited (12- to 15-sessions) intervention. Initially developed as an individual treatment, it has been adapted for use with groups (Daley, Baker, Donovan, Hodgkins, & Perl, 2011; Maude-Griffin et al., 1998; Seraganian, Brown, Tremblay, & Annies, 1998). In either format, TSF is a highly structured intervention whose sessions follow a prescribed sequence. Each session begins with a review of the patient's *recovery week*, including any 12-step meetings attended and reactions to them, episodes of drinking or drug use versus sober days, urges to drink or use drugs, reactions to any readings completed, and any journaling that the patient has done.

The second part of each session consists of presenting *new material*, consisting of material drawn from the core, elective, or conjoint programs. Each session ends with a wrapup that includes the assigning of *recovery tasks*: readings, meetings to be attended, and other prorecovery behavioral work that the patient agrees to undertake between sessions.

The various TSF interventions are grouped as follows:

Core (Basic) Program
- Introduction and assessment
- Acceptance
- People, places, and routines
- Surrender
- Getting active

Elective (Advanced) Program

- Genograms
- Enabling
- Emotions
- Moral inventories
- Relationships

Conjoint Program

- Enabling
- Detaching

Early Recovery

As mentioned above, early recovery has two goals: *acceptance* and *surrender*. "Acceptance" refers to the process in which the individual overcomes his or her denial of having a substance abuse problem and having lost the ability to effectively and reliably control substance use. Acceptance is also marked by a realization that life has become progressively more *unmanageable* because of alcohol or drug use, and that individual willpower alone is insufficient to sustain sobriety.

Insight alone is insufficient for recovery; it must be followed by surrender. "Surrender" means a willingness to take action, and specifically to embrace the 12 steps as a guide for recovery and spiritual renewal. AA and NA are programs of action as much as they are programs of insight and personal growth. Surrender represents the individual's commitment to making whatever changes in lifestyle are necessary in order to sustain recovery. For most people, it includes frequent attendance at AA and/or NA meetings, becoming active in meetings, reading AA/NA literature, getting a sponsor, making AA/NA friends, and giving up people, places, and routines that have become associated with substance abuse. In TSF, the actions that are the hallmarks of surrender are guided to some extent by the facilitator, but they are also heavily influenced by the individuals with whom the client will form relationships in the 12-step fellowships. One important relationship in early recovery is the relationship between the client and his or her sponsor.

Involvement in 12-step fellowships will inevitably expose both the patient and the therapist to a number of key 12-step concepts. These principles include the concept of a *higher power* (Alcoholics Anonymous, 2001, p. 50), the advocacy of fellowship over professionalism (Alcoholics Anonymous, 1952, p. 166), and the concepts of *group conscience* and *spiritual awakening* (Alcoholics Anonymous, 1952, pp. 106, 132). Because these concepts are central to the 12-step philosophy, the practitioner must not only be familiar with them but must be prepared to discuss them and their implications for action. Effective assignment of recovery tasks assumes that the therapist is familiar with the culture and traditions of 12-step fellowships. For this reason, we encourage therapists who have no personal knowledge of 12-step fellowships to familiarize themselves with the basic AA texts, such as *Alcoholics Anonymous* (Alcoholics Anonymous, 2001), *Twelve Steps and Twelve Traditions* (Alcoholics Anonymous, 1952), and *Living Sober* (Alcoholics Anonymous, 1975). When working with drug-using clients, the basic NA text (Narcotics Anonymous, 1982) is also useful. Finally, therapists who are unfamiliar with 12-step fellowships are encouraged to attend several open AA, NA, and/or Al-Anon meetings prior to implementing TSF.

Principles of TSF

TSF seeks to be both philosophically and pragmatically compatible with the 12 steps of AA. Accordingly, therapists are encouraged to reflect on the following concepts.

Locus of Change

TSF considers that the primary locus of change lies less in the hands of the therapist and more in the hands of 12-step fellowships. In other words, the goal is the patient's active participation and involvement in 12-step fellowships to support the patient's ongoing recovery. That is the main reason why we prefer the word *facilitation* to words such as *therapy* or *treatment*. The facilitator must possess not only good psychotherapy skills but also a working knowledge of 12-step fellowships. However, to be maximally effective, the therapist must also be able to resist becoming the client's recovery program. For example, the facilitator must develop skill in knowing when to provide advice and support personally versus when to encourage the client to seek these things through AA or NA. He or she must accept the idea that the patient's recovery is not dependent solely on the skills acquired through therapy; rather, sustained recovery is dependent on skills the patient acquires through active fellowship with other recovering persons. Such a therapeutic stance frames the therapist–patient relationship as one of collaboration to achieve the goal of involvement in AA and/or NA.

Motivation

From its inception, AA has described itself as a fellowship that is "based on attraction rather than promotion" (Alcoholics Anonymous, 1952, p. 180). Through this statement, AA established a tradition of not seeking to attract members through overt advertising or promotion, much less through coercive techniques. The historic rate of AA growth has been likened to a "social movement" (Room, 1993). This growth, in turn, has relied in great part on the notion of identification and attraction, and also on the 12th step, which states: *"Having had a spiritual awakening as the result of these steps, we tried to carry this message to alcoholics, and to practice these principles in all our affairs"* (Alcoholics Anonymous, 1952, p. 106).

AA assumed from the outset that if an alcoholic attended meetings, listened to the stories of other alcoholics, and identified with them, then eventually he or she would be motivated to try the program laid out in the 12 steps. Meanwhile, the 12th step supported the institution of sponsorship, in which individuals who have succeeded in sustaining recovery through AA or NA over a period of years, and who have remained active in it, will take newcomers under their wing for a period of time. They do so in order to support the newcomer and to teach him or her the traditions, etiquette, and other "rules of the road" that have evolved in 12-step fellowships.

The AA/NA philosophy of attraction has implications for the therapist who wishes to use TSF. Like AA itself, TSF eschews a heavily confrontational approach in favor of one that seeks to frame treatment as a collaborative endeavor. Typically, newcomers are greeted warmly. There is no "hard sell," but rather a low-key approach that is welcoming and emphasizes "giving it a try" and "keeping an open mind." Similarly, those attending 12-step meetings will rarely find themselves accused of being in denial or castigated for having a slip; rather, they are invariably welcomed back into a fellowship that seeks "progress, not perfection."

Spirituality

One aspect of 12 step recovery that clearly separates it from other models of intervention lies in its active promotion of spirituality. The guiding books of AA—*Alcoholics Anonymous* (2001) and *Twelve Steps and Twelve Traditions* (1952)—are replete with references to the importance of spirituality to recovery. In fact, AA asserts that a conscientious effort to follow the 12 steps will lead to a "spiritual awakening." Here are some examples of the way that 12-step fellowships speak of spirituality:

> We have learned that whatever the human frailties of various faiths, those faiths have given purpose and direction to millions. People of faith have a logical idea of what life is all about. (Alcoholics Anonymous, 2001 p. 49)

> On one proposition, however, these men and women [alcoholics] are strikingly agreed. Every one of them has gained access to, and believes in, a Power greater than himself. (Alcoholics Anonymous, 2001, p. 50)

... as a result of practicing all the Steps, we have each found something called a spiritual awakening. (Alcoholics Anonymous, 2001, p. 106)

Twelve-step fellowships regard spirituality as a force that provides direction and meaning to one's life. They equate spiritual awakening with a realignment of personal goals, specifically, with a movement away from radical individualism and the pursuit of the material toward community and the pursuit of serenity as core values.

At several different points in treatment (Nowinski, 2006, pp. 27–29; Nowinski & Baker, 2003, pp. 73–81) the facilitator engages the patient in a discussion of his or her spiritual beliefs. These discussions generally focus on issues of willpower, powerlessness, and faith, as well as on issues of personal values and goals.

Pragmatism

Although many people see AA and its sister fellowships primarily as spiritual programs (and sometimes confuse them with religions), historically pragmatism has been as central to AA as spirituality. One official AA publication is titled *Living Sober: Some Methods AA Members Have Used for Not Drinking* (Alcoholics Anonymous, 1975). This book contains a wealth of practical advice, such as:

- Using the 24-hour plan
- Changing old routines
- Making use of "telephone therapy"
- Getting plenty of rest
- Fending off loneliness
- Letting go of old ideas

In TSF, the facilitator attempts to educate the patient with practical methods for staying sober. The facilitator consistently advises the patient to focus on "one day at a time," and encourages the patient to solicit and follow advice from fellow AA members and his or her sponsor on issues ranging from the best ways to deal with difficult situations, to how to cope with cravings, to what to do after a slip. Every TSF session ends with the facilitator assigning one or more *recovery tasks*, which are specific suggestions for action, including meetings, readings, journaling, and the like.

A Collaborative Approach

In setting a tone for the intervention, the TSF facilitator relies on the third tradition: *the only requirement for AA membership is a desire to stop drinking* (Alcoholics Anonymous, 1952, p. 139). This tradition is deliberate in its wording. It means that it is not essential for the patient to embrace every tenet of AA or to adopt a particular spiritual philosophy. Indeed, AA states: "Alcoholics Anonymous does not demand that you believe anything. All of its Twelve Steps are but suggestions" (Alcoholics Anonymous, 1952, p. 26).

The TSF therapist seeks to be flexible in establishing a collaborative relationship with the patient on his or her pathway to recovery. Confrontation in TSF is common, but it never takes the form of threat. For example, the 12-step facilitator will never terminate treatment because a patient drinks or uses between sessions. On the other hand, the facilitator will consistently confront the patient about drinking or drug use and their connection to unmanageability. The facilitator also continues to ask for and encourage frequent attendance at meetings, but will never make attendance a *condition* of treatment. Similarly, the facilitator will talk frankly about any "slips" that the patient reports and what could have been done to prevent them.

Focus

The focus of TSF is on helping the patient *begin* the process of recovery—to help the patient bond to a 12-step fellowship by understanding its key concepts and learning how to utilize its resources for support and advice. Although collateral issues may (and frequently are) raised by patients in the course of treatment, facilitators are advised to avoid "drift," that is, a loss of focus on drinking or drug use and AA or NA, in favor of some other issue. Facilitators may validate patients' legitimate concerns about work, marriage, or family issues, but they avoid getting sidetracked by them. While concurrent therapies may be necessary at times (e.g., for an acutely depressed patient), the TSF model advocates prioritizing problems, with early recovery from alcohol or drug abuse being at the top of the list.

Objectives

TSF seeks to achieve a number of specific objectives that can be broken down broadly into two related categories: (1) active involvement and (2) identification and bonding.

Active Involvement

Active involvement in 12-step fellowships means going to meetings. But merely attending meetings does not qualify as *active* involvement. Very often, practitioners who are unfamiliar with the 12-step model may stop their intervention at this point. "I suggested that my patient go to an AA meeting," a clinician might say, "but she told me that she tried that once and didn't like it." Facilitating active involvement means helping the patient to examine and work through resistance to active involvement in AA and/ or NA just as much as any psychotherapy involves helping patients work through resistance to change. When working within a 12-step frame of reference, one is more likely to encounter the word "denial" instead of "resistance," even though the two are in fact conceptually equivalent.

"Getting active" begins with going to meetings. For the individual who is just beginning to give up alcohol or drugs, 12-step fellowships have traditionally advocated attending 90 meetings in 90 days (i.e., a meeting a day, if not more, as a minimum goal). The exact origins of this common wisdom are vague, as are the origins of much of the "culture" of AA. However, such advice squares well with research on relapse (Marlatt & Gordon, 1985), which shows consistently, across addictions, that the majority of relapses occur within 90 days of initial abstinence.

AA and NA meetings vary a great deal with respect to membership, tone, and format. By tradition, AA is deliberately decentralized (Alcoholics Anonymous, 1952, pp. 160, 172), so no two meetings will be exactly alike. The result is a fellowship that is eclectic in form, diverse in membership, and open to continual change. The facilitator should understand that there are discernable regional differences in the overall tone of meetings along with a growing trend toward various "specialty" meetings. It is common, for example, to find meetings for men, women, Latinos, gay men, and so on, in some communities.

As an organization, AA purposefully exerts no effort to ensure that meetings are organized or run in a prescribed way. However, there are a number of AA and NA traditions, as well as discernable types of meetings. An important tradition is anonymity. Only first names are used at meetings, and participants expect what transpires at meetings to be kept in confidence. Another tradition is a rule against *cross-talk*, meaning interrupting a speaker to question him or her. *Service work*, such as making coffee, setting up and taking down chairs, and passing the hat for voluntary contributions to pay for any costs associated with supporting the meeting is another tradition likely to be seen across groups. Finally, most groups will establish a series of rituals and rites, such as ways of starting and ending meetings, and ways of recognizing the achievement of certain landmarks, such as 1, 2, 5, and 10 years of sobriety.

There are also, by tradition, several different generic types of meetings. One is the *speaker meeting*, in which an individual tells his or her story of addiction and recovery: "How it was then, what happened, and how it is now." The common theme of these stories echoes the legend of the phoenix and captures the capacity of the human spirit to rise from the ashes of defeat. The key to this dramatic change in each case is the individual's courage to admit that alcohol or drugs has made life unmanageable (acceptance), and to replace individual willpower with fellowship and the 12 steps as a pathway to recovery and spiritual renewal (surrender). A second type of meeting is the *open discussion* meeting. Here a designated member or members raises an issue (e.g., resentment, loneliness, spirituality) that members respond to in turn, sharing their thoughts or experiences on the subject. A third type of meeting is a *step meeting*. Usually a group will focus on one of the 12 steps each month. At the beginning of the meeting, the step is read aloud. Members then respond to the step, explaining how they are "working" it in their daily lives. Some groups go through the entire 12 steps in this way; other groups may limit themselves to certain steps only— for example, the first three—and cycle through them repeatedly. A fourth type of meeting is an *open* meeting. One does not have to admit to having a problem with alcohol or drugs in order to attend. *Open* meetings are a good fit for patients who are not yet sure that they have a problem or that they need to stop drinking or using drugs. An appropriate "recovery task" in these cases is to ask the patient to simply sit and listen. *Open* meetings are also useful for therapists who want to learn more about 12-step fellowships before implementing TSF in their practices. The last type of meeting is a *closed* meeting, which should only be attended by persons who are ready to admit to alcoholism or addiction, and who say they want to stop.

In facilitating early recovery, the facilitator should monitor not only *how many* meetings a patient attends, but also *what kinds* of meetings he or she attends and *how active* he or she is in them. One tool for doing this is to ask patients to maintain a personal "recovery journal" in which they record meetings attended, the meeting type, and their own reactions to them. This will allow the therapist to review the patient's "recovery week" and to help maintain momentum in treatment.

Facilitators should make an effort to encourage patients to try out several different types of meetings. They should also encourage patients to attend one or two specialized meetings (e.g., a men's or a women's meeting). After the patient has attended a number of different meetings, he or she can be encouraged to begin thinking about making one of them his or her *home group*. This means making a commitment to attend that meeting regularly, to accept some service work responsibility at the meeting, and to find a sponsor from within that group. It also moves the newly recovering patient to a deeper level of active involvement and bonding to the fellowship. Another level is achieved as the patient begins to utilize *telephone therapy*, which means exchanging phone numbers and making contact with others outside of meetings. Today, the Internet offers an additional vehicle for connecting to other AA/NA members via e-mail and texting. There are even online AA and NA meetings that individuals can "attend." It is important for the therapist to normalize this tradition and explain its purpose, which is to build a support network of fellow AA/NA members who are sympathetic to the goal of not drinking or using drugs, and who can be contacted in times of need.

Using the phone and e-mail and becoming more active in meetings also serves to gradually reconstruct the patient's social circle and bond him or her to a new social network: one that supports sobriety as opposed to substance use. Over time it can lead to less contact with old, drinking or using friends and more contact with new, sober friends. Since research suggests that social support is a significant factor in substance use as well as recovery from addiction (Wu & Witkiewitz, 2008; Longabaugh et al., 1998; Sobell, Cunningham, Sobell, & Toneatto, 1993), this process of establishing a new social network can be thought of as a core objective of TSF.

The last objective with regard to facilitating active involvement in AA or NA concerns *sponsorship*. A sponsor is, by tradition, a sort of mentor: an individual who has traveled the road before you and who can serve as your guide. AA succinctly describes the role and significance of the sponsor in early recovery in this way: "Not every A.A. member has a sponsor. But thousands of us say we would not be alive were it not for the special friendship of one recovering alcoholic in the first months and years of our sobriety" (Alcoholics Anonymous, 1975, p. 26).

The sponsor–sponsee relationship is usually a close one. The facilitator encourages the patient to find a sponsor early in the recovery process, but, cannot become a patient's sponsor in order to maintain clear boundaries. For newcomers, sponsors will often establish a pattern of daily telephone or e-mail contact. They may meet the newcomer at meetings, introduce him or her to new people, and suggest meetings to attend. Sponsors try, to the best of their ability, to answer questions about the 12 steps or the fellowship itself. The issue of needing a sponsor is often brought up directly in meetings, as the individual chairing the meeting will usually ask if there are any newcomers present, and if anyone is in need of a sponsor.

Taken together, the above set of objectives serve to establish a broad basis of social support for sobriety while simultaneously breaking the patient away from people, places, and routines that have long been associated with alcohol or drug use.

Identification and Bonding

In AA, it is the similarities among alcoholics, not the differences, that are important. The similarity, of course, is not being able to control drinking. Bill Wilson expressed it this way:

> We are average Americans. All sections of this country and many of its occupations are represented, as well as many political, economic, social, and

religious backgrounds. We are people who normally would not mix. But there exists among us a fellowship, a friendliness, and an understanding which is indescribably wonderful. (Alcoholics Anonymous, 1952, p. 17)

It is common, indeed natural, for the newcomer to AA and NA to experience discomfort. After all, alcoholism and addiction still carry with them a significant social stigma. In addition, people who have little or no direct knowledge of 12-step fellowships are apt to hold many stereotyped attitudes and beliefs. For example, they may have the idea that AA and NA are religions or that their members are obsessed with God. Many worry that they will be asked to join a cult, or that they will find themselves surrounded by skid-row bums. Because of these preconceptions, patients may miss the essential similarity between their own experiences and those of everyone else in the room.

The facilitator needs to normalize and empathize with patient's initial reticence to identify with those attending a meeting. Reading the above quote can initiate a productive discussion of this issue, as can having the patient share entries from his or her recovery journal. The facilitator needs to remain alert and help the patient work through any resistance to identification. The first strategy for doing so is education: solicit and discuss any stereotypes the patient has about AA/NA, their members, or what happens at meetings; ask the patient to attend and listen to some open speaker and discussion meetings; and ask the patient to recount what he or she heard, being vigilant for stereotypes versus realities.

The facilitator should routinely ask the patient who is new to AA or NA if there was a person, or a particular part of a story or discussion, to which he or she could relate. Building on this foundation, the facilitator can gradually promote the patient's capacity for identification and bonding.

Other methods for facilitating identification are keeping a journal or reading AA and NA material. Two useful sources for promoting identification are the personal stories of addiction and recovery that appear in *Alcoholics Anonymous* (2001) and *Narcotics Anonymous* (1982). For patients with a great deal of social anxiety, attempting to identify through reading at home may be easier at first than identifying through listening at meetings.

However identification is achieved, it is a highly desirable outcome of TSF. Becoming active is a crucial part of the early stages of recovery. However, in order to sustain sobriety over the long run, a deeper sense of bonding may be crucial. It is in the context of this bonding that many AA members begin to pursue more advanced work such as creating moral inventories (Steps 4 and 5) and to experience firsthand some of the spiritual renewal that has long been associated with AA. Indeed, it may be impossible for an individual to experience the "spiritual awakening" that the 12th step speaks of in the absence of this bonding process.

Taken together, active involvement and identification form a solid basis for recovery. The more effective the facilitator is in collaborating with the patient, the more likely it is that the patient will sustain his or her sobriety.

Assessment

TSF begins in the same way as any good treatment for substance abuse: with a thorough assessment. The specific approach to assessment employed in TSF has been described in detail elsewhere (Nowinski, 2006; Nowinski & Baker, 2003) and for reasons of space will be described only briefly here.

One purpose for conducting a thorough alcohol and drug history, as well as a careful inventory of consequences, is to establish from the outset a collaborative therapeutic relationship with the patient and, ideally, to reach a *consensus* regarding diagnosis and treatment. This may require the facilitator to refer back frequently in subsequent sessions to data collected during the assessment. Toward this end, we recommend that the patient be given a copy of the assessment and be asked to review it as one of his or her first *recovery tasks* between sessions.

An alcohol–drug history is a graphical representation of chronological changes in the type and amount of substances used by the patient, along with correlated events and effects. Creating an alcohol–drug history is best done using a chart like the example shown in Figure 8.1.

In this hypothetical example, the patient reported first use of alcohol at age 11. At that time, he sipped from his father's supply of beer, primarily on weekends. Drinking made him feel "silly," but sometimes it made him feel sick. He also reported that his mother and father had fought often. By age 13, his use of alcohol had increased to two or three beers, two or three times a week. This made him feel "high," suggesting that he was experiencing some pleasurable affect as a consequence of his drinking, and was using alcohol primarily for its euphoric effects. At about this same time, his father left the home. By the time he was 14, our hypothetical patient was drinking beer as well as smoking marijuana three to four times a week. He reports that this made him feel "mellow," which suggests that he was at that point of using substances to control his mood and to create a sense of relaxation and calm. He also reports getting into trouble at school and having much conflict at home.

Although Figure 8.1 is necessarily brief for purposes of illustration, the clinician should take care to fill in a similar chart as completely as possible, adding as much detail as the patient will offer. The objective is to engage the patient in a collaborative effort in the creation of this autobiography, and most importantly to document the *progression* of substance use over time and all significant events correlated with that progression.

Substance/age	Type/amount	Frequency	Effects	Significant events
Alcohol/11	Beer: sips from Dad's supply	Weekends	"Silly" "Sick"	Mom and Dad fighting
Alcohol/13	Beer: 2–3 cans	2–3/wk	"High"	Dad left
Alcohol/14	Beer: 2–3 cans	3–4/wk	"Mellow"	Doing poorly in school/fighting at home
Marijuana/14	1–2 joints	3–4/wk		

FIGURE 8.1. Alcohol and drug history.

The second major part of the assessment is an inventory of *consequences* of alcohol and drug use. Again, both for purposes of clarity and to enhance motivation, this is best done chronologically. The facilitator can introduce this part of the assessment with an opening statement similar to the following: "Let's take some time to examine some of the issues, conflicts, and problems that you've experienced over your life, and let's see if any of them are connected in any way to your use of alcohol or drugs."

Negative consequences of alcohol or drug use should be explored both chronologically and categorically. Be sure not to leave out (or allow the patient to avoid) examining each of the following areas.

Physical Consequences

Included here (especially for older patients) are the physical consequences of long-term substance abuse, including diabetes, gastrointestinal problems, sleep disorders, weight loss, alcohol- or drug-related injuries and accidents, emergency room visits, liver disease, and so on. Keep in mind that it is estimated that approximately 50% of all general hospital beds in the United States are occupied by patients whose medical illnesses are alcohol- or drug-related (National Institute on Alcohol Abuse and Alcoholism, 1990).

Legal Consequences

Alcohol and drug use often lead to legal troubles such as charges for DWI (driving while intoxicated), disorderly conduct, and the like. There may also be other alcohol- or drug-related illegal activities (e.g., sale, theft, prostitution) for which the patient was either not arrested or convicted.

Social Consequences

Social consequences of alcohol or drug use include relationship, family, or job conflicts. People who abuse substances often alienate their partners, perform more poorly at work, and are dysfunctional as parents. They may destroy their marriages, lose their jobs, and alienate their friends. It is important to do a thorough inventory of such losses, in chronological order, and to connect them to the patient's alcohol–drug history as appropriate. Substance abuse can have severe deleterious effects on families. A companion program for treating families of substance abusers is available (Nowinski, 2011), which can be used together or apart from TSF.

Psychological Consequences

Habitual use of alcohol and drugs, even in the absence of clear dependency, often leads to negative psychological consequences such as anxiety and depression. Other consequences include poor anger control, irritability, apathy, and confused thinking. As habitual use gives way to dependency, and as negative consequences accrue, suicidal thinking and suicide attempts are not uncommon.

Sexual Consequences

Not only is alcohol and other substance abuse associated with sexual dysfunction in both males and females (Powell, 1984), but alcohol and drug use and dependency are often correlated with sexual victimization and exploitation. The facilitator should explore the patient's sexual history to determine if sexual dysfunction, victimization, or exploitation are present, and, if so, whether they are correlated with substance abuse. Frank discussion of sexuality is often omitted from assessment, despite being a strong motivator for recovery. Guidelines for conducting substance-abuse-related sexual histories have been published elsewhere (Nowinski, 2006; Nowinski & Baker, 2003).

Financial Consequences

It is a good idea to have the patient estimate how much money she or he has spent on alcohol or drugs in the 2 years prior to the assessment. Expenses should include both the cost of the substances themselves and the costs of any consequences. The latter include such costs as traffic tickets, legal defense or representation, and lost income.

Treatment

After completing both the alcohol–drug history and the inventory of consequences, the facilitator can share a diagnosis and treatment plan. This
should come as no surprise to the patient if the assessment process has been
a collaborative venture. Still, the patient and the clinician may disagree,
especially if the clinician thinks the patient is addicted, but the patient still
does not believe that he or she is addicted. It is important to note that it
is not essential for the patient to acknowledge alcoholism or addiction in
order to proceed with TSF. The sole criteria for making use of AA, and
therefore using TSF, is a *desire to stop drinking*. Acceptance of a label (e.g.,
"addicted") is not a prerequisite.

It is hoped that a successful assessment has not only confirmed a clinical diagnosis for both the clinician and the patient, but has also motivated
the patient to want to stop drinking or using drugs. In some cases, this
motivation will mean that the patient will be willing to follow the therapist's advice—for example, to begin attending meetings, doing some reading, keeping a journal, and so on.

Many patients acknowledge that drugs and/or alcohol have indeed
caused serious consequences, and may even express a desire to stop using
drugs or drinking; nonetheless, their behavior may reveal a resistance to
taking any of the actions that recovery requires. Others may produce a history replete with consequences, and appear to be leading an unmanageable
life, yet still deny addiction. In each of these situations, successful treatment
demands that the therapist be able to establish a collaborative relationship
with the patient. Within AA and other 12-step fellowships the transition
from outright denial, to passive acknowledgment of a problem, to active
participation in a 12-step fellowship is known as "working the steps." This
is also the crux of early recovery. It is a process wherein the patient could
be said to move from *denial*, to *acceptance*, to *surrender*.

Acceptance

The first step of AA and NA as it appears in their respective "Big Books"
read as follows: "We admitted we were powerless over alcohol—that our
lives had become unmanageable"(Alcoholics Anonymous, 2001, p. 59) and
"We admitted we were powerless over our addiction—that our lives had
become unmanageable" (Narcotics Anonymous, 1982, p. 8).

Although many individuals take issue with the word "powerless"
in these statements, it is important for clinicians to understand exactly
how that concept is used within the fellowships of AA and NA, which

is *contextual*. In other words, 12-step fellowships speak of powerlessness only in the context of alcohol or drug use. Step 1 refers specifically to *powerlessness over alcohol or drug use*; it does not imply any kind of generalized powerlessness or helplessness.

Twelve-step fellowships are built on acceptance of a simple recognition: that individual willpower can be gradually overwhelmed by the addiction process. Once addicted, efforts to control use will only lead to failure and frustration, and eventually to hopelessness. Furthermore, once addicted, individuals are not as likely to sustain sobriety alone as they are through mutual support. In order to stay sober, AA admonishes the alcoholic to "quit playing God" (Alcoholics Anonymous, 2001, p. 62), and to accept the notion that "any life run on self-will can hardly be a success" (Alcoholics Anonymous, 2001, p. 60).

In essence, then, the first step is a statement of humility. It reflects an acceptance of personal limitation: that life has become *unmanageable*, that this unmanageability is the result of substance abuse, and that willpower alone has not been enough to change that. Philosophically, the first step (and AA itself) has been seen as a challenge to the radical individualism that has long been a core theme in U.S. culture (Room, 1993).

In discussing Step 1 with patients, the therapist will find it extremely useful to have the alcohol–drug history and the chronology of consequences at hand. The focus of therapist–patient dialogue should be on the *progressive pattern of unmanageability in the patient's life and the limitations of personal willpower* (i.e., attempts to limit or stop use). If the patient's history and chronology do not make a case for total loss of control, it should at least show a pattern of growing unmanageability that can be pointed out. The patient can also be encouraged to describe some of the methods that he or she has used in the past in order to limit or stop his or her use of alcohol or drugs. In this regard, the facilitator would do well to share the following excerpt with the patient:

> Here are some of the methods we have tried: Drinking beer only, limiting the number of drinks, never drinking alone, never drinking in the morning, drinking only at home, never having it in the house, never drinking during business hours, drinking only at parties, switching from scotch to brandy, drinking only natural wines, agreeing to resign if ever drunk on the job, swearing off forever (with or without a solemn oath), taking more physical exercise, reading inspirational books, going to health farms and sanitariums, accepting voluntary commitment to asylums—we could increase the list ad infinitum. (Alcoholics Anonymous, 2001, p. 31)

A discussion of Step 1 can also proceed toward acceptance in a series of steps, as follows:

1. The patient acknowledges that he or she has a "problem" with alcohol or drugs—that life has become, or is becoming, progressively more unmanageable.
2. The patient acknowledges that individual efforts to limit or stop drinking or using have failed (i.e., accepting powerlessness in the context of substance use).
3. The patient acknowledges the need to give up alcohol and/or drugs as opposed to trying to limit or control their use.

As simple and straightforward as this sounds, clinicians find that moving a patient from denial to acceptance usually is more of a *process* than an *event*—and a painful one at that. For many individuals with alcohol or drug problems, acceptance represents an insight that is achieved gradually and only reluctantly. It is also an awareness that is frequently accompanied by intense emotional reactions such as anger or discouragement. As a rule, acceptance without emotion is suspect. More typically, patients will experience most or all of the emotional stages associated with grief and loss as they move through the stages of acceptance. The clinician does well to raise this issue of emotional responses to Step 1, to normalize it, and then to explore it with the patient.

People, Places, and Routines

With this topic, TSF moves on to help the patient prepare for change. The vehicle for this is the Lifestyle Contract, an example of which is shown in Figure 8.2. The Lifestyle Contract is based on the notion that addiction evolves into a virtual lifestyle that is supported by a range of "people, places, and routines." In order to support his or her recovery, the substance abuser must be prepared to make changes in each of these areas. The Lifestyle Contract, which is developed collaboratively by the patient and the therapist, becomes a blueprint for this life change.

	Dangerous to recovery	Supportive of recovery
People	Drinking friends	AA members Nondrinking friends
Places	Bars, casinos	AA meetings Nondrinking friends' homes
Routines	Drinks after work	Meeting AA friends Exercise

FIGURE 8.2. Lifestyle Contract.

The Lifestyle Contract also assumes that simply "giving things up" will not be a successful strategy for long-term change. To truly support recovery, people, places, and routines that are supportive of recovery must be substituted for those that pose a threat to recovery. Viewed another way, the Lifestyle Contract is an inventory of the lifestyle that supports drinking or drug use versus an alternative lifestyle that supports sobriety.

It is recommended that the therapist work with the patient to develop a Lifestyle Contract early in treatment, but only after the patient has achieved at least some degree of acceptance of the need to give up alcohol or drugs.

Surrender

Surrender follows acceptance and the development of the Lifestyle Contract. It represents the patient's decision to abandon personal willpower in favor of reaching out as a means of stopping use of alcohol or drugs and their consequences. Like acceptance, surrender is more typically a process than an event. Steps 2 and 3 of Alcoholics Anonymous reflect this:

> We came to believe that a Power greater than ourselves could restore us to sanity. We made a decision to turn our will and our lives over to the care of God *as we understood Him.* (Alcoholics Anonymous, 2001, p. 59)

The italics at the end of the third step appear in the original text and are emphasized in order to point out that the AA view of God or a higher power is a pluralistic one. There is no specific dogma within AA or NA. The closest thing to a dogma are the 12 steps themselves, which are framed not so much in religious terms as much as in terms of a pathway to character growth and personal renewal.

AA does have a long spiritual tradition to the extent that the 12 steps challenge us to believe in a center of power that is greater than our individual wills. Substituting faith in the group (or some other higher power) for faith in personal willpower has been construed as a form of spiritual conversion or awakening:

> Faith is a dynamic process of construal and commitment in which persons find and give meaning to their lives through trust in and loyalty to shared centers of value, images and realities of power, and core stories. Conversion in AA perspective begins when one reaches and acknowledges a state of helpless desperation in the effort to maintain the false self and the illusion that one can manage one's drinking. Gradually it comes to mean making a commitment to enter into the 12 steps and become part of the 12 traditions of Alcoholics Anonymous. (Fowler, 1993)

If Step 1 involves *accepting the problem* (i.e., alcoholism or drug addiction), then Steps 2 and 3 can be thought of as *accepting the solution*, which requires the addict to reach out. Within 12-step fellowships this is commonly referred to as "turning it over"—that is, moving away from self-centeredness and an excessive belief in the power of individual willpower toward a willingness to reach out to and accept the strength of fellowship. This is more than an abstract notion: it will be directly reflected in patients' *hope for recovery*, in their *willingness to become active in the fellowship*, and in their *openness to receiving advice*. When an individual begins to "surrender" in this fashion, he or she begins to appreciate that accepting powerlessness over alcohol or drugs does not in any way imply helplessness.

The clinician should engage the patient in a specific and ongoing dialogue about willpower, faith, and surrender. It is suggested that at least one entire session be devoted to reading Steps 2 and 3 and discussing the patient's reactions to them. Questions like the following can be used as a guideline for this discussion:

- "As a youth, who were your heroes, and who are they now?"
- "What are your most cherished values? In other words, what personal qualities in others do you admire most?"
- "How do you feel about people who ask others for help when they feel stuck, and why?"
- "Are you open to the idea that people struggling with similar problems can help each other more than each of those people can help themselves?"
- "Whose advice are you most likely to follow?"
- "Are you open to the idea that there are some personal problems that a person can solve only by reaching out for help and support from others?"
- "Do you believe that others could help you stay clean or sober?"
- "What is your idea of God?"
- "Who in the world do you trust the most, and why?"
- "Are you willing to do what someone else who has overcome alcoholism or drug addiction tells you to do? When would you, and when wouldn't you, follow his or her advice?"
- "How do you feel about using the support of people in AA or NA to help you stay clean and sober?"

This sort of dialogue is more than an intellectual exercise. It is central to introducing the patient to the spiritual foundation of 12-step fellowships. Not all therapists are equally comfortable engaging patients in this sort of dialogue. In fact, therapists would be wise to ponder such questions themselves before entering into this kind of dialogue. In the end, it can be very productive to venture down this road since it represents a highly effective route to working through patients' resistances to becoming active in AA or NA and making full use of their social and spiritual resources.

Getting Active

The fifth and final component of the TSF core program centers on facilitating patients' active participation in AA and/or NA. "Getting active," in 12-step parlance, means "working the steps." AA puts it this way:

> Just stopping drinking is not enough. Just not drinking is a negative, sterile thing. That is clearly demonstrated by our experience. To stay stopped, we've found we need to put in place of the drinking a positive program of action. (Alcoholics Anonymous, 1975)

A popular meditation book expresses similar sentiments in this way: "Work and prayer are the two forces which are gradually making a better world. We must work for the betterment of ourselves and other people. Faith without works is dead" (Anonymous, 1975, p. 83).

The message is clear: recovery requires faith, but it also requires action. Steps 1 and 2 in particular can be thought of as necessary but not sufficient conditions for staying clean or sober. To facilitate recovery, the clinician must be prepared to work with the patient toward the goal of becoming actively involved in a 12-step fellowship. This may include participating in frequent meetings, getting phone numbers and building a support network, finding people and places that support recovery, seeking a home group and a sponsor, and reading AA/NA material.

Two useful vehicles for pursuing the goal of getting active are keeping a *recovery journal* (described earlier) and doing *recovery tasks*. The latter are not unlike "homework" that is often employed in CBT which, like TSF, also involve patient–therapist collaboration and active work on the part of the patient. It is recommended that the clinician end each session with a series of specific recovery tasks and begin each session with a review of the patient's "recovery week," including progress made on recovery tasks.

Recovery tasks and the subsequent review should cover each of the following areas:

- Readings from AA and/or NA literature.
- Suggestions about specific meetings to attend.
- Progress made on the use of telephone therapy, selecting a home group, taking on responsibility, and getting a sponsor.

Clinicians may wish to employ techniques like role playing in order to facilitate reaching specific objectives (e.g., asking for a phone number or e-mail address, speaking up at meetings) that are difficult for patients who suffer from high social anxiety. Therapists must also be prepared to shape behavior—in this case, active participation—through positive reinforcement of the patient's efforts. It is not uncommon, for example, for patients to make several false starts when first "testing the waters" of AA or NA. They may get as far as the door of a meeting, for example, only to turn around at the last second. They may come to a meeting late and leave early. Or they may attend only one meeting after promising to attend three.

Obviously, to be able to shape behavior, the facilitator must first know about it. A blaming or unreceptive attitude on the part of the facilitator is likely to cloud communication when openness is needed. The patient should feel safe disclosing what he or she actually did between sessions. This is not inconsistent with his or her also knowing what the clinician would *like* him or her to have done.

Readings

Here are some suggestions for readings that might be assigned relative to the subjects of acceptance, the Lifestyle Contract, surrender, and getting active:

Acceptance

- *Twelve Steps and Twelve Traditions*: pp. 21–24.
- *Alcoholics Anonymous*: "The Doctor's Opinion," "Bill's Story," "More about Alcoholism."
- *Narcotics Anonymous*: "Who Is an Addict," "Why Are We Here?" "How It Works."
- *Living Sober*: pp. 7–10.

Surrender

- *Alcoholics Anonymous*: "There Is a Solution," "More About Alcoholism," "How It Works."
- *Narcotics Anonymous*: pp. 22–26.
- *Twelve Steps and Twelve Traditions*: pp. 25–41.
- *Living Sober*: pp. 77–87.

Lifestyle Contract/Getting Active

- *Alcoholics Anonymous*: Personal stories (to be selected by facilitator).
- *Living Sober*: Chapters 3, 6, 8, 10, 11, 13, 14, 15, 18, 22, 26, 27, 29.

Therapists should be familiar with any assigned readings and be prepared to discuss them at the outset of each TSF session. For patients who cannot read, audiotapes of AA publications are available through Alcoholics Anonymous World Services (www.AA.org). Similarly, most AA and NA texts are available in various translations.

Meetings

In order to know which meetings to suggest, the facilitator must obtain current AA and NA meeting schedules. These are available online at *www. aa.org*. Printed lists may also be available at some meetings. In addition, clinicians wishing to utilize TSF are encouraged to occasionally attend open AA, NA, and/or Al-Anon meetings and, if possible, to develop their own small network of AA and NA contacts who may be useful resources for getting shy newcomers to meetings, explaining the AA/NA "rules of the road," and so on. Many recovering persons express a great deal of gratitude to those first "friendly faces" encountered at meetings. Therapists should not hesitate to reach out to such people since it is an integral part of the AA culture to help those who need help.

Conjoint Programs

It is not uncommon for interventions based on a 12-step model to include a family and/or marital component. Such an inclusion recognizes that substance abuse affects not only the abuser but also his or her significant others. A detailed intervention for significant others of substance abusers is described elsewhere (Nowinski, 2011a).

TSF incorporates an abbreviated conjoint program into its model. The TSF conjoint program is consistent with the philosophy of Al-Anon, which is a 12-step fellowship for significant others of substance abusers (Al-Anon Family Group Headquarters, 1986).

The objectives of the TSF conjoint program, which generally spans two sessions, is to provide a spouse or significant other with an overview of the facilitation program that the patient is undergoing, to do an initial assessment of possible partner substance abuse, and to introduce the significant other to Al-Anon and two of its key concepts: enabling and detaching.

TSF recognizes that relationships, including marriages and parent–child relationships, are often rendered deeply dysfunctional and wounded as a result of addiction. It recognizes also that marital and/or family therapy are often much needed by alcoholics and addicts in recovery. At the same time, TSF is based on the idea that *early* recovery is best focused on acceptance, surrender, and getting active. In a similar vein, TSF seeks to help significant others get a *start* on recovering from the effects of addiction, and believes that programs like Al-Anon offer the best resources for that start. Accordingly, before a patient who is just beginning recovery and his or her partner or family are referred for marital or family therapy, TSF attempts to engage them in fellowships that can offer understanding, support, and advice.

Partner Substance Abuse

The issue of partner substance abuse cannot be ignored because it represents a threat to the early recovery of the primary patient. Accordingly, basic questions should be asked in order to determine whether a partner should also be referred to treatment:

- "Do you drink or use drugs at all? If so, what do you drink [use] and how often?"
- "Have you ever felt [or has anyone else ever suggested] that you have a problem with alcohol or drugs?"
- "Have you ever suffered any consequences of any kind related to alcohol or drug use?"
- "Has drinking or drug use ever interfered with your day-to-day life or made it 'unmanageable' in any way?

Based on this simple and brief inquiry a decision can usually be made about whether it should be suggested to a partner that he or she should also seek further help. At the same time the facilitator will know whether partner substance abuse should be taken into account when constructing the primary patient's Lifestyle Contract.

Introducing Al-Anon and/or Nar-Anon

Al-Anon and Nar-Anon are fellowships that parallel AA and NA. However, these fellowships were formed not to support recovering addicts or alcoholics, but rather to support those who are in relationships with them. Like AA and NA, both Al-Anon and Nar-Anon begin with statements of "powerlessness." In this case, however, it is the behavior of the alcoholic or addict over which the individual is powerless. Coming to terms with this personal limitation (Step 1 of Al-Anon) parallels the alcoholic's or addict's coming to terms with his or her powerlessness over alcohol or drugs. Similarly, the decision to reach out to others (Al-Anon) for support and guidance has its parallels in Steps 2 and 3 of AA.

Central to Al-Anon and Nar-Anon is an effort to stop doing things that either purposefully or inadvertently allow the alcoholic or the addict to continue drinking or using (*enabling*), and to let go of any illusion of being able to control the alcoholic or addict (*detaching*). It is only through this detachment that partners and family members can begin to recover their own mental health. Al-Anon and Nar-Anon provide both the social and the spiritual support for this process. Al-Anon expresses the overall goal this way:

> "Detach!" we are told in Al-Anon. This does not mean detaching ourselves, and our love and compassion, from the alcoholic. Detachment, in the Al-Anon sense, means to realize we are individuals. We are not bound morally to shoulder the alcoholic's responsibilities. (Al-Anon Family Group Headquarters, 1986, p. 54)

After giving partners an overview of TSF and inquiring into their own use of alcohol or drugs, the facilitator devotes the bulk of the conjoint program to discussing the issues of enabling and detaching and encouraging the partner to get active in Al-Anon or Nar-Anon. Examples include

- Making excuses to cover up for the patient when she or he would ordinarily experience consequences for alcohol or drug use.
- Providing money or other support for acquiring alcohol or drugs.
- Justifying (rationalizing) inappropriate or illegal behavior while under the influence of alcohol or drugs.

The significant other is asked to give specific examples of how he or she has enabled the patient to continue to drink or use. The motivation behind these actions is also explored. Typically, it is concern for the well-being of the patient, or fear of the consequences (e.g., to the family) of *not* enabling, that motivates it. For example, a spouse might fear the loss of income if she refused to call in "sick" for a drunk spouse. Others might fear physical abuse if they say no to a demand for money that they know will be spent on alcohol or drugs. Less often, enabling is motivated by a desire to avoid facing one's own alcohol or drug problem.

Detaching can be thought of as a process of learning not to enable, but it also can be conceptualized more positively as learning what to do *instead of* enabling. The facilitator engages the partner in some discussion of this change, using examples of enabling as a springboard. Following from the above example, instead of calling in "sick" for the alcoholic who in fact is hungover, the partner could sympathize with the drinker's dilemma but still refuse to make the call for him or her.

It takes courage to detach. It can be supported by the therapist, to be sure, but it is through the fellowships of Al-Anon and Nar-Anon that partners will find the greatest amount of support and comfort for their task. Toward this end, the facilitator should suggest several specific Al-Anon or Nar-Anon meetings that the partner could attend, and follow up on these suggestions at the outset of subsequent sessions. For family members who appear to have been severely negatively affected as a result of the client's substance abuse or addiction, a separate intervention, described elsewhere (Nowinski, 2011a) is available.

Termination of Treatment

If TSF has been successful, then termination essentially consists of "turning over" the patient to the care of a 12-step fellowship. The more successfully the patient and the therapist have collaborated toward this end, the more likely it is that the patient will continue his or her progress toward lasting sobriety. This prediction is based in part on AA member surveys, which show that the best predictor of future sobriety is current active participation in AA (Alcoholics Anonymous General Services Office, 2007; Fiorentine, 1999).

Because the overarching goal of TSF is involvement in AA and/or NA, termination should in part consist of an honest appraisal of how much progress has been made toward that end. Questions such as the following are in order:

- "How many meetings per month, on average, do you now attend? What kinds of meetings are they?"
- "Do you have a home group?"
- "On average, how many AA/NA friends do you call by phone each week? How many AA/NA people call you?"
- "Do you have a sponsor?"
- "Have you taken on any responsibility at a meeting—for example, making coffee, setting up, or cleaning up?"

Besides monitoring AA/NA activity, the facilitator should check to see whether the patient has absorbed key 12-step concepts, and whether his or her attitudes about addiction and recovery have changed as a result of participation in TSF. Questions such as the following can be useful for this purpose:

- "To what extent do you think that alcohol or drug use made your life unmanageable prior to coming to the program?"
- "Do you believe now that alcoholics and addicts can 'control' their drinking or drug use?"
- "Do you think that willpower is enough to achieve sobriety, or do addicts need to reach out to others?"
- "What do the following concepts mean to you: *denial, enabling, higher power?*"

- "What role, if any, has AA or NA played so far in your effort to stay clean and sober?"
- "What are your plans relative to AA (or NA) now that this program is coming to an end?"

Clinical experience suggests that the best the facilitator can hope to do is to introduce key concepts in ways in which the patient can understand them, actively encourage the patient to give 12-step fellowship a try, confront the patient constructively with the role that alcohol or drugs have played in making the patient's life unmanageable, and answer questions about AA or NA to the best of his or her ability. In the final analysis, the facilitator must be able to "turn over" the patient and his or her future to the care of whatever higher power in which the facilitator happens to believe.

Advanced Work

This chapter has focused on a structured, time-limited intervention for "early" recovery. It is unlikely that any more ground than what has been described here could reasonably be covered in brief therapy. Indeed, the goals of the TSF core program are ambitious.

TSF does include an advanced or "elective" program (Nowinski, 2006) that provides therapist guidelines for covering the following topics: genograms, enabling, emotions, moral inventories, and relationships. A discussion of this material is beyond the scope of this chapter; however, parts of the elective program may be appropriate for patients on an individual basis. For example, the TSF module on emotions would be appropriate for clients whose substance use appears to be "triggered" by a particular emotional state, such as anger, anxiety, loneliness, or boredom. As such, the elective topics can be incorporated into an individualized treatment plan.

Case Example

The following is an illustration of how the TSF intervention model may be applied.

Bob and Kathy, married for 20 years, came to see me ostensibly for help with long-standing marital difficulties that had reached crisis proportions since their youngest child had left home for college. Though it was initially obscured by discussions and arguments about money and sex, it became apparent after a while that Bob had a drinking problem that needed to be evaluated. He was asked to come in individually for two sessions to talk about this problem.

The assessment sessions revealed that Bob had several signs of alcohol dependence. He had a powerful tolerance, drank daily, and had experienced a number of drinking-related consequences, not the least of which was a seriously strained marriage. In addition, it was discovered that he was in trouble at work as a consequence of his drinking, a problem he'd kept secret from his wife.

Bob at first was reluctant to change the focus of therapy from his troubled marriage to his drinking. He was assured that his concerns about the marriage were legitimate and would be dealt with. But he was told that first he needed to examine his drinking and either take action about it or risk losing his job and/or his marriage.

The story of Bob's private struggle for control over alcohol was a testament to stubborn determination as much as it was a classic story of the power of addiction. Having started out sipping beers stolen from the refrigerator as a youth barely 12 years old, Bob had been drinking for nearly 30 years. Things didn't get "really bad," though, according to him, until after he was married and the kids were born. Two things happened then. First, he felt obligated to stay in a job that paid well but that he had intended to leave. Second, his relationship with Kathy, in his words, became "diluted" as a consequence of the demands of family life—meaning that sex between them became a very occasional thing, and that she paid much less attention to him in general than she did when they were a couple.

It was around this time that Bob developed the habit of having "a cocktail or two" every night after work and before dinner. For a long time Kathy went along with this, though she did notice that "a cocktail or two" eventually became three, four, or more. She didn't much care for alcohol herself, and she had little personal experience with it in her own family. Out of naiveté she took Bob's ability to "drink others under the table"— in other words, his tolerance—to be a good thing. Ironically, she believed that this ability to "hold his liquor" was actually a sign that Bob could *not* become addicted.

As time went on, the process of addiction gradually set in. Instead of eating lunch with his colleagues in the company cafeteria, Bob started going out alone for lunch two or three times a week to a local bar where he'd grab a sandwich and a couple of cocktails. By the time he got home he was anxious to "relax"—his euphemism for having more cocktails. Kathy and the kids soon found that anything that stood between Bob and his cocktails made him irritable. He didn't want to be bothered with problems until he was "relaxed." Of course, by that time he was also intoxicated, emotionally unstable, and prone to losing his temper. In time, the family learned to avoid him. Kathy took to solving most of the household problems by herself, or else she let them go. The kids, meanwhile, led their own lives and had minimal communication with their father.

Though he was very hesitant to admit it for a long time, privately Bob had struggled long (and ultimately unsuccessfully) to control his drinking. He hadn't wanted to be like his own father: a "quiet drunk" who was less flamboyant than Bob in his drinking, but who had "liked his liquor" no less, and who had also been a social isolate and a "nonfactor" (as Bob described both himself and his father) within the family.

The story of Bob's private efforts to control his drinking sounded like something out of the AA Big Book: drinking only wine, drinking only beer (no cocktails) at lunch, drinking from a smaller glass, adding more ice cubes to his cocktails, and so on. While he was conscious on some level of gradually losing control, he continued to tell himself that he was really all right. It was not until his boss smelled liquor on his breath that the shell of self-deceit that Bob had built was finally shattered. He was told that a second such incident would result in disciplinary action. It also affected, he felt sure, his subsequent performance evaluation, which was lukewarm to say the least.

By the time he and Kathy came for "marriage counseling," Bob had managed to fall 2 years behind on his tax returns and owed the government several thousand dollars. According to Kathy, the house in which they lived was falling apart because of maintenance projects that Bob refused to hire someone to do but kept putting off doing himself. Their son, who had just turned 18, was failing half of his courses in his freshman year in college; meanwhile their daughter "hated" Bob and alternately fought with and ridiculed him. On top of all this, Kathy had been sexually disinterested in Bob for some time, which left him feeling frustrated and filled with self-pity.

The assessment process involved carefully chronicling first the progression of Bob's drinking, from cocktails on weekends to cocktails at lunch, how he had built a tolerance, and how drinking affected him (i.e., making him irritable and withdrawn). We then proceeded to talk at length about the methods that Bob had used to "control" his drinking, followed by discussion of all the ways in which his life had become increasingly unmanageable. At the end of this process Bob was willing to admit that he had a drinking problem and "probably" needed to stop drinking altogether. At that point, however, he was not willing to entertain the idea of using AA as a resource for helping him implement his desire to stop drinking. On the other hand, he was willing to defer marriage counseling while he met with me to work on his drinking problem.

In subsequent sessions Bob reported that he was drinking less than before, but had not gone more than one day without a drink. At that point, I moved ahead to a discussion of Step 1, reading it aloud and then talking with Bob about it at length, making sure he covered the following points:

- "What does this statement mean to you? What is your initial reaction to it . . .
  o *Emotionally*: How does it make you feel?
  o *Intellectually*: What thoughts do you have in response to it?"
- "How do you relate to the concept of *powerlessness*? What kinds of things can people be powerless over in their lives?"
- "Can you see how some people might be 'powerless' over alcohol or drugs?"
- "Have you ever felt powerless over something in your life? What have you felt powerless over?"
- "At this point do you believe that you can still control your use of alcohol? What makes you believe this?"
- "In what ways has your life become more *unmanageable* over the past several years? Where are the areas of conflict? In what ways are things not going well for you?"

The *recovery tasks* discussed at this time focused on getting Bob to begin reading some of the material in the Big Book, especially "Bill's Story" and "We Agnostics." This material was particularly relevant to Bob, who was personally alienated from organized religion and who stereotyped AA as a religion. In addition, he was a strong believer in self-determination, to the point where it was almost impossible for him to find the humility necessary to admit that he'd been ultimately unsuccessful, on his own, in controlling his drinking.

Reluctantly, and only after a frank discussion and appeal to be more open-minded, Bob agreed to attend a few different AA meetings as an observer. He agreed to a recovery task that involved going to meetings, listening to the stories being told, and trying to focus on *identifying* as much as possible with the theme of progressive loss of control, acceptance, and surrender. He was not asked to speak or to participate in any other way. On the other hand, he was advised to avoid focusing his attention on how he was different from other people at these meetings—for example, in terms of background, education, or financial circumstances.

One frequent problem of alcoholics who resist trying AA is their internalized stigma about alcoholism. Bob was no exception to this. He held very negative stereotypes about alcoholics, and fully expected to discover himself in the company of derelicts and criminals when he went to AA. Of course, he discovered just the opposite, which made it easier to encourage him to continue. In fact, he made a friend at one of the very first meetings he went to, and this person eventually became his first sponsor.

The next focus of treatment was denial. Bob had attempted to avoid coming to terms with his loss of control over drinking as fiercely as any alcoholic. His first line of defense had always been to get angry whenever his wife brought up the subject. After blowing up, he would usually change the subject, either launching into an attack on Kathy, or else complaining long and loudly about some other problem, like finances, his in-laws, or their sex life. In response to the ever-growing list of household chores that went undone, he pleaded fatigue—after all, he said, he worked hard all week and needed the weekends to "unwind."

Not surprisingly, Bob's denial extended outwardly to his behavior, and even inwardly to his own thought processes. For example, he went out of his way to associate with men who drank as much or even more than he did, and then comforted himself by drawing the comparison between his own use and theirs. Of course, he concluded that he was merely "average" (and therefore "normal") among his peers. At times when he felt guilty pouring that fifth or sixth martini, he would tell himself that he "deserved" it—for example, because of the stress of having to endure an unsatisfying job. His trouble at work he tried writing off to a combination of bad luck and a vindictive boss; his increasing tendency toward sexual impotence he attributed to his wife's preoccupation with their children.

As is often the case, once Bob was able to admit to someone else (i.e., to me) the ways in which he had denied his drinking problem, the more open he became to accepting it. At this point, he was even willing to admit it to Kathy in a conjoint session. He continued to express reservations about whether he was a "true alcoholic," as he put it, but he was willing to keep going to AA on the premise that he did have the requisite desire to stop drinking.

As brief as this case example is, I hope it gives the reader a flavor for TSF as a mode of intervention. With respect to process, it incorporates elements of education, confrontation, interpretation, and suggestion. It is based on the 12-step model of addiction and recovery, and it relies upon sophisticated clinical skills for its successful implementation.

Conclusion

Although 12-step fellowships have been a mainstay of addictions treatment for many years, an individual counseling approach utilizing these principles has only recently been developed. TSF can help to engage a person in the beginning steps and to encourage them to join a 12-step fellowship. TSF can be used by practitioners who do not necessarily have extensive experience with 12-step fellowships, but who wish to connect clients to these important services. This chapter has presented the TSF sequence, including core, elective, and conjoint components. It has also highlighted the philosophical connection between TSF and 12-step ideas, such as locus of change, acceptance, and surrender. Whether used alone or in conjunction with other approaches, TSF strategies can provide an important bridge between individual psychotherapy and 12-step practices.

References

Al-Anon Family Group Headquarters. (1986). *Al-Anon faces alcoholism* (2nd ed.). New York: Author.

Alcoholics Anonymous. (1952). *Twelve steps and twelve traditions*. New York: Alcoholics Anonymous World Services.

Alcoholics Anonymous. (1975). *Living sober: Some methods A. A. members have used for not drinking*. New York: Alcoholics Anonymous World Services.

Alcoholics Anonymous. (2001). *Alcoholics Anonymous: The story of how many thousands of men and women have recovered from alcoholism* (4th ed.). New York: Alcoholics Anonymous World Services.

Alcoholics Anonymous General Services Office. (2007). *Alcoholics Anonymous 2007 membership survey*. New York: Author.

Anonymous. (1975). *Twenty-four hours a day*. Center City, MN: Hazelden.

Daley, D., Baker, S., Donovan, D., Hodgkins, C., & Perl, H. (2011). A combined group and individual 12-step facilitation intervention targeting stimulant abuse in the NIDA Clinical Trials Network: SAGE 12. *Journal of Groups in Addiction and Recovery, 6*, 228–244.

Fiorentine, R. (1999). After drug treatment: Are 12 step programs effective in maintaining abstinence? *American Journal of Drug and Alcohol Abuse, 25*(1), 93–116.

Fowler, J. W. (1993). Alcoholics Anonymous and faith development. In B. S. McCrady & W. R. Miller (Eds.), *Research on Alcoholics Anonymous: Opportunities and alternatives* (pp. 113–135). New Brunswick, NJ: Rutgers Center of Alcohol Studies.

Glassner-Edwards, S., Tate, S. R., McQuaid, J. R., Cummins, K., Granholm, E., & Brown, S. A. (2007). Mechanisms of action in integrated cognitive-behavioral treatment versus twelve step facilitation for substance-dependent adults with comorbid major depression. *Journal of Studies on Alcohol and Drugs, 68*, 663–672.

Kadden, R., Carroll, K., Donovan, D., Cooney, N., Monti, N., Abrams, D., et al. (1992). *Cognitive-behavioral coping skills therapy manual: A clinical research guide for therapists treating individuals with alcohol abuse and dependence*. (Project MATCH Monograph Series, Vol. 3). Rockville, MD: National Institute on Alcohol Abuse and Alcoholism.

Longabaugh, R., Wirtz, P. W., Zweben, A., & Stout, R. L. (1998). Network support for drinking, Alcoholics Anonymous, and long-term matching effects. *Addiction, 93*(9), 1313–1333.

Marlatt, G. A., & Gordon, J. R. (Eds.). (1985). *Relapse prevention: Maintenance strategies in the treatment of addictive behaviors*. New York: Guilford Press.

Maude-Griffin, P. M., Hohenstein, J. M., Humfleet, G. L., Reilly, P. M., Tusel, D. J., & Hall, S. M. (1998). Superior efficacy of cognitive-behavioral therapy for urban crack cocaine users: Main and matching effects. *Journal of Consulting and Clinical Psychology, 66*(5), 832–837.

Miller, W. R., & Rollnink, S. (2002). *Motivational interviewing: Preparing people for change* (2nd ed.). New York: Guilford Press.

Miller, W. R., Zweben, A., DiClemente, C. C., & Rychtarik, R. G. (1995). *Motivational enhancement therapy manual* (Project MATCH Monograph, No. 2). Rockville, MD: U.S. Department of Health and Human Services.

Moos, R. H., & Moos, B. S. (2005). Paths of entry into Alcoholics Anonymous: Consequences for participation and remission. *Alcohol: Clinical and Experimental Research, 29*(10), 1858–1868.

Narcotics Anonymous. (1982). *Narcotics Anonymous* (4th ed.). Van Nuys, CA: Narcotics Anonymous World Services.

National Institute on Alcohol Abuse and Alcoholism. (1990). *Alcohol and health.* Washington, DC: Author.

Nowinski, J. (2006). *The Twelve Step Facilitation Outpatient Program.* Center City, MN: Hazelden.

Nowinski, J. (2011a). *The Family Recovery Program: A professional's guide for treating families of alcoholics and addicts.* Center City, MN: Hazelden Publications.

Nowinski, J. (2011b). *Twelve-step facilitation for the dually diagnosed client.* Center City, MN: Hazelden Publications.

Nowinski, J., & Baker, S. (2003). *The twelve-step facilitation handbook: A systematic approach to recovery from alcoholism and addiction.* Center City, MN: Hazelden.

Powell, D. (Ed.). (1984). *Alcoholism and sexual dysfunction: Issues in clinical management.* New York: Haworth Press.

Project MATCH Research Group. (1997). Matching alcoholism treatments to client heterogeneity: Project MATCH posttreatment drinking outcomes. *Journal of Studies on Alcohol, 58*, 7–29.

Project MATCH Research Group. (1998). Matching alcoholism treatments to client heterogeneity: Project MATCH three-year drinking outcomes. *Alcohol: Clinical and Experimental Research, 22*(6), 1300–1311.

Room, R. (1993). Alcoholics Anonymous as a social movement. In B. S. McCrady & W. R. Miller (Eds.), *Research on Alcoholics Anonymous: Opportunities and alternatives* (pp. 167–187). New Brunswick, NJ: Rutgers Center of Alcohol Studies.

Seraganian, P., Brown, T. G., Tremblay, J., & Annies, H. M. (1998). *Experimental manipulation of treatment aftercare regimes for the substance abuser* (National Health Research and Development Program [Canada] Project No. 6605-4392-404). Unpublished paper, Concordia University, Montreal, Canada.

Sobell, L., Cunningham, J. A., Sobell, M., & Toneatto, T. (1993). A life-span perspective on natural recovery (self-change) from alcohol problems. In J. S. Baer, G. A. Marlatt, & R. J. McMahon (Eds.), *Addictive behaviors across the life span: Prevention, treatment and policy issues* (pp. 34–66). Thousand Oaks, CA: Sage.

Triffleman, E. (2000). Gender differences in a controlled pilot study of psychosocial treatments in substance dependent patients with post-traumatic stress disorder. *Alcoholism Treatment Quarterly, 18*, 113–126.

Walitzer, K. S., Dermen, K. H., & Barrick, C. (2009). Facilitating involvement in Alcoholics Anonymous during out-patient treatment: A randomized clinical trial. *Addiction, 104*, 391–401.

Wu, J., & Witkiewitz, K. (2008). Network support for drinking: An application of multiple groups growth mixture modeling to examine client-treatment matching. *Journal of Studies on Alcohol and Drugs, 69*, 21–29.

Chapter 9

Theoretical Bases of Family Approaches to Substance Abuse Treatment

Barbara S. McCrady
Benjamin O. Ladd
Kevin A. Hallgren

Social support is an important factor in the development and resolution of substance use disorders (SUDs). Social support is usually thought of in broad terms because it is likely to be a multidimensional construct, and historically has not been well defined within the substance abuse field. As a result, attempts have been made to narrow in on the sources of social support that are most influential. Most research shows that the family has a different impact on SUDs compared to the larger social network (Beattie & Longabaugh, 1997; Havassy, Hall, & Wasserman, 1991; McCrady, 2004; Mohr, Averna, Kenny, & Del Boca, 2001). As McCrady (2004) pointed out, consideration of the larger network in the etiology and treatment of SUDs is not necessarily contraindicated, but current research on these larger networks is limited. Because evidence suggests a strong influence of family, family models have received considerable attention in the substance abuse field. Additionally, family members of substance abusers often suffer considerably in their own right; for example, adult and child relatives experience medical and psychiatric disorders at higher rates than the general population (Moss, Mezzich, Yao, Gavaler, & Martin, 1995; Ray, Mertens, & Weisner, 2007).

This chapter briefly describes the historical roots of family approaches to conceptualizing the etiology, maintenance, and treatment of SUDs. The chapter focuses specifically on alcohol abuse and dependence, given the high prevalence of and abundant research in alcohol use disorders. The chapter then presents key theoretical elements that serve as the basis for family-based treatment approaches, which are described in Chapter 10.

Historical Overview

Psychodynamic Models

In the 1930s many alcoholics received treatment in state mental hospitals. Social workers in those facilities interviewed the spouses (most often, wives) of alcoholic patients, and observed their distress. Lewis (1937) noted that the women were anxious, depressed, and experiencing a variety of psychosomatic symptoms. From these observations, theoretical models were proposed. The earliest model, the *disturbed personality hypothesis*, derived from psychodynamic theory, postulated that wives of alcoholics were disturbed and resolved their neurotic conflicts through their marriages to alcoholic men. Although some authors postulated a single primary underlying conflict (e.g., with aggression or dependence), Whalen (1953) hypothesized four different kinds of conflicts that could be resolved through marriage to an alcoholic: conflicts with aggression ("Punitive Polly"), control ("Controlling Catherine"), masochism ("Suffering Susan"), and ambivalence ("Wavering Winifred").

A corollary to the disturbed personality hypothesis was the *decompensation hypothesis*. Central to psychodynamic models is the notion that neurotic conflicts serve as a defense against more basic or primitive conflicts. If defenses are removed, an individual would be expected to exhibit these more primitive conflicts and decompensate. For instance, if an alcoholic successfully stopped drinking, his wife would be expected to decompensate and exhibit more severe psychopathology. MacDonald (1956) studied 18 women hospitalized in a state mental hospital, all of whom were married to alcoholics. He found that 11 of these women had husbands who had decreased drinking recently, which he viewed as support for the decompensation hypothesis. Beyond this anecdotal report, evidence to support the decompensation hypothesis is lacking.

Stress and Coping Models

In the 1950s, Jackson (1954) proposed a stress and coping model based on interviews with women attending Al-Anon meetings. She suggested that living with an alcoholic is stressful, and that most of the symptoms that wives of alcoholics experienced were common to families living with long-term stressors such as a chronic illness or family absence for military service. She suggested that families go through stages in coping with alcoholism. Each stage is characterized by different psychological phenomena: (1) denial of the problem; (2) attempts to control the problem; (3) feeling hopeless and chaotic; (4) attempts to maintain stable family functioning with the alcoholic present; (5) attempts to escape from the problem through marital separation; (6) attempts to organize and maintain the family without the alcoholic present; and (7) readjustment if the alcoholic stopped drinking. Kogan and Jackson (1965) later tested this stress and coping model by comparing the psychological characteristics of women whose husbands were actively drinking, had stopped drinking, or who had never had drinking problems. They found that women whose husbands were actively drinking were significantly more distressed than women whose husbands had stopped drinking or had never had a drinking problem. Moos and colleagues (Moos, Finney, & Gamble, 1982) conducted a 2-year longitudinal study of alcoholics and their families, comparing their functioning to sociodemographically matched community controls. The results of this prospective design supported Jackson's model: 2 years after treatment, spouses whose alcoholic partners successfully resolved their drinking problems were indistinguishable on measures of psychological distress from spouses in the community control sample.

Research also has examined Jackson's (1954) view of wives of alcoholics as actively attempting to cope with their spouses' drinking. Hurcom, Copello, and Orford (2000) described a three-factor model of spouse coping that holds across cultures: (1) engagement with the drinker by using assertive, controlling, emotional, and supportive behaviors to change the husband's drinking; (2) tolerance of the drinking, including self-sacrifice and inactivity by the wife of the alcoholic; and (3) withdrawal, where the wife avoids the drinker and engages in independent activities. Tolerant or withdrawing coping styles appear to have particularly negative consequences for the family, and are associated with higher rates of depression in the nonalcoholic spouse, higher alcohol intake by the nonalcoholic spouse, and more arguments between the partners. Tolerant and withdrawal coping also are associated with poorer drinking outcomes for the alcoholic, whereas assertive anti-alcohol messages by the wife are associated with a reduction in drinking levels in the husband (reviewed in Hurcom et al., 2000). Thus, a confrontational yet supportive coping style seems likely to lead to better drinking outcomes.

Family Systems Models

By the 1970s, family systems models began to influence the alcohol field. Steinglass and his colleagues observed the behavior of alcoholics hospitalized in an experimental unit, noting repetitive, patterned sequences of family interaction (Steinglass, Davis, & Berenson, 1977; Steinglass, Weiner, & Mendelson, 1971), as well as significant differences in their patterns of interaction when sober or intoxicated. These observations led to the hypothesis that alcohol performed certain positive functions in a family. For instance, alcohol might help to stabilize family roles, allow for the expression of affect, allow for greater intimacy among family members, or assist in the exploration of topics that the family might avoid when sober. This set of positive functions was called the "adaptive consequences of alcoholism" (Davis, Berenson, Steinglass, & Davis, 1974). Steinglass (1981) later reported observable differences in home-based functioning among families with an alcoholic family member who was drinking, abstinent, or in transition from one drinking status to another. Families with a sober alcoholic were most flexible in their functioning, having a balance between time together and time apart when at home. In laboratory studies, sober families showed greater flexibility in solving structured tasks (Steinglass, 1979). Conversely, drinking families showed the most rigidity of family roles and interactions, while transitional families were intermediate in their functioning.

Wolin, Bennett, Noonan, and Teitelbaum (1980) provided a second family systems perspective on alcoholism, focusing primarily on the intergenerational transmission of alcoholism. Their work examined family "rituals" such as how families vacation, have dinner, or celebrate holidays. They observed three types of ritual patterns: *intact rituals* that were maintained despite drinking, *subsumptive ritual patterns* that were modified to incorporate drinking, and *disrupted rituals* that were not maintained in the presence of drinking. They reported that those families whose rituals were intact were least likely to have offspring who became alcoholic, while those families whose rituals were most disrupted were most likely to have alcoholic offspring.

Later research examined other family systems concepts. For example, research suggests that the acquisition or loss of roles can change the overall functioning of the family system as well as individual members' drinking patterns. Hajema and Knibbe (1998) assessed changes in drinking patterns following changes in familial and social roles among a Dutch community sample. Adult men who married reduced their drinking overall, and men and women who became parents decreased the frequency of their heavy drinking. The only significant change in drinking following a role loss was for women, who increased heavy drinking following any loss of the spouse role (through divorce or death).

Later research also examined ways that drinking might serve various functions within a family system, with implications for the quality of the marital relationship. Roberts and Leonard (1998) identified five distinct drinking patterns among a community sample of newlywed couples, three of which varied considerably in terms of relationship functioning. They found that couples with compatible drinking styles generally reported more marital intimacy than couples with elevated male drinking levels. Heavy out-of-home drinking was characterized by marital conflict, alcohol dependence, risky drinking styles, and increased adverse consequences for both husband and wife. Couples with heavy drinking husbands also suffered relationship problems, and the wives in these partnerships reported higher levels of depression than any of the other wives.

Behavioral Models and Marital Interaction Research

The fourth category of major theoretical family models to evolve was behavioral models. Model development began with observational studies of the interactions between alcoholic men and their wives in a structured problem-solving task (Becker & Miller, 1976; Billings, Kessler, Gomberg, & Weiner, 1979; Hersen, Miller, & Eisler, 1973). Careful coding of behavior during the interactions revealed that the wives looked at their husbands more when the husbands were discussing alcohol than when they were discussing a more neutral topic, and that alcoholic husbands spoke more during alcohol-related conversations. These findings suggested that discussing alcohol was reinforced in the couple's interaction. Frankenstein, Hay, and Nathan (1985) found that alcoholics spoke more when intoxicated than when sober, that couples emitted more positive verbal behaviors during drinking sessions than sober sessions, and that spouses were more verbally positive in the alcohol session. Moreover, objective raters and the couples themselves rated the alcoholic as more dominant when drinking than when sober (Frankenstein, Nathan, Sullivan, Hay, & Cocco, 1985).

More refined research on the possible ways that family interactions might reinforce drinking was conducted by Jacob and colleagues (Jacob, Ritchey, Cvitkovic, & Blane, 1981). Jacob et al. (1981) initially reported that alcoholic couples became more negative when drinking, and that the wives of male alcoholics expressed more disagreements during drinking than during sober sessions. However, they later identified two subtypes of alcoholics: steady, at-home drinkers and binge, out-of-home drinkers. In steady, at-home drinkers, alcohol consumption was associated with positive familial consequences, but in binge, out-of-home drinkers, drinking was associated with negative consequences (Dunn, Jacob, Hummon, & Seilhamer, 1987; Jacob, Dunn, & Leonard, 1983). Leonard and Jacob (1997) found that wives of episodic drinkers were more likely to reciprocate negativity from their husbands in a drinking session than in a nondrinking session. The reverse was true of steady drinkers' wives, who were less negative when their husbands were drinking than not. However, when the episodic husbands used problem-solving behaviors during the interaction, their wives' negativity was tempered. It may be that wives of episodic alcoholics learn skills to protect themselves when their husbands are drinking because binge drinking is less predictable and causes greater disruption and stress to the family system (Leonard & Jacob, 1997). Thus, research from Jacob's group supported the view that family interactions might reinforce alcohol-related behaviors; however, the nature of the reinforcers might vary depending on the drinker's style of drinking.

In addition to interactional research, beginning in the early 1970s, clinical treatment models based on behavioral principles were developed (e.g., Corder, Corder, & Laidlaw, 1972) and evidence accrued from these clinical trials (reviewed below) that lent support to behavioral models.

Family Disease Models

The family has been a focus of the disease model almost from the beginning of Alcoholics Anonymous (AA). For example, the primary publication of AA (Alcoholics Anonymous, 1976) includes a chapter with advice to family members. Early AA meetings, held in members' homes, often included husbands and wives together in the meetings, leading to the development of Al-Anon, which began in 1949 as an organization to assist the family and friends of alcoholics. The contemporary family focus of disease model approaches began with Cork's (1969) book on children of alcoholics, followed by Black's (1982) and Wegsheider's (1981) books about children in alcoholic families and the adult sequelae of their early experiences. Later, authors focused on the partners of alcoholics (e.g., Beattie, 1987; Cermak, 1986). Although controlled research related to disease model conceptualizations is limited, these models have had a substantial impact on both treatment and popular thinking.

Contemporary disease model approaches describe alcoholism as a "family disease." Family members are seen as suffering from codependence, which is considered a disease itself. *Codependence* has been described as a "recognizable pattern of personality traits, predictably found within most members of chemically dependent families" (Cermak, 1986, p. 1). Proposed symptoms of codependence (Cermak, 1986) include investing self-esteem in controlling self and others in the face of serious adverse circumstances; assuming responsibility for meeting the needs of others before one's own; experiencing anxiety and distortions of boundaries around issues of intimacy and separation; being enmeshed in relationships with persons with personality disorders or alcohol or drug problems; and having other signs and symptoms such as denial, constricted emotions, depression or anxiety, or hypervigilance.

Family members who are codependent are assumed to engage in a variety of behaviors that serve to maintain substance use. *Enabling* refers to patterns of behavior that perpetuate the substance use, either by making it easier for the person to use or by providing positive responses to use and avoiding negative or limit-setting responses. Although clinical descriptions of codependency are common, empirical support for the concept is limited. Correlational studies find relationships between hypothesized codependency characteristics and depression, problems with reality testing, and a history of sexual abuse (Carson & Baker, 1994). Studies comparing subjects in relationships with substance-abusing partners to normal controls find that the former group is higher on stress owing to the substance abuse, higher on other life stressors, and lower on measures of relationship functioning than the latter (Wright & Wright, 1990). One study reported that subjects who had an alcoholic father were more likely to want to help an exploitive person (Lyon & Greenberg, 1991). To date, although there is substantial correlational literature demonstrating that spouses of substance abusers experience distress when their partner is actively using, there are no compelling empirical data indicating causal evidence for the full construct of codependency.

Current Status of Family Theory

Three models dominate contemporary family substance abuse treatment: family disease models, family systems models, and behavioral models. Research now examines constructs derived from more than one of these models, and the focus has shifted away from large theories to a focus on more specific realms related to family functioning and alcoholism: biology, affect, cognition, behavior, the environment, and how these interact.

Most treatments provide some amalgam of the three dominant models. For example, contemporary family disease models emphasize codependency, alcoholism as a disease, and family members learning to focus on changing themselves—concepts deriving from disease models. At the same time, many disease model treatment programs that include the family also emphasize communication, dysfunctional family roles, and family equilibrium—concepts derived from family systems theory.

Similarly, family systems models examine the functions that substance use serves for the family. These models attempt to change family roles, rules, and boundaries through communication, problem solving, and direct behavioral treatments to facilitate abstinence.

Behavioral family models examine family behaviors as antecedents to substance use and as reinforcing consequences, and utilize treatments to modify antecedents and consequences of substance use. Behavioral therapists also examine repetitive relationship themes, communication, and the functions that alcohol may play in maintaining the stability of the relationship – concepts derived from family systems theory.

The next section describes how historical trends in understanding substance use and family functioning, and the terminology of behavioral, systemic, and disease models are integrated into our model of the functioning of families with substance abuse.

Key Elements in Theory

Etiology and Development of SUDs

The etiology of SUDs is generally thought to be a complex phenomenon (Hill, 1994; Schuckit, 1998) with multiple determinants. Family models of substance abuse are useful when considering the etiology and development of SUDs. At this point, the familial heritability of SUDs has been well established. However, questions concerning the confluence of genetic and environmental factors affecting the familial transmission of SUDs abound. The empirical findings on variation in the presentation of substance use problems are important to consider in order to create a comprehensive theory of substance abuse from a family perspective. A family therapist who adopts a simplistic model of substance abuse and does not consider etiological determinants of substance use problems will lose a great deal of valuable information that would help conceptualize the case and develop treatment strategies.

Relatives of individuals with a SUD are eight times more likely to have a SUD of their own compared to relatives of controls (Merikangas et al., 1998). Although the evidence is mixed, research suggests that the impact of familial transmission of addictive disorders differs depending on whether one considers alcohol use disorders (AUDs) versus other SUDs. One study found that AUD rates were elevated in family members of alcoholic patients but not of other substance abusers (Hill, 1994, p. 128), indicating "alcoholism appears to breed 'true to type' even among the substance abuse disorders." Other findings suggest that the heritability of drug abuse is greater than that of alcohol abuse (Jang, Livesley, & Vernon, 1995). The development of AUDs and other SUDs is likely to operate through separate mechanisms (Chassin, Flora, & King, 2004; Zhou, King, & Chassin, 2006); thus, it is important that clinicians and researchers distinguish between the etiological pathways of AUDs and other SUDs.

Adoption and twin research suggest that transmission of substance abuse involves some genetic mediation (Hesselbrock, 1995; Kendler, Heath, Neale, Kessler, & Eaves, 1992; King, Burt, Malone, McGue, & Iacono, 2005). McGue, Iacono, Legrand, and Elkins (2001) found that early alcohol use is genetically heritable, at least in males. Additionally, the heritable influence of heavy drinking has been found to be relatively stable from late adolescence into young adulthood (King et al., 2005), a developmental transition period when environmental factors are hypothesized to begin to exert additional influences over genetic factors. Research also suggests that there are gender differences in the genetic transmission of SUDs, such that genetic factors may be more important for males than for females (King et al., 2005; McGue et al., 2001).

In addition to biological factors affecting the familial transmission of SUDs, the family environment plays a significant role in the etiology and development of SUDs. Familial transmission of alcoholism is posited to result from the function drinking serves within the family. For instance, nontransmitter families did not tolerate the "intrusion of intoxicated behavior" during family rituals, while transmitter families did not automatically and consistently reject the intoxicated family member from participating in family rituals (Steinglass, Bennett, Wolin, & Reiss, 1987, p. 321). Multiple studies also have found associations between parental behavior and children's problematic substance use. Not surprisingly, parental alcohol use is a strong predictor of children's alcohol use (Chassin, Pillow, Curran, Molina, & Barrera, 1993; Eitle, 2005; White, Johnson, & Buyske, 2000) and intentions to use alcohol (Tildesley & Andrews, 2008). Additionally, non-substance-related parental influences (such as monitoring or attachment) have been linked to offspring drinking behavior (van der Vorst, Engels, Meeus, Dekovic, & Vermulst, 2006; Wood, Read, Mitchell, & Brand, 2004). Although this chapter is on family models, it is useful to briefly discuss the importance of peer influences in the development of SUDs. Considerable research has indicated the importance of peer influences on substance use (e.g., Borsari & Carey, 2001). Of interest for this chapter, some investigators have shown mediating effects of familial factors on peer influence. For example, higher levels of parental involvement were shown to weaken the relationship between peer influences and alcohol use problems (Wood et al., 2004). While deficits in both perceived parental and peer support are associated with the development of substance abuse, only deficits in parental support predicted substance abuse when both sources of support were entered into a multivariate model, along with depressive symptoms and negative emotionality (Measelle, Stice, & Springer, 2006).

In summary, both genetic and environmental familial influences are important to the etiology and development of SUDs. While the complexities of such gene-by-environment interactions have yet to be fully elucidated, the evidence suggests the impact of genetic factors often is mediated by environmental factors (McGue et al., 2001; Walden, McGue, Iacono, Burt, & Elkins, 2004). Thus, it appears that to gain a comprehensive understanding of the etiological pathways of SUDs from a family models perspective, clinicians and researchers must consider the interaction of genetic and environmental influences, rather than merely summing the two sources.

Maintenance of Substance Abuse

Just as etiology is multiply determined, so is maintenance. In this chapter we adopt a cognitive–behavioral–systemic framework to describe factors that maintain drinking, regardless of etiological underpinnings. This model views maintenance as a complex interplay of environmental, biological, social, cognitive, and familial factors.

The cognitive–behavioral–systemic model of maintenance empha-sizes the role of family interaction patterns and problems as both anteced-ents and consequences of alcohol use. These family interactions maintain drinking both directly and indirectly, both intentionally and without the family's awareness of the process. Several basic assumptions are central to the model: (1) external antecedents to drinking have a lawful relationship to subsequent alcohol consumption, through repeated associations with reinforcement or anticipation of reinforcement; (2) cognitive and affec-tive events mediate the relationship between external antecedents and drinking; (3) drinking is maintained by physiological, psychological, and/ or interpersonal consequences; and (4) reciprocal interactions between the drinker and his or her environment determine repetitive, stressful intra- and interpersonal behavioral patterns (Epstein & McCrady, 2002; McCrady, 2001).

Antecedents to Use

Although a variety of antecedent events and stimuli may precede drink-ing, including individual, dyadic, or other factors, this chapter will focus specifically on familial antecedents to drinking. Specific spouse coping behaviors form one class of drinking antecedents. The three-factor model of spouses' coping styles discussed previously is one way to explain how spouse coping behaviors affect the alcoholic's drinking (described in Hur-com et al., 2000). Wives often withdraw from their drinking husbands because they believe withdrawal will encourage their husbands' abstinence, but empirical studies show that the opposite may be true, with assertive and engaged spouse coping styles correlated with reductions in the male spouse's drinking (Moos, Finney, & Cronkite, 1990; Orford et al., 1975). Qualitative research similarly has found that problem users see withdrawal and avoidance strategies on the part of family members to be unsupportive (Krishnan, Orford, Bradbury, Copello, & Velleman, 2001). Thus, family treatment programs should emphasize assertive but supportive communi-cation to address concerns about the drinking, rather than withdrawal.

A second class of familial antecedents is negative interactions. The cognitive–behavioral–systemic model of maintenance is based in part on a series of findings that alcoholic families are more negative, conflicted, and estranged than control families (Halford, Bouma, Kelly, & Young, 1999; Moos & Moos, 1984; Rotunda & O'Farrell, 1997). These negative familial qualities point to a series of interactional deficits that character-ize communication and behaviors in an alcoholic family. These negative interactions are a source of stress for alcoholic families, and probably serve as one antecedent to drinking and relapse. Interactional styles found to be characteristic of alcoholic families, such as demand–withdraw interac-tions (Shoham, Rohrbaugh, Stickle, & Jacob, 1998) and hostile or critical expressed emotion (O'Farrell, Hooley, Fals-Stewart, & Cutter, 1998), help perpetuate the drinking and problems in the relationship. Because lower initial marital satisfaction predicts poorer treatment outcomes (McCrady, Hayaki, Epstein, & Hirsch, 2002; Moos et al., 1990), it is important to understand the sources and patterns of dissatisfaction in the maintenance of alcoholism. The nonalcoholic spouse's criticism and disappointment, when directed at the alcoholic spouse, may lead to more marital distress, dissatisfaction and, ultimately, more drinking. Subsequently, a more severe drinking problem may lead to more expressed negative emotion as well as to a greater probability of relapse. Examples of family-level antecedents to substance use are presented in Figure 9.1.

Consequences of Use

The spouse and other family members may unwittingly supply positive consequences of drinking, for instance, by taking care of the intoxicated family member, pampering him or her when sick from drinking too much, or protecting the drinker from negative consequences (e.g., calling in sick for the drinker). As noted earlier, drinking often is associated with an increase in positive interactions. For example, in female alcoholic couples with nonalcoholic male partners, drinking appears to decrease conflict and regulate

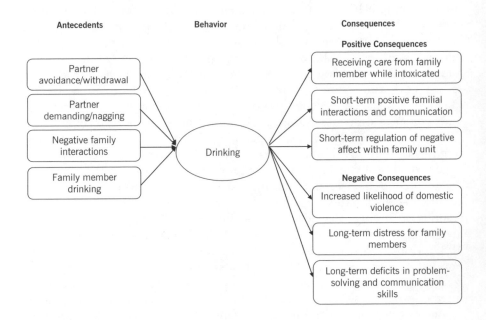

FIGURE 9.1. Example of drinking behavior chain from a cognitive–behavioral–systemic approach.

affect, a desirable consequence that reinforces and perpetuates drinking (Haber & Jacob, 1997).

Although families may provide positive consequences for drinking, drinking has major negative consequences for the family. Ultimately, awareness of these negative consequences could motivate a drinker to change. Marital violence is a serious negative consequence associated with AUDs that is influenced by the family system. Among a community sample of newlywed couples, the husband's drinking during the first year of marriage was found to predict marital violence in subsequent years (Quigley & Leonard, 2000). The highest levels of marital violence were seen in couples where the husband was a heavy drinker and the wife was not. Violence was not seen in couples where the wife was a heavy drinker and the husband was not. Acute alcohol consumption also has been linked to violent domestic conflicts (Leonard & Quigley, 1999; Murphy, Winters, Fals-Stewart, O'Farrell, & Murphy, 2005). In addition, increased rates of child abuse have been linked to problems with drugs and alcohol (Bays, 1990).

To summarize, the effect of alcohol on family and marital interaction is complex, but negative consequences are often quite prominent. Family members may avoid or criticize the drinker. In some cases, family members find it difficult to tolerate the drinking or the behavior of the intoxicated individual, and verbal or even physical assaults ensue. Typically, these negative consequences serve only to exacerbate the problem. Finally, since the alcoholic with a moderate to severe problem may spend an inordinate amount of time seeking, consuming, or recovering from the effects of alcohol, he or she typically is unable to contribute fully to the daily functioning of the household. Other family members must then take on more responsibilities, leading to increased resentment and stress. Reciprocal interactions between the drinker and his or her social environment typically tend to worsen drinking and drinking-related consequences over time, and dysfunctional patterns of individual and family interactions become overlearned and "automatic" through repetition. Families experiencing substance abuse also may be experiencing other individual and family problems. Examples of family-level consequences of substance use are presented in Figure 9.1.

Systemic Variables

According to family systems theories, the ways in which substance use preserves stability within the family unit contribute to the continued use of substances despite negative consequences. For example, alcohol- and nicotine-dependent individuals are more likely to communicate positively, make more problem-solving statements, and experience positive emotions with their partners when they are under the influence of alcohol or nicotine than when they are not under the influence of these substances (Frankenstein et al., 1985; Shoham, Butler, Rohrbaugh, & Trost, 2007). Substance use may have particularly strong, short-term positive effects on emotion regulation within family systems with multiple substance users (e.g., Rohrbaugh, Shoham, Butler, Hasler, & Berman, 2009).

At the same time, substance use is associated with poorer long-term family functioning and increased psychological distress for family members and romantic partners (Halford et al., 1999). Couples in which one or both partners has an alcohol or drug problem are more likely to have lower relationship satisfaction, deficits in problem-solving skills, negative communication patterns, and domestic violence (Jacob & Leonard, 1992; Keller, El-Sheikh, Keiley, & Liao, 2009; Kelly, Halford, & Young, 2002; Marshal, 2003).

The short-term positive and long-term negative consequences of substance use may interact in reciprocal patterns that serve to maintain substance use. For example, long-term substance use may cause relationship dissatisfaction and deficits in problem-solving skills, and substance use in turn may temporarily aid communication and dysregulated emotion and restore stability within the family system. In this manner, patterns of substance use are maintained by short-term positive consequences to the family while proliferating long-term problems that may subsequently serve as antecedents to substance use.

Relationship between Substance Abuse and Other Psychopathology

Rates of comorbid psychopathology are elevated in substance-abusing populations. Estimates of lifetime drug use disorders comorbid with alcohol dependence are as high as 80% (Carroll, 1986; Ross, Glaser, & Germanson, 1988). In general population studies, estimates of co-occurring personality disorders are about 28–29% for persons with AUDs and 47–48% among those with other SUDs (Burckell & McMain, 2008). In studies of clinical populations, estimates range widely from as low as 2% to as high as 84% (Burckell & McMain, 2008). Borderline personality disorders are more common in females with SUDs; antisocial personality disorders are more often comorbid with SUDs in males. Estimated comorbidity of mood disorders among those with SUDs in the general population range from 19–34% for major depression, with lower rates for other mood disorders (Goldstein, 2008). Comorbidity rates are higher in clinical samples, with estimates ranging from 18–54% for major depression (Goldstein, 2008). Rates of comorbidity between SUDs and anxiety disorders in population samples are estimated at 10–23% for phobias, 4–9% for panic disorder, and 9% for generalized anxiety disorder (GAD; Goldstein, 2008). In clinical samples, estimates of co-occurring anxiety disorders and SUDs range widely, from 0.1–32% for GAD, 2–20% for social phobia, 1–19% for panic disorders, 3–7% for simple phobias (Goldstein, 2008), and up to 50% for posttraumatic stress disorders (Ouimette, Coolhart, Funderburk, Wade, & Brown, 2007).

Most major theoretical models of family and addictions are silent about the relations among psychopathology, substance use, and family functioning. However, since family systems models view psychopathological symptoms as serving particular functions in the family interaction, the presence of more than one form of psychopathology would not inherently be conceptualized differently from the presence of one form of psychopathology. Thus, any psychopathological symptoms would be viewed similarly as having the functions of maintaining family identity and homeostatic balance and expressing dysfunctional interactions and structures within the family.

Most research on the relations among family functioning, SUDs, and comorbid psychopathology has focused on individuals with or without comorbid antisocial personality (ASP) characteristics. For example, Jacob and colleagues (Jacob, Leonard, & Haber, 2001; Jacob, Haber, Leonard, & Rushe, 2000) found that families with one member who had an AUD and who also was high on ASP characteristics were less positive and less instrumental in their communications. These families also expressed more negativity when the alcoholic member was drinking, with more of the spouse negativity being a contingent response to the drinker's negative communications. Ichiyama, Zucker, Fitzgerald, and Bingham (1996) examined how men with AUDs and ASP characteristics viewed themselves in their intimate relationship, and found that people with high ASP characteristics were more likely than others to trust their wives less, blame them more, and view their wives as sulking in response to their husband's blame.

In one of the few studies to examine the impact of family-based treatment on persons with SUDs and co-occurring disorders, McCrady, Epstein, Cook, Hildebrandt, and Jensen (2009) found more positive drinking outcomes for women with AUDs who had co-occurring Axis I or Axis II disorders if they received conjoint therapy rather than individual therapy. McCrady et al. (2009) did not probe the possible mechanisms by which conjoint treatment effected better outcomes with these populations, but it may be that intimate partners learned a generalized set of skills to support the women in dealing with individual problems, that changes in the intimate relationship had a positive impact on individual problems, or that shifts in the family system decreased the need for dysfunctional symptoms in general.

In summary, both Axis I and Axis II disorders commonly occur with SUDs, particularly in clinical populations, but family theoretical models have not developed an explicit way to conceptualize the complex interactions among these different domains of presenting problems. Family models have been used in treatment for a range of other types of psychopathology (e.g., mood disorders, anxiety disorders, schizophrenia), and some research suggests that although the presence of certain co-occurring disorders may imply greater family dysfunction, family-based treatments may still be appropriate and efficacious. However, despite a lack of conceptual models and a strong evidence base, clinicians still need to be cognizant of the high comorbidity rates between SUDs and other Axis I and Axis II psychopathologies, as well as the need to assess for and treat these other disorders.

Impact of Family Involvement on Treatment Engagement and Outcomes

A number of randomized clinical trials have provided evidence that partner- and/or family-involved treatments are equally or more efficacious compared to individually involved treatments in improving substance use, domestic violence, and relationship satisfaction. Family-involved treatment modalities also may provide a unique benefit for improving treatment engagement for identified clients.

Behavioral couple therapy (BCT) has been shown to be more efficacious than individual behavior therapy at reducing the frequency and intensity of drug and alcohol use and increasing the length of abstinence periods (Fals-Stewart, O'Farrell, & Birchler, 2001;[1] McCrady et al., 2009; McCrady, Noel, Abrams, & Stout, 1986; McCrady, Stout, Noel, & Abrams, 1991; O'Farrell, Cutter, Choquette, & Floyd, 1992). Couple therapy may be effective for males and females, patients in heterosexual and same-sex relationships, and criminal-justice-referred patients (Fals-Stewart, Birchler, & O'Farrell, 1996; Fals-Stewart, O'Farrell, & Lam, 2009; McCrady et al., 2009; Winters, Fals-Stewart, O'Farrell, Kelley, & Birchler, 2002).

In addition to improving substance-using outcomes, BCT has been shown to be more efficacious than individual-focused therapies at improving relationship satisfaction, enhancing family and child functioning, and decreasing domestic violence (Fals-Stewart, Kashdan, O'Farrell, & Birchler, 2002; Kelley & Fals-Stewart, 2002; McCrady et al., 1986; McCrady et al., 1991; O'Farrell, Murphy, Stephan, Murphy, & Fals-Stewart, 2004).

A meta-analysis of 12 randomized clinical trials with 754 couples found favorable results for behavioral couple therapy compared to individual-based therapy for the treatment of AUDs and other SUDs (Powers, Vedel, & Emmelkamp, 2008). The results of this meta-analysis showed that BCT produced better results with medium effect sizes at follow-up for

---

[1]Questions have been raised about the validity of research on BCT supported by grants to William Fals-Stewart as Principal Investigator (see *www.ag.ny.gov/media_center/2010/feb/feb16a_10.html*). However, even without Fals-Stewart's published studies, the body of work supporting BCT is very strong.

relationship satisfaction (d = 0.51), drinking frequency (d = 0.50), and negative consequences from drinking (d = 0.50).

Evidence suggests that BCT is particularly efficacious at maintaining changes in substance use and relationship satisfaction for longer periods of time compared to individual-based treatment. Whereas abstinence rates generally decrease over the first year after receiving individual-based treatment, abstinence rates tend to decrease more slowly or not at all after receiving BCT (Fals-Stewart, Birchler, & Kelley, 2006; McCrady et al., 2009; Powers et al., 2008). Evidence supporting the long-term effects of BCT is generally consistent. However, one study has found that the incremental effect of BCT compared to individual therapy diminished over time (O'Farrell et al., 1992). Additional work has suggested that family-involved relapse prevention sessions delivered after treatment may provide small incremental benefits by reducing the length of subsequent relapse episodes (McCrady, Epstein, & Hirsch, 1999) and by increasing the use of Antabuse contracts (O'Farrell, Choquette, & Cutter, 1998), but the incremental effect of relapse prevention on frequency of abstinent days has been mixed (McCrady et al., 1999; O'Farrell, Choquette, et al., 1998). Individuals with Axis I or Axis II diagnoses, lower baseline relationship satisfaction, or demand–withdraw communication patterns with their partners may be most likely to fare better in spouse-involved than individual treatment (McCrady et al., 2009; Shoham et al., 1998).

Family-involved treatments may offer unique opportunities for engaging clients in therapy. In a study of men entering treatment for an AUD, about half of the clients said their spouses and/or family members were a major reason for entering treatment, with this being the most commonly reported motive (Steinberg, Epstein, McCrady, & Hirsch, 1997). Relationship problems are relatively common among people with SUDs and thus engaging clients into treatment by first focusing on relationship problems may be helpful for some clients who are resistant to entering treatment for substance use problems (McCrady et al., 1986).

Family members also may motivate clients to enter treatment by arranging environmental antecedents and consequences to change reinforcement patterns for substance use or by changing their communication with the identified patient. Community reinforcement and family training (CRAFT; Smith & Meyers, 2004) trains family members of treatment-refusers to disrupt the patterns that maintain substance use. Strategies include introducing enjoyable outside activities to compete with substance use, improving positive interpersonal exchanges with the identified client, and avoiding interfering with the naturally occurring negative consequences of substance use. A meta-analysis of four randomized clinical trials showed that CRAFT was more effective at getting identified clients to enter substance abuse treatment than Johnson Institute interventions or Al-Anon involvement, and led to greater improvements in psychological well-being for concerned family members (Roozen, de Waart, & van der Kroft, 2010).

Finally, family-involved treatments may be particularly useful for youth with heavy drug involvement. In two randomized clinical trials comparing multidimensional family therapy (MST) to individual cognitive-behavioral therapy with ethnically diverse drug-using adolescents, adolescents with less drug use had similar outcomes between the individual- and family-based interventions, but heavier drug-using adolescents had better outcomes in the family-based intervention than in the individual-based intervention (Henderson, Dakof, Greenbaum, & Liddle, 2010).

Therapeutic Tasks Required for Treatment to Be Successful

Clinicians often need to be flexible in planning and sequencing therapy. Therapeutic plans may involve a dynamic interplay among different levels of intervention at different points in the therapy. There are at least three different reasons to involve families in treatment: (1) to help the user change his or her substance use, (2) to change family members' own behavior and patterns of coping, and (3) to modify dysfunctional patterns of interaction. As reviewed in the previous section, empirical studies support treatment interventions in each of these domains.

Several family-involved therapeutic tasks may help the individual change his or her substance use. The first family role may be to foster treatment engagement. Family members may be engaged in treatment prior to the user, as in unilateral family therapy (Thomas & Ager, 1993) or the CRAFT model (Smith & Meyers, 2004). A second family therapeutic role may be in facilitating therapeutic compliance. Here, behavioral-contracting procedures appear to be particularly effective, both for treatment attendance and for compliance with medication. A third family role is to assist in user-focused cognitive-behavioral treatment. During treatment, the family provides valuable information to help identify antecedent stimuli for use, mediating variables, and consequences of use. Family members may play an active role in helping the user identify high-risk situations, cognitions and affects associated with use, and positive and negative consequences of use.

In individually focused treatment, behavioral techniques may be used to achieve abstinence or nonproblem use, and pharmacological adjuncts may be considered as well. Family members also play an important role in effecting change in substance use by learning about necessary individual change efforts, and ways to support and participate in these changes.

Treatment also may focus on the individual difficulties of family members. At times, family members may be sufficiently distressed that they need separate treatment. However, the distress of family members often is linked directly to the active substance use, and will abate as the use decreases or stops. Family members also may have dysfunctional coping styles, so another task of treatment is to facilitate the development of more effective coping responses such as reacting to the substance use rather than the user, being assertive and clear in reactions to the use, decreasing control behaviors, and detaching from alcohol- or drug-related interactions.

The third major area of therapeutic work involves modifying patterns of family interaction; improving communication and problem-solving skills; and considering family themes, rules, and roles that interfere with effective family functioning. Specific family problems, such as financial, child, or sexual problems, may serve as antecedents to alcohol or drug use, and may respond to direct family-level interventions. In addition, recent research has identified several patterns of interaction that appear particularly toxic, including polarized demand–withdrawal interactions and hostile and critical expressed emotion from family members (O'Farrell, Hooley, et al., 1998). The clinician also is challenged to identify ways in which alcohol or other substance use may serve to stabilize family interactions, for example, by decreasing negative interactions (particularly in women and in certain subtypes of alcoholics), or by facilitating regulation and dampening down of negative affect. Modification of family interactions to facilitate more effective means of dealing with intense affect in the family may be a particularly crucial family-level intervention.

Finally, there is a high probability of some level of physical aggression in families where a member is abusing alcohol or drugs. Therapists must address this issue through a direct assessment, development of appropriate safety plans, and utilization of effective treatments for domestic violence.

Mechanisms of Behavior Change

Family Systems Therapies

Family systems models typically focus on ways that family system dynamics influence environmental antecedents, consequences, and cognitions related to substance use. For example, substances may be used to cope with disturbances to the homeostasis of the family unit when poor coping skills may prevent adaptive, non-substance-using behaviors. Additionally, misperceived substance-using norms and low self-efficacy to refuse substance use within the social system may perpetuate substance-use behavior (Moos, 2007).

One hypothesized mechanism of behavior change in family systems therapies for adolescents is the increase in parental monitoring of adolescent activities. Greater parental monitoring is thought to decrease adolescents' affiliation with substance-using peers and subsequently reduce their substance use. One study has supported parental monitoring as a mediator of change in MST (Henderson, Rowe, Dakof, Hawes, & Liddle, 2009).

Similarly, treatment effects for multisystemic therapy, a systems-based therapy shown to reduce delinquent behavior among adolescents, have been shown to be mediated by improved family cohesion, family functioning, parental monitoring, and decreased affiliation with delinquent peers (Huey, Henggeler, Brondino, & Pickrel, 2000). Self-efficacy to resist smoking in social situations also may be an important mediator of change for adolescents (Bricker et al., 2010), and efforts to increase self-efficacy in social situations may be incorporated into family systems treatment models. These findings suggest that family systems can influence social affiliation and social cognition, which may be a particularly important target for evoking change with adolescents.

SUD treatments that draw on family systems theories have most commonly been used to treat adolescent substance abuse. With adult populations, treatments based on family systems theories typically have focused on larger social networks rather than just families. Research has consistently provided evidence that quantity of substance use with adults is positively correlated with substance use among families and social network members (Beattie, 2001; Broome, Simpson, & Joe, 2002; Groh, Jason, Davis, Ferrari, & Olson, 2007; Litt, Kadden, Kabela-Cormier, & Petry, 2009; Manuel, McCrady, Epstein, Cook, & Tonigan, 2007; McAweeney, Zucker, Fitzgerald, Puttler, & Wong, 2005; Velleman, 2006; Warren, Stein, & Grella, 2007). Research on social system-based treatment has shown that change in social network composition, for example, by becoming more involved with AA, is a mediating factor between the treatment and substance use outcomes (Groh, Jason, & Keys, 2008; Litt et al., 2009).

In general, however, linkages between family systems variables and substance use behavior have mostly been established in studies using non-mediational designs. Thus, further work is necessary to test these variables within meditational frameworks to determine which family systems components may be mechanisms of change and to specify how they may cause change.

Behavioral Couple Therapy for AUDs

Behavioral couple therapy for AUDs (ABCT) draws from three major theoretical perspectives: (1) cognitive-behavioral models that conceptualize drinking as a learned behavior; (2) interactional models that conceptualize drinking as occurring in and influenced by social–interpersonal systems, and (3) social exchange models. This theoretical framework conceptualizes relationships in terms of the balance of and exchange of reinforcers in the relationship (as described in McCrady's section of Longabaugh et al., 2005). The model articulates changes in identified client-, partner-, and dyad-level behaviors as necessary mechanisms by which the treatment works. Figure 9.2 summarizes the hypothesized mechanisms of change in ABCT.

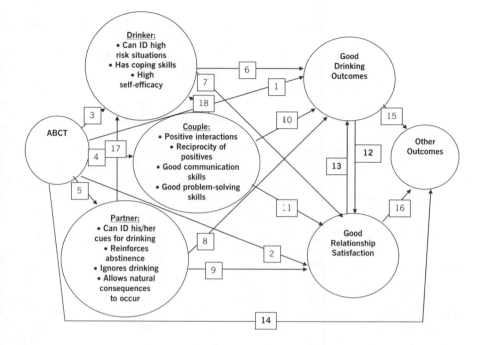

FIGURE 9.2. Hypothesized mechanisms of change in ABCT. Adapted from Long-abaugh et al. (2005). Adapted with permission.

At the level of the identified client, ABCT should lead to a greater ability to identify high-risk situations, better skills to cope with these high-risk situations, and greater self-efficacy to use these coping skills. Hunter-Reel, McCrady, and Hildebrandt (2009) have proposed that social support in general, and partner support in particular, may contribute to these mechanisms of behavior change at the level of the identified client. Pathways 17 and 18 in Figure 9.2 show the general hypothesized relationships between partner- and couple-level skills and identified client mechanisms of change.

At the partner level, ABCT should result in greater partner ability to identify behaviors that may serve as cues for drinking, better skills to cope with drinking-related high-risk situations, better skills to support the drinker's efforts at change, more frequent reinforcement of abstinence, and less attention to drinking. In general, ABCT should result in increases in partner support for change and decreases in partner support for drinking.

At the couple level, ABCT should result in a greater frequency of positive interactions, greater positive reciprocity in interactions, increased positive and supportive communication in the dyad, decreased negative communication, and better problem-solving skills.

There is support for most components of the ABCT model, both in the impact of ABCT on individual- and couple-level skills, and in the impact of these skills on treatment outcome. There is good evidence that ABCT leads to positive drinking and relationship outcomes (Figure 9.2, pathways 1 and 2). No research has examined the impact of ABCT on drinker coping skills (pathway 3), so there also are no data about the relations between drinker coping skills and either drinking or relationship functioning outcomes (pathways 6 and 7).

O'Farrell, Choquette, et al. (1998) have reported some evidence suggesting a positive impact of ABCT on partner coping, specifically reinforcement of abstinence (pathway 5), but less research has focused on other aspects of partner coping skills. The limited research on the relations between partner coping and outcomes suggests that partner reinforcement of abstinence (pathway 8) is associated with better drinking outcomes, but no research has examined the relations between partner coping and relationship outcomes (Figure 9.2, pathway 9).

Evidence suggests that ABCT leads to increases in positive interactions in couples (McCrady et al., 1991) (pathway 4). Data suggest a positive relation between couple-level behaviors and drinking outcomes, specifically finding that positive interactions and reciprocal positive interactions both are associated with better drinking outcomes (e.g., McCrady et al., 2002) (pathway 10). However, no study has examined the relations between changes in couple behaviors and relationship satisfaction (pathway 11).

Two other major research approaches have contributed to understanding how ABCT works. First, O'Farrell et al. (2004) looked at the sequencing of change to determine whether ABCT is effective because it leads first to reduced drinking, which then positively impacts relationship functioning, or because ABCT leads first to improved relationship functioning, which leads to improvements in drinking. O'Farrell et al. (2004) found fairly strong support for the hypothesis that improved relationship functioning leads to improvements in drinking (pathway 12), with some evidence suggesting that the reciprocal relation is also true but weaker (pathway 13). In contrast, McCrady, Epstein, and Kahler (2004) looked at the relation between relationship satisfaction and drinking after ABCT. They reported a strong concurrent relation between the two variables, but did not find either that relationship satisfaction predicted subsequent drinking in the next 3 months, or that drinking predicted relationship satisfaction. Second, recent research has examined the impact of ABCT on other outcomes, such as domestic violence, child well-being, and behaviors that increase risk for HIV infection. Available evidence (Kelley & Fals-Stewart, 2002; O'Farrell et al., 2004) suggests that couples show significant decreases in domestic violence after ABCT and that child well-being increases (pathway 14). It seems that decreased drinking and improved relationship satisfaction both contribute to improvements in violence and child functioning (pathways 15 and 16).

Advantages and Disadvantages of a Family-Based Approach

There are several advantages to a family-based approach to conceptualizing and treating substance use disorders. Most important is the strong empirical base for the theoretical models and for treatments derived from family models. Family models also direct the theoretician's attention to the environmental contexts in which alcohol and other drug use occur, and direct the clinician to consider maintaining factors beyond the individual. Family involvement is associated with better engagement, greater compliance with treatment, and better treatment outcome. There is clear evidence that family-based models result in decreases in intimate partner violence (e.g., O'Farrell et al., 2004), and preliminary evidence that child functioning is improved when couples participate in conjoint alcohol or drug treatment. By directing attention to the family, the clinician increases the probability that the identified client will comply with treatment and have a successful outcome. In addition, ample research supports the negative impact that substance use has on the functioning of the rest of the family; thus involving the family in treatment may ease familial distress. Family models provide a framework for conceptualizing the interrelationships between substance use and family functioning, and can be used as a guide for treatment with any part of the family that is available for treatment.

One disadvantage of family models is their greater complexity, both conceptually and in the delivery of the treatments. Theoreticians must account for multiple interactive relationships, and clinicians must be able to attend to the complexities inherent in dealing with several individuals and the interactions among them. Thus, working with families requires specialized skills and training that many frontline clinicians may not have, and they also may feel intimidated by the complexity of the treatment. Clinicians and treatment programs that use a family-based model also must be able to provide flexible clinical hours to accommodate family schedules, and may have difficulty in obtaining third-party reimbursement for family-based services. Additionally, behavioral and systemic family models, which give primacy to treatment that includes more than one patient in the room, are not consistent with disease model-based treatment, which emphasizes the primacy of individual change prior to any treatment that might involve family members.

Family models also have some limits from a theoretical perspective. The models lack a conceptualization of the limits of family treatment. The models do not address the complexities introduced by families with multiple substance-abusing members, families with members who have other kinds of psychopathology, or families characterized by an extremely high degree of disorganization or destructive interactions. The models also give no explicit attention to the relative importance of the needs of various family members. For example, although the presence of a supportive spouse might increase the probability of a successful treatment outcome, continuing in a relationship might have adverse consequences for the non-substance-abusing partner. Family models also have no explicit theory to facilitate decision making about the focus of intervention (e.g., individual, familial, or other social systems).

Conclusion

A large body of evidence has consistently demonstrated bidirectional associations between substance use and family factors. In one direction, substance use influences positive and negative consequences to the family unit such as short-term improvements in communication and affect regulation, long-term decreases in relationship satisfaction, and an increased likelihood of domestic violence and child abuse. In the other direction, substance use may arise from antecedents involving family members such as conflict, withdrawal strategies, or expressed emotion.

The relationship between substance use and family factors is most commonly explained by three non-mutually-exclusive family models that each focus on somewhat different components and levels of interaction. Family systems models focus on the function of substance use within the family system and how substance use maintains homeostasis for the family system; family behavioral models focus on how family members' behavior and interactions create or modify antecedents and consequences to substance use; and family disease models focus on codependence within other family members and how this may lead to substance use through behaviors such as enabling.

It is important to note that family systems do not exist in isolation, but instead are embedded within a larger network of community, societal, and cultural systems. While most family research in the substance abuse field has focused on the isolated family system, it is important to consider how each of these larger systems may influence the context of the family system. Family structures and functions may vary cross-culturally, and while these differences do not preclude the use of a family approach to SUD treatment, it is important that these factors are attended to by clinicians and researchers alike. For example, families in collectivist and Latino cultures may differ structurally from families in individualist and Caucasian cultures by incorporating more extended family members into the family system. They may likewise differ functionally by placing greater importance on sacrificing one's individual needs to attend to the needs of the family unit. Thus, the interrelationships among the identified client, the family system, and substance use may vary due to the larger context of the cultural system. Cross-cultural differences may be further complicated within family models when the boundaries of what constitutes a family become less clear. For example, an immigrant with no biological family in his or her country of residence may adopt a secondary "family" of other people with a similar background while still maintaining contact with his or her biological family. In this case, the distinction of who is and is not considered to be a part of the family system becomes blurred, which can complicate family models of SUD treatment. Further care also must be taken to understand how acculturating to the values of the new culture may impact the individual's relationships with his or her original and secondary family, and how this may impact substance use within a family model.

The bidirectional manner in which substance use and family functioning affect one another suggests that incorporating family members into treatment may provide additional benefit to identified clients and their family members. Several randomized clinical trials have shown that family member involvement leads to better substance use outcomes that are longer lasting compared to individual treatment, and that clients and family members also experience improvements in relationship satisfaction, domestic violence, and child functioning. These data suggest a significant advantage for the use of family-based treatment approaches to SUD treatment, particularly when there are relationship problems, mild or moderate domestic violence, or the identified client is reluctant to engage in treatment. Current models hypothesize that better substance use outcomes are mediated by improvements in family functioning and family cohesion. While there is some preliminary evidence to support this hypothesis, future work is necessary to better understand the specific factors within family therapies that contribute to changes in substance use.

Acknowledgments

Preparation of this chapter was supported in part by Grant Nos. R37 AA07070 and T32 AA018108 from the National Institute on Alcohol Abuse and Alcoholism.

References

Alcoholics Anonymous. (1976). *Alcoholics Anonymous: The story of how many thousands of men and women have recovered from alcoholism* (3rd ed.). New York: Alcoholics Anonymous World Services.

Bays, J. (1990). Substance abuse and child abuse: Impact of addiction on the child. *Pediatric Clinics of North America, 37*(4), 881–904.

Beattie, M. (1987). *Co-dependent no more*. Minneapolis, MN: Hazelden.

Beattie, M. C. (2001). Meta-analysis of social relationships and posttreatment drinking outcomes: Comparison of relationship structure, function and quality. *Journal of Studies on Alcohol, 62*(4), 518–527.

Beattie, M.C., & Longabaugh, R. (1997). Interpersonal factors and post-treatment drinking and subjective wellbeing. *Addiction, 92*, 1507–1521.

Becker, J. V., & Miller, P. M. (1976). Verbal and nonverbal marital interaction patterns of alcoholics and nonalcoholics. *Journal of Studies on Alcohol, 37*, 1616–1624.

Billings, A. G., Kessler, M., Gomberg, C. A., & Weiner, S. (1979). Marital conflict resolution of alcoholic and nonalcoholic couples during drinking and non-drinking sessions. *Journal of Studies on Alcohol, 40*, 183–195.

Black, C. (1982). *It will never happen to me!* Denver: M.A.C.

Borsari, B., & Carey, K. (2001). Peer influences on college drinking: A review of the research. *Journal of Substance Abuse, 13(4)*, 391–424.

Bricker, J. B., Liu, J., Comstock, B. A., Peterson, A. V., Kealey, K. A., & Marek, P. M. (2010). Social cognitive mediators of adolescent smoking cessation: Results from a large randomized intervention trial. *Psychology of Addictive Behaviors, 24(3)*, 436–445.

Broome, K. M., Simpson, D. D., & Joe, G. W. (2002). The role of social support following short-term inpatient treatment. *American Journal on Addictions, 11(1)*, 57–65.

Burckell, L. A., & McMain, S. (2008). Concurrent personality disorders and substance use disorders in women. In K. T. Brady, S. E. Back, & S. F. Greenfield (Eds.), *Women and addiction: A comprehensive handbook* (pp. 269–285). New York: Guilford Press.

Carroll, J. F. X. (1986). Treating multiple substance abuse clients. *Recent Developments in Alcoholism, 4*, 85–103.

Carson, A. T., & Baker, R. C. (1994). Psychological correlates of codependency in women. *International Journal of the Addictions, 29*, 395–407.

Cermak, T. (1986). *Diagnosing and treating co-dependence.* Minneapolis: Johnson Institute Books.

Chassin, L., Flora, D., & King, K. M. (2004). Trajectories of alcohol and drug use and dependence from adolescence to adulthood: The effects of familial alcoholism and personality. *Journal of Abnormal Psychology, 113*, 483–498.

Chassin, L., Pillow, D., Curran, P., Molina, B., & Barrera, M. (1993). Relation of parental alcoholism to early adolescent substance use: A test of three mediating mechanisms. *Journal of Abnormal Psychology, 102*, 3–19.

Corder, B. F., Corder, R. F., & Laidlaw, N. D. (1972). An intensive treatment program for alcoholics and their wives. *Quarterly Journal of Studies on Alcohol, 33*, 1144–1146.

Cork, M. (1969). *The forgotten children.* Toronto: Addiction Research Foundation.

Davis, D. I., Berenson, D., Steinglass, P., & Davis, S. (1974). The adaptive consequences of drinking. *Psychiatry, 37*, 209–215.

Dunn, N. J., Jacob, T., Hummon, N., & Seilhamer, R. A. (1987). Marital stability in alcoholic-spouse relationships as a function of drinking pattern and location. *Journal of Abnormal Psychology, 96*, 99–107.

Eitle, D. (2005). The moderating effects of peer substance use on the family structure–adolescent substance use association: Quantity versus quality of parenting. *Addictive Behaviors, 30*, 963–980.

Epstein, E. E., & McCrady, B. S. (2002). Couple therapy in the treatment of alcohol problems. In A. S. Gurman & N. S. Jacobson (Eds.), *Clinical handbook of couple therapy* (3rd ed., pp. 597–628). New York: Guilford Press.

Fals-Stewart, W., Birchler, G. R., & Kelley, M. L. (2006). Learning sobriety together: A randomized clinical trial examining behavioral couples therapy with alcoholic female patients. *Journal of Consulting and Clinical Psychology, 74*(3), 579–591.

Fals-Stewart, W., Birchler, G. R., & O'Farrell, T. J. (1996). Behavioral couples therapy for male substance-abusing patients: Effects on relationship adjustment and drug-using behavior. *Journal of Consulting and Clinical Psychology, 64*(5), 959–972.

Fals-Stewart, W., Kashdan, T. B., O'Farrell, T. J., & Birchler, G. R. (2002). Behavioral couples therapy for drug-abusing patients: Effects on partner violence. *Journal of Substance Abuse Treatment, 22*(2), 87–96.

Fals-Stewart, W., O'Farrell, T. J., & Birchler, G. R. (2001). Behavioral couples therapy for male methadone maintenance patients: Effects on drug-using behavior and relationship adjustment. *Behavior Therapy, 32*(2), 391–411.

Fals-Stewart, W., O'Farrell, T. J., & Lam, W. K. K. (2009). Behavioral couple therapy for gay and lesbian couples with alcohol use disorders. *Journal of Substance Abuse Treatment, 37*(4), 379–387.

Frankenstein, W., Hay, W. M., & Nathan, P. E. (1985). Effects of intoxication on alcoholics' marital communication and problem solving. *Journal of Studies on Alcohol, 46*(1), 1–6.

Frankenstein, W., Nathan, P. E., Sullivan, R. F., Hay, W. M., & Cocco, K. (1985). Asymmetry of influence in alcoholics' marital communication: Alcohol's effects on interaction dominance. *Journal of Marital and Family Therapy, 11*, 399–411.

Goldstein, R. B. (2008). Comorbidity of substance use disorders with independent mood and anxiety disorders in women: Results from the National Epidemiologic Survey on Alcohol and Related Conditions. In K. T. Brady, S. E. Back, & S. F. Greenfield (Eds.), *Women and addiction: A comprehensive handbook* (pp. 173–192). New York: Guilford Press.

Groh, D. R., Jason, L. A., Davis, M. I., Ferrari, J. R., & Olson, B. D. (2007). Friends, family, and alcohol abuse: An examination of general and alcohol-specific social support. *American Journal on Addictions, 16*(1), 49–55.

Groh, D. R., Jason, L. A., & Keys, C. B. (2008). Social network variables in Alcoholics Anonymous: A literature review. *Clinical Psychology Review, 28*(3), 430–450.

Haber, J. R., & Jacob, T. (1997). Marital interactions of male versus female alcoholics. *Family Process, 36*, 385–402.

Hajema, K. J., & Knibbe, R. A. (1998). Research report: Changes in social roles as predictors of changes in drinking. *Addiction, 93*, 1717–1727.

Halford, W. K., Bouma, R., Kelly, A., & Young, R. M. (1999). Individual psychopathology and marital distress: Analyzing the association and implications. *Behavior Modification, 23*(2), 179–216.

Havassy, B. E., Hall, S. M., & Wasserman, D. A. (1991). Social support and relapse: Commonalities among alcoholics, opiate users and cigarette smokers. *Addictive Behaviors, 16*, 235–246.

Henderson, C. E., Dakof, G. A., Greenbaum, P. E., & Liddle, H. A. (2010). Effectiveness of multidimensional family therapy with higher severity substance-abusing adolescents: Report from two randomized controlled trials. *Journal of Consulting and Clinical Psychology, 78*(6), 885–897.

Henderson, C. E., Rowe, C. L., Dakof, G. A., Hawes, S. W., & Liddle, H. A. (2009). Parenting practices as mediators of treatment effects in an early-intervention trial of multidimensional family therapy. *American Journal of Drug and Alcohol Abuse, Research Translation, 35*(4), 220–226.

Hersen, M., Miller, P. M., & Eisler, R. M. (1973). Interactions between alcoholics and their wives: A descriptive analysis of verbal and nonverbal behavior. *Quarterly Journal of Studies on Alcohol, 34,* 516–520.

Hesselbrock, V. (1995). The genetic epidemiology of alcoholism. In H. Begleiter & B. Kissin (Eds.), *The genetics of alcoholism* (pp. 17–39). New York: Oxford University Press.

Hill, S. (1994). Etiology. In J. Langenbucher, B. McCrady, W. Frankenstein, & P. Nathan (Eds.), *Annual review of addictions research and treatment* (Vol. 3, pp. 127–148). Elmsford, NY: Pergamon Press.

Huey, S. J., Henggeler, S. W., Brondino, M. J., & Pickrel, S. G. (2000). Mechanisms of change in multisystemic therapy: Reducing delinquent behavior through therapist adherence and improved family and peer functioning. *Journal of Consulting and Clinical Psychology, 68*(3), 451–467.

Hunter-Reel, D., McCrady, B. S., & Hildebrandt, T. (2009). Emphasizing interpersonal factors: An extension of the Witkiewitz and Marlatt relapse model. *Addiction, 104,* 1281–1290.

Hurcom, C., Copello, A., & Orford, J. (2000). The family and alcohol: Effects of excessive drinking and conceptualizations of spouses over recent decades. *Substance Use and Misuse, 35,* 473–502.

Ichiyama, M. A., Zucker, R. A., Fitzgerald, H. E., & Bingham, C. R. (1996). Articulating subtype differences in self and relational experience among alcoholic men using structural analysis of social behavior. *Journal of Consulting and Clinical Psychology, 64,* 1245–1254.

Jackson, J. (1954). The adjustment of the family to the crisis of alcoholism. *Quarterly Journal of Studies on Alcohol, 15,* 562–586.

Jacob, T., Dunn, N. J., & Leonard, K. (1983). Patterns of alcohol abuse and family stability. *Alcoholism: Clinical and Experimental Research, 7,* 382–385.

Jacob, T., Haber, J. R., Leonard, K. E., & Rushe, R. (2000). Home interactions of high and low antisocial male alcoholics and their families. *Journal of Studies on Alcohol, 61,* 72–80.

Jacob, T., & Leonard, K. (1992). Sequential analysis of marital interactions involving alcoholic, depressed, and nondistressed men. *Journal of Abnormal Psychology, 101*(4), 647–656.

Jacob, T., Leonard, K. E., & Haber, J. R. (2001). Family interactions of alcoholics as related to alcoholism type and drinking conditions. *Alcoholism: Clinical and Experimental Research, 25,* 835–843.

Jacob, T., Ritchey, D., Cvitkovic, J. F., & Blane, H. T. (1981). Communication styles of alcoholic and nonalcoholic families when drinking and not drinking. *Journal of Studies on Alcohol, 42,* 466–482.

Jang, K. L., Livesley, W. J., & Vernon, P. A. (1995). Alcohol and drug problems: A multivariate behavioural genetic analysis of co-morbidity. *Addiction, 90,* 1213–1221.

Keller, P. S., El-Sheikh, M., Keiley, M., & Liao, P. (2009). Longitudinal relations between marital aggression and alcohol problems. *Psychology of Addictive Behaviors, 23*(1), 2–13.

Kelley, M. L., & Fals-Stewart, W. (2002). Couples- versus individual-based therapy for alcohol and drug abuse: Effects on children's psychosocial functioning. *Journal of Consulting and Clinical Psychology, 70*(2), 417–427.

Kelly, A. B., Halford, W. K., & Young, R. M. (2002). Couple communication and female problem drinking: A behavioral observation study. *Psychology of Addictive Behaviors, 16*(3), 269–271.

Kendler, K. S., Heath, A. C., Neale, M. C., Kessler, R. C., & Eaves, L. C. (1992). A population-based twin study of alcoholic women. *Journal of the American Medical Association, 14*, 1877–1882.

King, S. M., Burt, A., Malone, S.M., McGue, M., & Iacono, W. G. (2005). Etiological contributions to heavy drinking from late adolescence to young adulthood. *Journal of Abnormal Psychology, 114*, 587–598.

Kogan, K. L., & Jackson, J. (1965). Stress, personality and emotional disturbance in wives of alcoholics. *Quarterly Journal of Studies on Alcohol, 26*, 486–495.

Krishnan, M., Orford, J., Bradbury, C., Copello, A., & Velleman, R. (2001). Drug and alcohol problems: The user's perspective on family members' coping. *Drug and Alcohol Review, 20*, 385–393.

Leonard, K. E., & Jacob, T. (1997). Sequential interactions among episodic and steady alcoholics and their wives. *Psychology of Addictive Behaviors, 11*, 18–25.

Leonard, K. E., & Quigley, B. M. (1999). Drinking and marital aggression in newlyweds: An event-based analysis of drinking and the occurrence of husband marital aggression. *Journal of Studies on Alcohol, 60*, 537–545.

Lewis, M. L. (1937). Alcoholism and family casework. *Social Casework, 35*, 8–14.

Litt, M. D., Kadden, R. M., Kabela-Cormier, E., & Petry, N. M. (2009). Changing network support for drinking: Network Support Project 2–year follow-up. *Journal of Consulting and Clinical Psychology, 77*(2), 229–242.

Longabaugh, R., Donovan, D. M., Karno, M. P., McCrady, B. S., Morgenstern, J., & Tonigan, J. S. (2005). Active ingredients: How and why evidence-based alcohol behavioral treatment interventions work. *Alcoholism: Clinical and Experimental Research, 29*, 235–247.

Lyon, D., & Greenberg, J. (1991). Evidence of codependency in women with an alcoholic parent: Helping out Mr. Wrong. *Journal of Personality and Social Psychology, 61*, 435–439.

MacDonald, D. E. (1956). Mental disorders in wives of alcoholics. *Quarterly Journal of Studies on Alcohol, 17*, 282–287.

Manuel, J. K., McCrady, B. S., Epstein, E. E., Cook, S., & Tonigan, J. S. (2007). The pretreatment social networks of women with alcohol dependence. *Journal of Studies on Alcohol and Drugs, 68*(6), 871–878.

Marshal, M. P. (2003). For better or for worse?: The effects of alcohol use on marital functioning. *Clinical Psychology Review, 23*(7), 959–997.

McAweeney, M. J., Zucker, R. A., Fitzgerald, H. E., Puttler, L. I., & Wong, M. M. (2005). Individual and partner predictors of recovery from alcohol-use disorder over a nine-year interval: Findings from a community sample of alcoholic married men. *Journal of Studies on Alcohol, 66*(2), 220–228.

McCrady, B. S. (2001). Alcohol use disorders. In D. H. Barlow (Ed.), *Clinical handbook of psychological disorders* (3rd ed., pp. 376–433). New York: Guilford Press.

McCrady, B. S. (2004). To have but one true friend: Implications for practice of research on alcohol use disorders and social networks. *Psychology of Addictive Behaviors, 18*, 113–121.

McCrady, B. S., Epstein, E. E., Cook, S., Hildebrandt, T., & Jensen, N. (2009). A randomized trial of individual and couple behavioral alcohol treatment for women. *Journal of Consulting and Clinical Psychology, 77*(2), 243–256.

McCrady, B. S., Epstein, E. E., & Hirsch, L. S. (1999). Maintaining change after conjoint behavioral alcohol treatment for men: Outcomes at 6 months. *Addiction, 94*(9), 1381–1396.

McCrady, B. S., Epstein, E. E., & Kahler, C. W. (2004). AA and relapse prevention as maintenance strategies after conjoint behavioral alcohol treatment for men: 18 month outcomes. *Journal of Consulting and Clinical Psychology, 72*, 870–878.

McCrady, B. S., Hayaki, J., Epstein, E. E., & Hirsch, L. S. (2002). Testing hypothesized predictors of change in conjoint behavioral alcoholism treatment for men. *Alcoholism: Clinical and Experimental Research, 26*, 463–470.

McCrady, B. S., Noel, N. E., Abrams, D. B., & Stout, R. L. (1986). Comparative effectiveness of three types of spouse involvement in outpatient behavioral alcoholism treatment. *Journal of Studies on Alcohol, 47*(6), 459–467.

McCrady, B. S., Stout, R., Noel, N., & Abrams, D. (1991). Effectiveness of three types of spouse-involved behavioral alcoholism treatment. *British Journal of Addiction, 86*(11), 1415–1424.

McGue, M., Iacono, W. G., Legrand, L. N., & Elkins, I. (2001). Origins and consequences of age at first drink: II. Familial risk and heritability. *Alcoholism: Clinical and Experimental Research, 25*, 1166–1173.

Measelle, J. R., Stice, E., & Springer, D. W. (2006). A prospective test of the negative affect model of substance abuse: Moderating effects of social support. *Psychology of Addictive Behaviors, 20*, 225–233.

Merikangas, K. R., Stolar, M., Stevens, D. E., Goulet, J., Preisig, M. A., Fenton, B., et al. (1998). Familial transmission of substance use disorders. *Archives of General Psychiatry, 55*, 973–979.

Mohr, C. D., Averna, S., Kenny, D. A., & Del Boca, F. K. (2001). "Getting by (or getting high) with a little help from my friends": An examination of adult alcoholics' friendships. *Journal of Studies on Alcohol, 62*, 637–645.

Moos, R. H. (2007). Theory-based active ingredients of effective treatments for substance use disorders. *Drug and Alcohol Dependence, 88*(2), 109–121.

Moos, R. H., Finney, J. W., & Cronkite, R. C. (1990). *Alcoholism treatment: Context, process and outcome.* Oxford, UK: Oxford University Press.

Moos, R. H., Finney, J. W., & Gamble, W. (1982). The process of recovery from alcoholism: II. Comparing spouses of alcoholic patients and matched community controls. *Journal of Studies on Alcohol, 43*, 888–909.

Moos, R. H., & Moos, B. S. (1984). The process of recovery from alcoholism: III.

Comparing functioning in families of alcoholics and matched control families. *Journal of Studies on Alcohol, 45(2)*, 111–118.

Moss, H. B., Mezzich, A., Yao, J. K., Gavaler, J., & Martin, C.S. (1995). Aggressivity among sons of substance-abusing fathers: Association with psychiatric disorder in the father and son, paternal personality, pubertal development, and socioeconomic status. *American Journal of Drug and Alcohol Abuse, 21(2)*, 195–208.

Murphy, C. M., Winters, J., Fals-Stewart, W., O'Farrell, T. J., & Murphy, M. (2005). Alcohol consumption and intimate partner violence by alcoholic men: Comparing violent and nonviolent conflicts. *Psychology of Addictive Behaviors, 19(1)*, 35–42.

O'Farrell, T. J., Choquette, K. A., & Cutter, H. S. (1998). Couples relapse prevention sessions after behavioral marital therapy for male alcoholics: Outcomes during the three years after starting treatment. *Journal of Studies on Alcohol, 59*, 357–370.

O'Farrell, T. J., Cutter, H. S., Choquette, K. A., & Floyd, F. J. (1992). Behavioral marital therapy for male alcoholics: Marital and drinking adjustment during the two years after treatment. *Behavior Therapy, 23(4)*, 529–549.

O'Farrell, T. J., Hooley. J., Fals-Stewart, W., & Cutter, H. Q. (1998). Expressed emotion and relapse in alcoholic patients. *Journal of Consulting and Clinical Psychology, 66*, 744–752.

O'Farrell, T. J., Murphy, C. M., Stephan, S. H., Murphy, M., & Fals-Stewart, W. (2004). Partner violence before and after couples-based alcoholism treatment for male alcoholic patients: The role of treatment involvement and abstinence. *Journal of Consulting and Clinical Psychology, 72(2)*, 202–217.

Orford, J., Guthrie, S., Nicholls, P., Oppenheimer, E., Egert, S., & Hensman, C. (1975). Self-reported coping behavior in wives of alcoholics and its association with drinking outcome. *Journal of Studies on Alcohol, 36*, 1254–1267.

Ouimette, P., Coolhart, D., Funderburk, J. S., Wade, M., & Brown, P. J. (2007). Precipitants of first substance use in recently abstinent substance use disorder patients with PTSD. *Addictive Behaviors, 32(8)*, 1719–1727.

Powers, M. B., Vedel, E., & Emmelkamp, P. M. G. (2008). Behavioral couples therapy (BCT) for alcohol and drug use disorders: A meta-analysis. *Clinical Psychology Review, 28(6)*, 952–962.

Quigley, B. M., & Leonard, K. E. (2000). Alcohol and the continuation of early marital aggression. *Alcoholism: Clinical and Experimental Research, 24*, 1003–1010.

Ray, G. T., Mertens, J. R., & Weisner, C. (2007). The excess medical cost and health problems of family members of persons diagnosed with alcohol or drug problems. *Medical Care, 45(2)*, 116–122.

Roberts, L. J., & Leonard, K. E. (1998). An empirical typology of drinking partnerships and their relationship to marital functioning and drinking consequences. *Journal of Marriage and the Family, 60*, 515–526.

Rohrbaugh, M. J., Shoham, V., Butler, E. A., Hasler, B. P., & Berman, J. S. (2009). Affective synchrony in dual-and single-smoker couples: Further evidence of "symptom–system fit"? *Family Process, 48(1)*, 55–67.

Roozen, H. G., de Waart, R., & van der Kroft, P. (2010). Community reinforcement and family training: An effective option to engage treatment-resistant substance-abusing individuals in treatment. *Addiction, 105*(10), 1729–1738.

Ross, H. E., Glaser, F. B., & Germanson, T. (1988). The prevalence of psychiatric disorders in patients with alcohol and other drug problems. *Archives of General Psychiatry, 45*, 1023–1031.

Rotunda, R. J., & O'Farrell, T. J. (1997). Marital and family therapy of alcohol use disorders: Bridging the gap between research and practice. *Professional Psychology: Research and Practice, 28*, 246–252.

Schuckit, M. A. (1998). Biological, psychological, and environmental predictors of the alcoholism risk: A longitudinal study. *Journal of Studies on Alcohol, 59*, 485–494.

Shoham, V., Butler, E. A., Rohrbaugh, M. J., & Trost, S. E. (2007). Symptom–system fit in couples: Emotion regulation when one or both partners smoke. *Journal of Abnormal Psychology, 116*(4), 848–853.

Shoham, V., Rohrbaugh, M. J., Stickle, T. R., & Jacob, T. (1998). Demand–withdraw couple interaction moderates retention in cognitive–behavioral versus family-systems treatments for alcoholism. *Journal of Family Psychology, 12*(4), 557–577.

Smith, J. E., & Meyers, R. J. (2004). *Motivating substance users to enter treatment: Working with family members.* New York: Guilford Press.

Steinberg, M. L., Epstein, E. E., McCrady, B. S., & Hirsch, L. S. (1997). Sources of motivation in a couples outpatient alcoholism treatment program. *American Journal of Drug and Alcohol Abuse, 23*(2), 191–205.

Steinglass, P. (1979). The alcoholic family in the interaction laboratory. *Journal of Nervous and Mental Disease, 167*, 428–436.

Steinglass, P. (1981). The alcoholic family at home: Patterns of interaction in dry, wet, and transitional stage of alcoholism. *Archives of General Psychiatry, 38*, 578–584.

Steinglass, P., Bennett, L. A., Wolin, S. J., & Reiss, D. (1987). *The alcoholic family.* New York: Basic Books.

Steinglass, P., Davis, D. I., & Berenson, D. (1977). Observations of conjointly hospitalized "alcoholic couples" during sobriety and intoxication: Implications for theory and therapy. *Family Process, 16*, 1–16.

Steinglass, P., Weiner, S., & Mendelson, J. H. (1971). Interactional issues as determinants of alcoholism. *American Journal of Psychiatry, 128*, 275–280.

Thomas, E. J., & Ager, R. D. (1993). Unilateral family therapy with spouses of uncooperative alcohol abusers. In T. J. O'Farrell (Ed.), *Treating alcohol problems: Marital and family interventions* (pp. 3–33). New York: Guilford Press.

Tildesley, E. A., & Andrews, J. A. (2008). The development of children's intentions to use alcohol: Direct and indirect effects of parent alcohol use and parenting behaviors. *Psychology of Addictive Behaviors, 22*, 326–339.

van der Vorst, H., Engels, R. C. M. E., Meeus, W., Dekovic, M., & Vermulst, A. (2006). Parental attachment, parental control, and early development of alcohol use: A longitudinal study. *Psychology of Addictive Behaviors, 20*, 107–116.

Velleman, R. (2006). The importance of family members in helping problem drinkers achieve their chosen goal. *Addiction Research and Theory, 14*(1), 73–85.

Walden, B., McGue, M., Iacono, W. G., Burt, S. A., & Elkins, I. (2004). Identifying shared environmental contributions to early adolescent substance use: The respective roles of parents and peers. *Journal of Abnormal Psychology, 113,* 440–450.

Warren, J. I., Stein, J. A., & Grella, C. E. (2007). Role of social support and self-efficacy in treatment outcomes among clients with co-occurring disorders. *Drug and Alcohol Dependence, 89*(2), 267–274.

Wegsheider, S. (1981). *Another chance: Hope and health for the alcoholic family.* Palo Alto, CA: Science and Behavior Books.

Whalen, T. (1953). Wives of alcoholics: Four types observed in a family service agency. *Quarterly Journal of Studies on Alcohol, 14,* 632–641.

White, H. R., Johnson, V., & Buyske, S. (2000). Parental modeling and parenting behavior effects on offspring alcohol and cigarette use: A growth curve analysis. *Journal of Substance Abuse, 12,* 287–310.

Winters, J., Fals-Stewart, W., O'Farrell, T. J., Kelley, M. L., & Birchler, G. R. (2002). Behavioral couples therapy for female substance-abusing patients: Effects on substance use and relationship adjustment. *Journal of Consulting and Clinical Psychology, 70*(2), 344–355.

Wolin, S. J., Bennett, L. A., Noonan, D. L., & Teitelbaum, M. A. (1980). Disrupted family rituals: A factor in the intergenerational transmission of alcoholism. *Journal of Studies on Alcohol, 41,* 199–214.

Wood, M.D., Read, J. P., Mitchell, R. E., & Brand, N. H. (2004). Do parents still matter?: Parent and peer influences on alcohol involvement among recent high school graduates. *Psychology of Addictive Behaviors, 18,* 19–30.

Wright, P. H., & Wright, K. D. (1990). Measuring codependents' close relationships: A preliminary study. *Journal of Substance Abuse, 2,* 335–344.

Zhou, Q., King, K. M., & Chassin, L. (2006). The roles of familial alcoholism and adolescent family harmony in young adults' substance dependence disorders: Mediated and moderated relations. *Journal of Abnormal Psychology, 115,* 320–331.

Chapter 10

Family Therapy Techniques for Substance Abuse Treatment

Wendy K. K. Lam
Timothy J. O'Farrell
Gary R. Birchler

Over the last half century the family treatment model has been rapidly accepted as a critical component of substance abuse treatment. The treatment literature from the 1950s and early 1960s primarily conceptualized substance abuse as an individual problem that was best treated on an individual basis (Jellinek, 1960). However, during the 1960s this view was supplanted by what is now the prevailing clinical wisdom that family members can play a central role in the treatment of alcoholics and drug abusers (Stanton & Heath, 1997). By the early 1970s couple and family therapies were described by the National Institute on Alcohol Abuse and Alcoholism as "one of the most outstanding current advances in the area of psychotherapy of alcoholism" (Keller, 1974, p. 161). By the late 1970s family therapy was embraced by the majority of substance abuse treatment programs and community mental health settings (Coleman & Davis, 1978). During the last three decades, family-based assessment and intervention has become widely viewed as part of standard care for alcoholism and drug abuse (Center for Substance Abuse Treatment, 2004). In fact, many have argued that the only reason not to include family members in the treatment of a substance-abusing patient is refusal by the patient or members of the family involved (O'Farrell, 1993).

In addition, the popular literature on families and substance abuse has grown into a cottage industry of sorts, with a wide range of books on codependency, enabling, and adult children of alcoholics appearing on bookstore shelves. Thus, the role of family factors in the etiology and maintenance of addictive disorders and the application of family therapy in substance abuse treatment has indeed come a long way.

Historically, the family interventions used to treat alcoholism grew out of couple therapy approaches, while family-based treatments to treat drug abuse evolved from systemic family therapy approaches that targeted the patient's spouse, children, parents, siblings, and so forth. More recently, this distinction has blurred, with both alcoholism and drug abuse treatment programs often providing a wide array of family therapy services for the patients and their family members. Moreover, the definition of what constitutes "family members" has been broadened to include other members of the substance abuser's social network, including employers, close friends, and other concerned persons (Kaufman, 1985).

This chapter provides an overview of different systems and techniques of family therapy commonly used to treat alcoholism and drug abuse. These interventions are as diverse as the variety of family functioning theories from which they evolved. In this chapter, we focus on the use of family-involved treatments to (1) help the family cope when the substance abuser refuses to get help; (2) help the family initiate change for loved ones who are resistant to seeking help; and (3) facilitate treatment and aid recovery when the substance abuser has sought help.

Helping the Family When the Substance Abuser Refuses to Get Help

Spouses and other family members often experience many stressors and heightened emotional distress caused by the negative consequences of the substance abuser's drinking and drug use. Stress is highest for the family when the substance abuser refuses to get help. The therapist can help family members cope with their emotional distress and concentrate on their own motivations for change by helping the family members use the concepts and resources of Al-Anon or by teaching coping skills.

Al-Anon Facilitation and Referral

Al-Anon is a widely used 12-step program that advocates that family members detach themselves from the substance abuser's drinking and drug use in a loving way, accept that they are powerless to control the substance abuser, and seek support from other members of the Al-Anon program (Al-Anon Family Groups, 1981). There are two ways in which an addictions professional might use Al-Anon to help family members. The first is *referral of family members to Al-Anon*. This includes providing information about times and locations of nearby Al-Anon meetings and discussing any concerns the family members may have about Al-Anon. It can be particularly effective to arrange for them to attend their first meetings with an established Al-Anon member. The second is *Al-Anon facilitation therapy* (AFT), a therapist-delivered counseling method designed to encourage involvement in Al-Anon. Nowinski (1999) developed and tested a 10- to 12-session program designed to engage the family member in the program and concepts of Al-Anon. Each session explores one of the Al-Anon 12 steps (e.g., admitting one is powerless over another person's addiction) or a closely related Al-Anon concept (e.g., detaching with love). AFT also asks the family member to complete recovery tasks between sessions, including attending Al-Anon meetings and reading Al-Anon literature.

Coping Skills Therapy

Coping skills therapy (CST) teaches family members how to deal with alcohol- and drug-related situations involving the substance abuser. Rychtarik and McGillicuddy (2005) developed and tested an eight-session CST group for spouses and family members of substance abusers. Based on a family stress and coping perspective, CST helps group members to apply a problem-solving approach to problem situations commonly experienced by families of substance abusers (e.g., dealing with intoxicated behavior, partner violence, failure to maintain household responsibilities). In each CST session, a group leader presents a stressful situation, leads the group in problem-solving exercises, and provides situation-specific skill hints. For example, the situation might involve the substance abuser asking for money when in the past he has used these occasions to go out and drink. The group discusses possible responses, which might range from passive acquiescence to assertively declining the request. The therapist then models the recommended response, group members role-play the situation, and the therapist and group provide feedback. As part of the treatment, participants keep a diary of personal situations they have found to be problematic, and discuss and role-play these situations with the group.

Evidence for Family Therapy When the Substance Abuser Refuses Help

Controlled studies have found that Al-Anon referral, AFT, and CST all produce improvements in family members' emotional distress and coping that are greater than in a wait-list control group (Barber & Gilbertson,

1998; Miller, Meyers, & Tonigan, 1999). Although they produce similar improvements in emotional distress, CST leads to less drinking and less violence by the alcoholic than does AFT. Specifically, compared with female spouses of alcoholics who participated in AFT, female spouses who participated in CST experienced less violence from their male partners and had male partners who drank less in the year after treatment (Rychtarik & McGillicuddy, 2005). These advantages of CST over AFT are important because as many as one-half of male substance abusers have been violent toward a female partner in the past year (O'Farrell, Murphy, Stephan, Fals-Stewart, & Murphy, 2004). In addition, reduced drinking by the alcoholic who was not in treatment is an important indirect effect of CST. Although CST is not widely used, these findings suggest it should receive more attention from clinicians and program administrators.

Family-Based Methods to Initiate Change When the Substance Abuser Refuses to Get Help

Many substance abusers seek treatment in response to some form of external pressure from a spouse, other family members, a physician, the legal system, and so forth (Krampen, 1989). Thus, in many instances, one or more family members or concerned significant others (CSOs) recognize the need to get help for the substance abuser and are the first persons to contact the substance abuse treatment system. With the possible exception of coercion from the legal system, pressure to enter treatment by a family member or CSO is the most powerful inducement for substance abusers to enter and engage in treatment (Stanton, 1997).

Several family-based intervention methods try to motivate resistant substance abusers to enter treatment: (1) the Johnson Institute Intervention; (2) A Relational Intervention Sequence for Engagement (ARISE); and (3) Community Reinforcement and Family Training (CRAFT). Although these interventions share a common goal, the techniques used within each vary considerably, particularly with respect to the level of coercion prescribed.

The Johnson Institute Intervention

Without question, the most well-known of these family-involved motivational techniques is the Johnson Institute intervention (Faber & Keating-O'Connor, 1991). This method was originally developed to motivate resistant alcoholics to enter treatment, but has been applied more broadly to individuals with other psychoactive substance use disorders. The Johnson Institute intervention, or the "intervention" as it is commonly called, involves three to four educational and rehearsal sessions with a trained therapist to prepare family and key support network members (e.g., employers, neighbors, friends) for a confrontation meeting. After a CSO contacts the therapist, the therapist assesses the nature and severity of the substance use problem, as well as the composition and structure of the substance abuser's social network. The therapist then determines which family members and CSOs should participate in the intervention meeting.

Those who agree to take part in the intervention are brought together initially to meet with the therapist to form the intervention team. The therapist orients the team members about the intervention process, and asks them to list specific incidents and behaviors caused by the substance abuser's drinking or drug use that have affected them directly. With therapist coaching, they practice how to deliver their concerns and feelings to the substance abuser in a sincere and nonjudgmental fashion. The intervention team needs to agree about what treatment the substance abuser needs; firmly insist that the substance abuser enter into and engage in the prescribed treatment; outline the specific consequences for the substance abuser if he or she fails to engage in the treatment; and follow through on these consequences if the substance abuser decides not to follow these treatment recommendations.

The intervention team then meets with the substance abuser, who typically does not know the agenda of the group. Once the substance abuser is in their midst, members share their concerns and feelings. Intervention team members also express their hope that the substance abuser will enter treatment, outline the consequences if the substance abuser refuses, and openly discuss the desired outcome of both the intervention and the recommended treatment. Often, at a later date, intervention team members meet with the therapist to discuss next steps for the family members and others in the substance abuser's social network.

Some have raised ethical concerns about the Johnson Institute intervention (Faber & Keating-O'Connor, 1991; Miller et al., 1999). For example, confidentiality is certainly an issue, given that the substance abuser does not participate in the decision about who becomes part of the intervention team and what information is disclosed during the intervention meeting. Additionally, there is potential for significant harmful effects of the intervention, particularly if the substance abuser refuses to enter treatment and the consequences are imposed. In addition, the therapist who is overseeing the intervention may have a conflict of interest, particularly when the team recommends treatment for the substance abuser at a facility where the therapist is employed.

A Relational Intervention Sequence for Engagement

As a partial response to these concerns about the Johnson Institute intervention approach, ARISE (Landeau & Garrett, 2006) emerged as a less coercive alternative to motivate resistant substance abusers to engage in treatment.

ARISE is a three-stage family-based approach designed to encourage reluctant substance abusers to seek help, with each stage involving greater family involvement, greater therapist involvement, and more pressure.

In the first stage, a CSO contacts the treatment agency to obtain information about treatment options. During one or more telephone sessions, the therapist assesses the nature and severity of the substance abuser's problem, the circumstances surrounding it, and the social support system of the substance abuser. The therapist invites the network of CSOs to attend an initial meeting at the clinic, as well as additional meetings as needed. These meetings serve to review efforts of network members to individually engage and confront the substance abuser; develop strategies to motivate the substance abuser to engage in treatment; and prepare network members to handle possible crises that may arise. The goal of these sessions is to mobilize members of the social network in support of treatment for the substance abuser.

Although these sessions may provide CSOs enough information and coaching to help them motivate the substance abuser to enter treatment, the process often requires a second stage, which involves an informal intervention with the CSO network and therapist present. The network members invite the substance abuser to attend, although these meetings can still occur without the substance abuser present. In these meetings, the members collectively consider possible approaches that they might use to motivate the substance abuser to enter treatment.

If, after repeated attempts, the substance abuser remains unwilling to seek help, the process moves to the third and final stage, use of an intervention similar to the Johnson Institute Intervention approach. Thus, the ARISE model advocates the use of less coercive steps early in the process and gradually proceeds to the use of greater therapist and family involvement if the lower intensity steps are not successful in motivating the substance abuser to engage in treatment.

The Community Reinforcement and Family Training Approach

The CRAFT approach (Smith & Meyers, 2004) is an outgrowth of the community reinforcement approach (CRA) for alcoholism (Azrin, 1976). Both of these interventions draw heavily on learning theory. In CRAFT, a CSO participates in a multifaceted intervention designed to encourage the substance-abusing family member to stop drinking or using drugs and to enter treatment. CRAFT employs several steps. With help from the CRAFT therapist, the CSO gauges the severity of the substance use problem (by measuring the quantity and frequency of use) and outlines the problems caused by the substance use. The therapist also asks the CSO to complete two exercises. First, the CSO identifies the substance abuser's triggers for using alcohol or drugs and the consequences of such use. Second, the CSO identifies the substance abuser's triggers for other, more prosocial behaviors and their resulting consequences.

CRAFT teaches the CSO how to use positive reinforcement and negative consequences to discourage drug use or drinking by the substance abuser. For example, the CSO would engage in pleasant activities (e.g., discussing enjoyable topics, giving gifts) with the substance abuser when the substance abuser is not drinking or using drugs while explicitly stating that it is because the substance abuser is not drinking or using drugs. Alternatively, the CSO would use negative consequences when the substance abuser is intoxicated. Such consequences might include withholding reinforcements, explaining why, and ignoring the substance abuser during periods of intoxication. CRAFT also teaches the CSO strategies to decrease stress in general and to increase positive aspects of his or her own life. These strategies might include establishing new friendships, engaging in positively rewarding activities outside of the relationship with the substance abuser, or joining a therapy group.

Another important aspect of CRAFT is to identify potentially dangerous situations that might emerge as behavioral changes are introduced at home. The CRAFT therapist teaches the CSO how to identify and anticipate potentially violent situations by recognizing their "cues" so that he or she can take immediate action before getting hurt. The CSO also develops a specific plan for leaving these situations until it is safe to return.

Finally, CRAFT also teaches the CSO the most effective ways to suggest to the substance abuser that he or she enter treatment. This may involve picking a time and situation when the substance abuser may be highly motivated to enter treatment because substance use has caused unacceptable behavior, such as embarrassment or arrest for drunk driving. The therapist teaches the CSO to have treatment options ready for when the substance abuser has agreed to enter treatment, regardless of time of day or day of the week.

Evidence for Family Therapy to Initiate Change
When the Substance Abuser Refuses Help

Of these family-based methods to promote change and treatment entry by the resistant substance abuser, CRAFT has the strongest evidence base. Across four randomized trials with alcoholics (Miller et al., 1999; Sisson & Azrin, 1986) and drug abusers (Kirby, Marlowe, Festinger, Garvey, & LaMonaca, 1999; Meyers, Miller, Smith, & Tonigan, 2002), the average treatment engagement rate for CRAFT was 68% (ranging from 59 to 85%), which was significantly and substantially higher than corresponding rates for AFT or Al-Anon referral (20%) or the Johnson Institute intervention (30%). Thus, CRAFT is a more effective alternative to engage substance abusers in treatment than popular confrontational or detachment approaches.

The Johnson Institute intervention showed a disappointing treatment engagement rate of 30% in the first randomized, controlled study of this popular method (Miller et al., 1999). This finding was similar to the 25% rate in an uncontrolled study (Liepman, Nirenberg, & Begin, 1989), not much higher than for Al-Anon, which does not specifically target the substance abuser's behavior. The reason for these disappointing findings is that 70% of families in these two studies who started the intervention process *did not go through with the family confrontation meeting*. Among families who completed the confrontation in these two studies (a small minority), around 90% succeeded in getting their substance abuser into treatment.

ARISE, as a less coercive multistep process, should lead to better engagement rates than the Johnson intervention. However, although ARISE has shown promise in uncontrolled studies (Landau et al., 2004), controlled studies have not been published. Table 10.1 summarizes key points about family-based methods to initiate change when the substance abuser refuses to get help.

Family-Based Methods to Aid Recovery When the Substance Abuser Has Sought Help

Preceding sections have described interventions to help the family and support the substance abuser's entry into treatment. Regardless of the impetus for seeking help, once the substance abuser has entered treatment, therapists often use family therapy interventions as a primary or adjunctive component of treatment. The family treatment model will typically dictate the degree of spouse or family member involvement, ranging from little involvement (e.g., providing assessment information only) to being an equal partner in the treatment process (e.g., couple therapy).

Although several systems of family therapy have been used with substance-abusing patients, five major approaches have guided treatment strategies most often used with substance abusers. The *family disease approach* views alcoholism and other drug abuse as an illness of the family, suffered not only by the substance abuser, but also by family members. The *family systems approach* applies the principles of general systems theory to families, with particular attention paid to ways in which families maintain a dynamic balance between substance use and family functioning and whose interactional behavior is organized around alcohol or drug use. *Behavioral approaches* assume that family interactions serve to reinforce alcohol- and drug-using behavior. *Social network therapy* involves the patient's social network in treatment to support the patient's recovery. *Ecological approaches* assume that substance abuse results from many sources

TABLE 10.1. Family-Based Interventions When the Substance Abuser Resists and Seeks Help

Major approaches	Description	Evidence
Substance abuser resisting help		
Johnson Institute intervention	• Therapist helps family plan and conduct surprise family confrontation meeting called an "intervention."	• 25–30% treatment engagement rate • Most families do not follow through with confrontation.
A Relational Intervention Sequence for Engagement (ARISE)	• Three-step model starting with low-pressure methods and ending with Johnson Institute intervention if needed.	• No controlled studies to date.
Community reinforcement and family training (CRAFT)	• Teaches family member(s) to use positive reinforcement and negative consequences to discourage substance use and encourage treatment.	• Average 68% treatment engagement rate. • Four randomized clinical trials (RCTs).
Substance abuser seeking help		
Family disease approach	• Views substance abuse as a family disease, best treated by AA or NA for the patient and Al-Anon for the family.	• AA and Al-Anon counseling, respectively, reduced patient drinking and spouses' distress.
Family systems therapy (FST)	• Joining with the family and restructuring family alliances and interactions to eliminate substance abuse.	• FST for adult drug abuse shows better outcomes than control groups. • Small number of studies.
Behavioral couple therapy (BCT)	• Adult cohabitating or married couples. • Recovery Contract with daily trust discussion supports abstinence; positive activities and communication skills improve relationship.	• BCT couples demonstrate strong and consistent evidence for greater abstinence, relationship, and family outcomes than IBT. • Multiple RCTs and meta-analytic reviews.
Network therapy	• Involves patient's social network in treatment to support the patient's recovery.	• Network therapy for adult alcoholism shows better outcomes than control groups. • Small number of studies.
Ecological approach	• Multisystemic family therapy (MST) and multidimensional family therapy (MDFT) for adolescent substance users • Multisystem intervention (e.g., family, school) to create an environment for the adolescent that is conducive to abstinence.	• MST and MDFT for adolescent substance abusers have strong evidence base showing greater improvements in youth substance use, mental health, sexual risk, juvenile delinquency than standard control groups.

of influence from the multiple systems in the substance abuser's life. This approach aims to modify these systems of influence to create an environment that is conducive to abstinence. The following sections describe the hallmark therapy techniques identified with all these approaches.

Family Disease Approach

This perspective views substance abuse as a "family disease" that affects most family members. In this perspective, family members of substance abusers suffer from the disease of "codependence." This term is often used to describe the process underlying the various problems observed in families affected by substance abusers. *Enabling* is a major feature of codependency. As the term implies, codependency includes any set of behaviors that help maintain the substance use. These include making it easier for the alcoholic or drug abuser to engage in substance use, or shielding the substance abuser from the negative consequences of drinking and drug use.

Although the problem of substance abuse exists within the family, the solution from this perspective is for each family member to recognize that they have a disease, to detach from the substance abuser, and to engage in their own program of recovery. The family disease approach typically involves separate treatment for family members without the substance abuser present. Treatment may consist of psychoeducational groups about the disease concept of addiction and codependency; referrals to Al-Anon, Al-Ateen, or Adult Children of Alcoholics groups; and individual and group therapy to address various psychological issues. (As described earlier in this chapter, Al-Anon may be used to help the family when the substance abuser has not sought help.)

Family members are taught that they must cease enabling in order to help the substance abuser stop using. In general, the family disease approach advocates that family members should not actively intervene to try to change the substance abuser's drinking or drug use, but should focus on themselves to reduce their own emotional distress and improve their own coping (Al-Anon Family Groups, 1981).

Family Systems Therapy

The family systems therapy model incorporates many core concepts of family systems theory as applied to substance abuse (Stanton, Todd, & Associates, 1982; Steinglass, Bennett, Wolin, & Reiss, 1987). Therapy focuses on the interactional rather than the individual level, using different techniques to affect interactions within the family. Emphasis is placed on identifying and changing family interaction patterns that are associated with problematic substance use.

The family systems approach views substance abuse as a major organizing principle for interaction patterns of behavior within the family. A reciprocal relationship exists between family functioning and substance use. According to family systems theory, substance abuse in adults and adolescents often evolves during periods in which an individual family member is having difficulty with an important developmental issue (e.g., leaving home) or when the family is facing a significant crisis (e.g., marital discord). During these periods, substance abuse can serve to (1) distract family members from their central problem or (2) slow down or stop transition to a different developmental stage that is being resisted by the family or by one of its members.

From a family systems perspective, substance abuse represents a maladaptive attempt to deal with difficulties that develop a homeostatic life of their own and regulate family transactions. Substance abuse serves an important role in the family. Once the therapist understands the function of the substance use for the family, the therapist can explain how the behavior has come about and the function it serves. In turn, treatment attempts to restructure the interaction patterns associated with the substance use, thereby making the substance abuse unnecessary to maintain the family system functioning. Family systems therapists use a variety of techniques to accomplish this goal. The therapist may alternate between joining that supports the family system and restructuring that challenges the system.

Joining as a Family Systems Therapy Technique

Joining consists of techniques designed to promote the therapeutic alliance and increase the therapist's leverage within the family. First, the therapist must make a connection with each family member engaged in treatment and instill confidence in his or her commitment to working together with family members on identified problems and convey the importance of each family member's viewpoint. In the joining process, the therapist typically solicits each family member's perspective and feelings about the problems in the family, thus promoting the view that disagreements about the identity, nature, and severity of problems are acceptable. The therapist attempts to communicate to each family member that he or she understands the family member's perceptions of the problems and has a clear idea about how to address the issues raised by him or her.

As part of the joining process, the therapist highlights areas of strength in the family, supports threatened members of the family, and uses the family member's methods of communicating (e.g., humor, touching) to introduce new ideas and concepts (Minuchin, 1974). Of course, joining is an ongoing process, which emerges as the therapist demonstrates understanding and helpfulness throughout the course of treatment.

Restructuring as a Family Systems Therapy Technique

Restructuring involves challenging the family's homeostasis through modifications in the family's bonding and power alignments among individuals and subsystems in the family (Haley, 1976; Minuchin, 1974). Several different techniques are used in the process of restructuring, including contracting, enactment, reframing, restructuring, and marking boundaries. *Contracting* is an agreement to work on agreed-upon issues, with an emphasis on helping the substance abuser with his or her problems before addressing other issues. The therapist develops the contract at the end of the first interview and maintains the agreement throughout treatment. As part of the contract, the family must choose to develop a family system that is conducive to abstinence by the substance abuser and agree to adhere to the contract once all family members agree to it. *Enactment* involves having family members describe recurring behavioral sequences to each other. By requiring family members to talk to each other about problems, rather than to the therapist during sessions, the therapist can carefully observe, interrupt, and destabilize the behavioral exchanges. *Reframing* involves helping family members to understand the interrelatedness of their behaviors and to see and understand how the substance use (and any other dysfunctional behavior) serves an important function in the family. *Restructuring* consists of shifting family interaction patterns and establishing new, healthier behaviors (e.g., changing seating arrangements to strengthen the role of parents in the family, restating problems in solvable form, teaching methods of communication and problem solving that preclude triangulation or conflict avoidance). Finally, the therapist *marks boundaries* by clearly delineating individual and subsystem boundaries. For example, to strengthen and protect the parental subsystem from intrusion by children and other adults, the therapist might conduct some parent-only sessions.

Family systems therapy is more than a set of techniques. It is a framework that explains puzzling clinical phenomena (e.g., a family member seeming to sabotage a patient's newfound sobriety) and guides interventions. From this perspective, substance abuse by a family member serves an important function for the family, helping to maintain the equilibrium of the family system. Thus, if a family has functioned as a stable unit with a substance-abusing member, subsequent sobriety would likely threaten equilibrium and may be resisted on some level. The family systems approach has been used widely in treatment settings with adult (Stanton et al., 1982) and adolescent substance abusers (Rowe, in press).

Behavioral Approach

Behavioral family therapy treatment models draw heavily on operant and social learning theories to understand the substance abuser's behavior within the family context. Viewed from this approach, substance use is a behavior learned in the context of social interactions (e.g., observing peers, parents, role models in the media) and reinforced by contingencies in the individual's environment (Akers, Krohn, Lanza Kaduce, & Radosevich, 1979). Thus, from a behavioral family perspective, substance use is maintained, in part, by the antecedents and consequences that are operating in the family environment.

Following these operant and social learning principles, treatment emphasizes contingency management designed to reward sobriety, reduce reinforcement of drinking or drug use, and increase prosocial behaviors that may be incompatible with substance use. The substance abuser and involved family members are trained in methods to increase positive interactions, improve problem solving, and enhance communication skills. By using these newly developed skills, family members can reduce the likelihood of continued drinking or drug use by the substance-using member.

Family-based behavioral treatment models have been used most frequently with alcoholic and drug-abusing couples. Three general reinforcement patterns are typically observed in substance abusers' families: (1) reinforcement for substance-using behavior in the form of attention or caretaking, (2) shielding the substance abuser from experiencing the negative consequences of his or her drinking or drug use, and (3) punishing drinking behavior (e.g., making negative or disparaging remarks or avoiding the substance abuser) (McCrady, 1986). In turn, behaviorally oriented treatment generally focuses on changing spousal or family interactions that serve as stimuli for abusive substance use or trigger relapse, improving communication and problem-solving abilities, and strengthening coping skills that reinforce sobriety.

Behavioral Couple Therapy with Adult Substance Abusers

Behavioral couple therapy (BCT; McCrady & Epstein, 2008; O'Farrell & Fals-Stewart, 2006) works directly to increase relationship factors conducive to abstinence. A behavioral approach assumes that family members can reward abstinence—and that alcoholic and drug-abusing individuals from happier, more cohesive relationships with better communication will be at lower risk of relapse. The substance-abusing patient and the spouse are seen together in BCT, typically for 15–20 outpatient couple sessions over 5 to 6 months. Generally, couples are married or have been cohabiting for at least 1 year, have no current psychosis, and one member of the couple has a current problem with alcoholism and/or drug abuse. The couple starts BCT soon after the substance abuser seeks help.

BCT sees the substance-abusing patient with the spouse to build support for sobriety. The therapist arranges a *Recovery Contract* that includes a "trust discussion" in which the substance abuser states his or her intent not to drink or use drugs that day (in the tradition of "one day at a time" from Alcoholics Anonymous), and the spouse expresses support for the patient's efforts to stay abstinent. For substance-abusing patients who are medically cleared and willing, daily ingestion of recovery medication (e.g., disulfiram, naltrexone) is also witnessed and verbally reinforced by the spouse as part of the trust discussion. The spouse records the performance of the daily contract on a calendar provided by the therapist. To prevent substance-related conflicts, both partners agree not to discuss past substance use or fears about future substance use at home, but instead reserve these discussions for the therapy sessions.

At the start of each BCT session, the therapist reviews the Recovery Contract calendar to see how well each spouse has done his or her part. If the Recovery Contract includes 12-step meetings or urine drug screens, these are also marked on the calendar and reviewed. The calendar provides a record of progress that the therapist rewards verbally at each session. The couple performs the trust discussion in each session to highlight its importance and to let the therapist observe this important ritual.

Because relationship factors are conducive to sobriety, BCT uses a series of behavioral assignments to increase positive feelings, shared activities, and constructive communication. *Catch Your Partner Doing Something Nice* has each spouse notice and acknowledge one pleasing behavior performed by his or her partner each day. In the *Caring Day* assignment, each partner plans ahead to surprise their spouse with a day when they do special things to show their caring. Planning and doing *shared rewarding activities* is important because many substance abusers' families have stopped the kind of shared activities that are associated with positive recovery outcomes (Moos, Finney, & Cronkite, 1990). Teaching *communication skills* can help the substance abuser and spouse to deal with stressors in their relationship and in their lives. Relapse prevention (Marlatt & Gordon, 1985) is the final activity of BCT. At the end of weekly BCT sessions, each couple completes a *Continuing Recovery Plan* that is reviewed at quarterly follow-up visits for an additional 2 years.

Other Behavioral Methods When the Substance Abuser Has Sought Help

Building on the successful outcomes of BCT with adult married or cohabiting couples, other behavioral methods have been developed for different groups of patients and different goals:

1. Behavioral family counseling adapts BCT for use with a family member other than a spouse (e.g., mother and young adult substance abuser) (O'Farrell, Murphy, Alter, & Fals-Stewart, 2010).
2. Behavioral family therapy is designed for use with adolescent substance abusers and their parents (Azrin, Donohue, Besalel, Kogan, & Acierno, 1994).

3. Couple relapse prevention sessions help maintain gains after weekly BCT ends, especially for those with more severe substance problems who may be vulnerable to relapse (O'Farrell, Choquette, & Cutter, 1998).
4. Behavioral contracting and family meetings can promote aftercare plan compliance following formal treatment (O'Farrell, Murphy, Alter, & Fals-Stewart, 2008; Ossip-Klein & Rychtarik, 1993).

Social Network Therapy Approach

Social network therapy (Galanter, 1999) is an approach to substance abuse treatment in which the therapist enlists the help of selected family members and friends to provide ongoing support for the substance abuser. Network members serve a supporting role for the therapist, but the emphasis of treatment is placed squarely on the identified patient. Social network therapy aims for the substance abuser's abstinence with relapse prevention within a drug- and alcohol-free lifestyle. The network (i.e., supportive family members and CSOs) is a crucial resource both to the substance abuser in his or her attempt to achieve sustained abstinence, and to the therapist helping the substance abuser achieve this objective.

In social network therapy, the network is chosen from among family members and CSOs who have a long-standing relationship with the substance abuser. The therapist uses the network to obtain an accurate, multifaceted substance use history, to exert social pressure on the substance abuser to engage in the treatment process, to facilitate compliance with treatment objectives, and to increase positive social support during and after treatment. In addition, network members can receive counseling about how they can better cope with having a substance abuser in their social sphere.

Typically, the substance abuser is also involved in individual counseling, while the therapist meets separately with network members. However, eventually the substance abuser is involved in the network meetings as well.

Ecological Approach

In ecological treatment models, interventions focus on assessing and changing multiple system influences that affect the substance abuser. These influences may include intrapersonal variables, the interpersonal system of the family and larger social network, and the extrapersonal system, such as the school and community at large. These approaches have much in common with family systems methods, but typically target youth and are broader in scope. Ecological approaches focus not only on the individual patient and his or her family, but also on extrafamilial factors (e.g., peer, school, and neighborhood) that may influence drinking and drug use. Two of the most promising and well-known ecologically based family approaches are multisystemic family therapy (MST; Henggeler et al., 1991), and multidimensional family therapy (MDFT; Liddle, 2002), both of which are well-established treatment approaches for adolescent substance abusers.

MST typically includes sessions or parts of sessions held conjointly with the adolescent substance abuser and other family members. The implicit goal of MST is to identify and restructure multiple risk factors in the youth's environment to reduce antisocial behavior. MST therapists work to empower parents in family sessions with the adolescent substance abuser. These sessions draw upon therapeutic techniques from other treatment models, including family systems therapy, behavioral approaches, and general counseling interventions. Therapists evaluate the factors in the adolescent's ecological environment that contribute to the substance use, and may implement interventions at comparatively broad levels (e.g., in the school system, through juvenile delinquency programs) to affect change. At the same time, the therapist may conduct one-on-one sessions with the adolescent to focus on decision making, emotion regulation, and other intrapersonal factors that may be related to substance-using and delinquent behaviors.

MDFT views adolescent substance abuse as a result of multifactorial, interacting systems. As such, it integrates multiple theoretical approaches in its interventions, such as family therapy, individual therapy, drug counseling, and multiple-systems-oriented intervention approaches. While an adolescent's substance abuse is the primary presenting problem, MDFT interventions typically have four primary target domains: the adolescent (intrapersonal and relational issues), the parent(s) (individual functioning as well as parenting role), the family environment (family interaction patterns), and extrafamilial systems of influence on the adolescent and family (e.g., peers, schools, social service agencies, juvenile justice system). Engaging and establishing alliances with members across each of these domains is critical to achieving high retention rates with target adolescents and their families. MDFT is a flexible approach. Treatment length is determined by the therapist, family, and setting, and may include a combination of individual and family sessions. MDFT begins with a thorough multisystem assessment of both developmental ecological risk and protective factors. The therapist uses this information to conceptualize the case and identify strengths and weaknesses in the adolescent's multiple systems, which then becomes the basis of the intervention.

Evidence for Family Therapy to Aid Recovery When the Substance Abuser Has Sought Help

With adult married or cohabiting substance abusers, BCT has a strong evidence base showing more abstinence and better relationship outcomes for BCT than for individual-based treatment (IBT). A meta-analysis of 12 controlled studies showed that BCT produced better outcomes than more typical individual-based treatment for married or cohabiting alcoholic and drug-abusing patients, with a medium effect size favoring BCT over IBT (Powers, Vedal, & Emmelkamp, 2008). More specifically, patients who received BCT had less substance use, fewer substance-related problems, and better relationship functioning through 12-month follow-up than patients who received IBT (Epstein & McCrady, 1998; O'Farrell & Clements, 2011).

For adolescent substance abusers, MST and MDFT have a strong evidence base showing greater improvements in multiple outcome domains than treatment as usually practiced. MST and MDFT have been particularly effective at reducing co-occurring problem behaviors among youth experiencing multiple comorbid problems such as delinquency (Letourneau et al., 2009), mental health symptoms (Liddle & Dakof, 2002), and sexual risks (Letourneau et al., 2009; see also Rowe, in press; Marvel, Rowe, Colon, DiClemente, & Liddle, 2009).

The other family approaches for use when the substance abuser has sought help have a less substantial evidence base than BCT, MST, or MDFT. Recent literature reviews of network therapy and FST have identified a small number of studies showing improved outcomes over control groups for adult alcoholism and drug abuse (O'Farrell & Clements, 2011; Rowe, in press). Finally, family disease approach studies show that 12-step facilitation based on AA and Al-Anon facilitation based on Al-Anon, respectively, produced improvements in drinking for alcoholic patients (Project MATCH Research Group, 1997) and reduced emotional distress for family members (Miller et al., 1999). However, family disease approach studies have not examined relationship outcomes. Table 10.1 summarizes key points about family-based methods to aid recovery when the substance abuser has sought help.

Case Example

To illustrate some of the techniques described, we present a case example of a married couple treated with BCT. This example is a composite of cases treated by O'Farrell.

Stephen was a 37-year-old white male who was referred to outpatient substance abuse treatment by his physician for alcohol dependence. Stephen had agreed to come to treatment only after a confrontation with his wife, Ellen, who was concerned with her husband's abusive drinking. During a detailed psychosocial assessment conducted as part of his intake assessment, Stephen described an extensive history of problematic alcohol use since his early 20s.

Stephen reported that he had entered a 28-day inpatient treatment program about 3 years before the present evaluation and had stayed sober for roughly 1 year after treatment. Financial problems, arguments with his wife, and stress at work contributed to his relapse. He also noted that, during the last 2 years, he drank daily, but that there had been a steady increase in daily drinking throughout that time period, going from two to three drinks a day, and rising more recently to six to eight drinks each day. Stephen admitted that he drove his car while intoxicated on "too many nights to count." The assessment revealed that Stephen met criteria for alcohol dependence.

The therapist asked Stephen if he was willing to participate in a marital assessment with Ellen. Although Stephen acknowledged that he was reluctant to participate, he reported that Ellen very much wanted to be involved in the treatment in some capacity. He signed a release-of-confidentiality form to allow his therapist to discuss the possibility of participation with Ellen. She agreed to come to the clinic with Stephen. The therapist described the planned assessment procedures, and emphasized that the assessment did not commit either the couple or the therapist to treatment.

During the assessment, Ellen reported that she knew Stephen drank "heavily," but was not aware of the extent of his drinking until he entered inpatient treatment. Both partners described their relationship as unstable and mentioned that they had recently discussed divorce.

Ellen said she felt "neglected" because Stephen spent so much time drinking with his friends. From her report, the partners rarely spoke, showed little affection toward each other, and had not spent much time engaging in shared recreational activities (e.g., going to the movies, eating out). Neither partner reported any episodes of physical aggression, although both acknowledged that Stephen was verbally abusive on several occasions when he was drunk.

As part of the assessment, the therapist asked the partners to discuss a problem they both agreed existed in their relationship while the therapist observed. The partners chose the topic of "financial problems." As part of this conflict resolution task, the therapist asked the partners to describe the problem and work toward a solution. The following is a partial transcript of the partners' discussion, occurring about 3 minutes after the task was initiated:

ELLEN: Why is it that you spend all of our money on your friends, going out getting loaded, and not saving one f**king dime for our future? You are never home, never here . . .

STEPHEN: Why would I want to stay home? When I'm there, you give me s**t about drinking, bringing up everything I've ever done wrong. I go out, and you complain about that. That's it . . . you just b**ch.

ELLEN: That's how you see it, but I want you to stop drinking and care about me more than you care about your drinking buddies, who really don't give a damn about you anyway.

STEPHEN: I've tried to stop . . . you know I have . . . but even when I stop, you just bark at me about why I didn't do it before. Do you know how much that sucks? How long you gonna carry that across?

ELLEN: For a while. Can you blame me? You come home drunk, go to sleep, go to work . . . we don't talk, we don't have sex. . . . I swear, I don't know you at all anymore.

STEPHEN: I know, but at least I went to the doctor as you wanted and came here. I don't like it either.

ELLEN: I know you say you have stopped drinking, but I don't believe it and have never believed it. You do nothing around the house, you don't fix the car, or lift a finger for anything.

STEPHEN: Christ, I stopped drinking and you don't believe me and call me a liar. I drink and I am a drunk and a liar. F**k the house, f**ck the car . . .

ELLEN: Don't you see . . . I sit alone all the time. Please just stop. I want to get our lives back.

STEPHEN: Yeah, me too . . . that's why I'm in this place. But I am not here to have this turn into a place where you can just yell at me and I take it. . . . I won't take it, be warned. I'd rather start over with someone who doesn't know the past and can't use it as a weapon.

ELLEN: It won't take a rocket scientist to figure out your past, no matter who you are with.

This exchange reflects not only significant deficits in these partners' communication patterns, but also deficits in their relationship commitment and ability to resolve conflict. Although the topic was "financial problems," they engaged in "kitchen sinking," that is, introducing several other conflict areas without addressing the problem at hand. This communication sample reveals the negative effects of alcohol and related behaviors on the marriage, with Stephen's drinking appearing to interfere greatly with important relationship activities (e.g., saving money, talking to each other, making love).

The partners agreed to participate in BCT. Early sessions involved introducing and following through with a negotiated Recovery Contract, which included five primary components: (1) Stephen agreed to allow Ellen to observe him take his prescribed disulfiram; (2) the couple agreed to a "trust discussion" when Stephen took the disulfiram (i.e., Stephen reporting he had stayed sober during the last day and promising to remain sober for the next day, and Ellen thanking him for remaining sober); (3) Ellen agreed not to bring up negative past events about Stephen's drinking; (4) Stephen agreed to attend AA meetings daily; and (5) the partners agreed they would not threaten to divorce or separate while at home and would, for the time being, bring these thoughts into the sessions.

The partners reported Stephen's use of disulfiram was very helpful to both of them. Stephen did not entertain the idea of drinking while taking disulfiram. Ellen, because she observed Stephen take the disulfiram, trusted he was not drinking (for the first time in many months), and thus had much greater peace of mind. The positive trust discussion between the partners made the daily Recovery Contract a caring behavior rather than a "checking-up" procedure. Stephen said there was substantially less stress in the home because Ellen did not bring up his past drinking and did not call him a liar when he reported he was not drinking. Stephen's AA involvement gave him a support network that did not include friends with whom he drank. Ellen reported sometimes attending an Al-Anon group for wives of alcoholics, which gave her a support group to discuss her marriage.

Communication skills training focused on slowing down the partners' verbal exchanges, reminding them to discuss one issue at a time. The partners learned to make positive specific requests and to use "I" statements as a way to own their feelings rather than attributing how they feel to their spouse.

Later sessions addressed identified relationship problems. Assignments such as Catch Your Partner Doing Something Nice and Shared Rewarding Activities increased positive verbal exchanges and mutual caring by the partners, along with reestablishing a long-term commitment to the relationship. Toward the end of therapy, the partners reported that BCT helped them learn to "enjoy each other again." They noted that their sex life had improved dramatically and, with a referral, they had sought help from a credit counselor to address some of their financial problems.

After completing primary treatment, the couple entered the aftercare phase of treatment. In this stage, the partners came to treatment once every other month for a year to stabilize Stephen's sobriety and the couple's relationship satisfaction. During this period, Stephen reported he had remained sober and continued to take disulfiram. Both partners reported that they made a point of doing something together that was mutually rewarding at least once per week. Stephen was attending AA meetings three times weekly and was generally "working the steps" of AA. Although the partners continued to have money problems, Ellen received a work promotion, which helped to alleviate some of the financial stress.

This case example highlights some important issues. First, with some coaching from a therapist, Ellen confronted her husband about his alcohol use and encouraged him to get an evaluation. The physician's evaluation increased his motivation to enter into formal treatment. The interrelatedness of Stephen's alcohol use and the relationship difficulties suggested that a couple-based treatment, addressing both sets of problems concurrently, would be helpful. Lastly, the couple continued to participate in aftercare treatment effectively to solidify their treatment gains.

Conclusion

As is evidenced by the breadth of interventions described in this chapter, there is no shortage of family-based treatment methods for therapists treating substance abusers. Although family treatment was, at one time, frowned upon by the treatment community, it is now an integral part of all phases of the treatment process, from motivating reluctant substance abusers, through primary treatment, to helping maintaining long-term sobriety after treatment. In many cases, failure to involve family members in the treatment process is considered substandard care.

The most recent decade has witnessed significant advances in research examining the generally robust effects of family-involved treatment for substance abuse. More recently, reviews of family therapy approaches applied to drug abuse (Rowe, in press) and alcoholism (O'Farrell & Clements, 2011) are identifying which of the family approaches demonstrate the strongest empirical effects for treating substance abuse, as well as other interrelated outcomes.

Despite increased recognition of the importance of involving the family in treatment, findings from other studies indicate that many effective family-based methods are not widely used in community-based treatment programs. For example, BCT appears to be a very effective treatment for married or cohabiting substance-abusing patients, but is rarely used by substance abuse treatment providers in nonresearch settings (McGovern, Fox, Xie, & Drake, 2004). Anecdotal observations suggest that at least some treatment programs involving families do so in one or two sessions only, rather than as an active component of treatment. The added burden of involving family members in these sessions adds to time, scheduling, and therapeutic complexity, though these additional expenses are typically not reimbursed by insurance companies.

Issues of cost have become more pressing in the current era of U.S. health care reform. A recent cost-effectiveness analysis (Morgan & Crane, 2010) underscores the need for providers to consider outcomes not in isolation, but in the context of rising service delivery costs. It currently is unclear whether the benefits yielded by more inexpensive modalities, such as individual-based therapy, are "sufficient" for certain patients given the lower costs. Research examining effects and costs of family-involved treatments must explore further both short-term and long-term outcomes. Effects on both primary and secondary behavior targets and persons, effects relative to other treatment modalities, and use of family approaches in stepped-care models may help determine when family-involved treatment is needed given its higher cost and intensity to deliver.

Acknowledgment

Preparation of this chapter was supported, in part, by the Department of Veterans Affairs.

References

Akers, R., Krohn, M., Lanza Kaduce, L., & Radosevich, M. (1979). Social learning and deviant behavior: A specific test of a general theory. *American Sociology Review, 44*, 636–655.

Al-Anon Family Groups. (1981). *This is Al-Anon.* New York: Author.

Azrin, N. (1976). Improvements in the community-reinforcement approach to alcoholism. *Behaviour Research and Therapy, 14*, 339–348.

Azrin, N., Donohue, B., Besalel, V., Kogan, E., & Acierno, R. (1994). Youth drug abuse treatment: A controlled outcome study. *Journal of Child and Adolescent Substance Abuse, 3*, 1–16.

Barber, J., & Gilbertson, R. (1998). Evaluation of a self-help manual for the female partners of heavy drinkers. *Research in Social Work Practice, 8*, 141–151.

Center for Substance Abuse Treatment. (2004). *Substance abuse treatment and family therapy* (Treatment Improvement Protocol Series, No. 39). Rockville, MD: Substance Abuse and Mental Health Services Administration.

Coleman, S., & Davis, D. (1978). Family therapy and drug abuse: A national survey. *Family Process, 17*, 21–29.

Epstein, E., & McCrady, B. (1998). Behavioral couples treatment of alcohol and drug use disorders: Current status and innovations. *Clinical Psychology Review, 18*, 689–711.

Faber, E., & Keating-O'Connor, B. (1991). Planned family intervention: Johnson Institute method. *Journal of Chemical Dependency Treatment, 4*, 61–71.

Galanter, M. (1999). *Network therapy for alcohol and drug abuse.* New York: Guilford Press.

Haley, J. (1976). *Problem-solving therapy.* San Francisco: Jossey-Bass.

Henggeler, S., Borduin, C., Melton, G., Mann, B., Smith, L., Hall, J., et al. (1991). Effects of multisystemic therapy on drug use and abuse in serious juvenile offenders: A progress report from two outcome studies. *Family Dynamics of Addiction Quarterly, 1*, 40–51.

Jellinek, E. (1960). *The disease concept of alcoholism.* New Haven, CT: Hillhouse Press.

Kaufman, E. (1985). Family therapy in the treatment of alcoholism. In E. T. Bratter & G. G. Forrest (Eds.), *Alcoholism and substance abuse: Strategies for clinical interventions* (pp. 376–397). New York: Free Press.

Keller, M. (1974). Trends in treatment of alcoholism. In *Second special report to the U.S. Congress on alcohol and health* (pp. 145–167). Washington, DC: Department of Health, Education, and Welfare.

Kirby, K., Marlowe, D., Festinger, D., Garvey, K., & LaMonaca, V. (1999). Community reinforcement training for family and significant others of drug abusers: A unilateral intervention to increase treatment entry of drug users. *Drug and Alcohol Dependence, 56*, 85–96.

Krampen, G. (1989). Motivation in the treatment of alcoholism. *Addictive Behaviors, 14*, 197–200.

Landau, J., & Garrett, J. (2006). *Invitational intervention: A step-by-step guide for clinicians helping families engage resistant substance abusers in treatment.* New York: Haworth.

Landau, J., Stanton, M., Ikle, D., Garrett, J., Shea, R., Browning, A., et al. (2004). Outcomes with the ARISE approach to engaging reluctant drug- and alcohol-dependent individuals in treatment. *American Journal of Drug and Alcohol Abuse, 30*, 711–748.

Letourneau, E., Henggeler, S., Borduin, C., Schewe, P., McCart, M., Chapman, J., et al. (2009). Multisystemic therapy for juvenile sexual offenders: 1–year results from a randomized effectiveness trial. *Journal of Family Psychology, 23*, 89–102.

Liddle, H. (2002). Advances in family-based therapy for adolescent substance abuse: Findings from the multidimensional family therapy research program. In L. Harris (Ed.), *Problems of Drug Dependence 2001: Proceedings of the 63rd Annual Scientific Meeting* (NIDA Research Monograph No. 182, pp. 113–115). Bethesda, MD: National Institute on Drug Abuse.

Liddle, H., & Dakof, G. (2002). A randomized controlled trial of intensive outpatient, family based therapy vs. residential drug treatment for co-morbid adolescent drug abusers. *Drug and Alcohol Dependence, 66*(Suppl.), S103.

Liepman, M., Nirenberg, T., & Begin, A. (1989). Evaluation of a program designed to help family and significant others to motivate resistant alcoholics into recovery. *American Journal of Drug and Alcohol Abuse, 15*, 209–221.

Marlatt, G., & Gordon, J. (Eds.). (1985). *Relapse prevention.* New York: Guilford Press.

Marvel, F., Rowe, C., Colon, L., DiClemente, R., & Liddle, H. (2009). Multidimensional family therapy HIV/STD risk-reduction intervention: An integrative family-based model for drug-involved juvenile offenders. *Family Process, 48*, 69–83.

McCrady, B. (1986). The family in the change process. In W. Miller & N. Heather (Eds.), *Treating addictive behaviors: Process of change* (pp. 305–318). New York: Plenum Press.

McCrady, B., & Epstein, E. (2008). *Overcoming alcohol problems: A couples-focused program therapist guide.* New York: Oxford University Press.

McGovern, M., Fox, T., Xie, H., & Drake, R. (2004). A survey of clinical practices and readiness to adopt evidence-based practices: Dissemination research in an addiction treatment system. *Journal of Substance Abuse Treatment, 26*, 305–312.

Meyers, R., Miller, W., Smith, J., & Tonigan, J. (2002). A randomized trial of two methods for engaging treatment-refusing drug users through concerned significant others. *Journal of Consulting and Clinical Psychology, 70,* 1182–1185.

Miller, W., Meyers, R., & Tonigan, J. (1999). Engaging the unmotivated in treatment for alcohol problems: A comparison of three strategies for intervention through family members. *Journal of Consulting and Clinical Psychology, 67,* 688–697.

Minuchin, S. (1974). *Families and family therapy.* Cambridge, MA: Harvard University Press.

Moos, R., Finney, J., & Cronkite, R. (1990). *Alcoholism treatment: Context, process, and outcome.* New York: Oxford University Press.

Morgan, T., & Crane, D. (2010). Cost-effectiveness of family-based substance abuse treatment. *Journal of Marital and Family Therapy, 36,* 486–498.

Nowinski, J. (1999). *Family recovery and substance abuse: A twelve-step guide for treatment.* Thousand Oaks, CA: Sage.

O'Farrell, T. (Ed.). (1993). *Treating alcohol problems: Marital and family interventions.* New York: Guilford Press.

O'Farrell, T., Choquette, K., & Cutter, H. (1998). Couples relapse prevention sessions after behavioral marital therapy for male alcoholics: Outcomes during the three years after starting treatment. *Journal of Studies on Alcohol, 59,* 357–370.

O'Farrell, T., & Clements, K. (2011). Review of outcome research on marital and family therapy for treatment of alcoholism. *Journal of Marital and Family Therapy.* Available at doi: 10.1111/j.1752-0606.2011.00242.x

O'Farrell, T., & Fals-Stewart, W. (2006). *Behavioral couples therapy for alcoholism and drug abuse.* New York: Guilford Press.

O'Farrell, T., Murphy, C., Stephan, S., Fals-Stewart, W., & Murphy, M. (2004). Partner violence before and after couple-based alcoholism treatment for male alcoholic patients: The role of treatment involvement and abstinence. *Journal of Consulting and Clinical Psychology, 72,* 202–217.

O'Farrell, T., Murphy, M., Alter, J., & Fals-Stewart, W. (2008). Brief family treatment intervention to promote continuing care among alcohol-dependent patients in inpatient detoxification: A randomized pilot study. *Journal of Substance Abuse Treatment, 34,* 363–369.

O'Farrell, T., Murphy, M., Alter, J., & Fals-Stewart, W. (2010). Behavioral family counseling for substance abuse: A treatment development pilot study. *Addictive Behaviors, 35,* 1–6.

Ossip-Klein, D., & Rychtarik, R. (1993). Behavioral contracts between alcoholics and family members: Improving aftercare participation and maintaining sobriety after inpatient alcoholism treatment. In T. O'Farrell (Ed.), *Treating alcohol problems: Marital and family interventions* (pp. 281–304). New York: Guilford Press.

Powers, M., Vedel, E., & Emmelkamp, P. (2008). Behavioral couples therapy (BCT) for alcohol and drug use disorders: A meta-analysis. *Clinical Psychology Review, 28,* 952–962.

Project MATCH Research Group. (1997). Matching alcoholism treatments to client heterogeneity: Project MATCH posttreatment drinking outcomes. *Journal of Studies on Alcohol, 58,* 7–29.

Rowe, C. (in press). Family therapy for drug abuse: Review and updates, 2003–2010. *Journal of Marital and Family Therapy.*

Rychtarik, R., & McGillicuddy, N. (2005). Coping skills training and 12–step facilitation for women whose partner has alcoholism: Effects on depression, the partner's drinking, and partner physical violence. *Journal of Consulting and Clinical Psychology, 73,* 249–261.

Sisson, R., & Azrin, H. (1986). Family-member involvement to initiate and promote treatment of problem drinkers. *Journal of Behavior Therapy and Experimental Psychiatry, 17,* 15–21.

Smith, J., & Meyers, R. (2004). *Motivating substance abusers to enter treatment: Working with family members.* New York: Guilford Press.

Stanton, M. (1997). The role of family and significant others in the engagement and retention of drug-dependent individuals. In L. Onken, J. Blaine, & F. Boren (Eds.), *Beyond the therapeutic alliance: Keeping the drug dependent individual in treatment* (pp. 157–180). Rockville, MD: National Institute on Drug Abuse.

Stanton, M., & Heath, A. (1997). Family and marital treatment. In J. Lowinson, P. Ruiz, R. Millman, & J. Langrod (Eds.), *Substance abuse: A comprehensive textbook* (3rd ed., pp. 448–454). Baltimore: Williams & Wilkins.

Stanton, M., Todd, T., & Associates. (1982). *The family therapy of drug abuse and addiction.* New York: Guilford Press.

Steinglass, P., Bennett, L., Wolin, S., & Reiss, D. (1987). *The alcoholic family.* New York: Basic Books.

Chapter 11

Neurobiological Bases of Addiction Treatment

Philip H. Chung
Julie D. Ross
Sidarth Wakhlu
Bryon Adinoff

Over the past two decades stunning progress has been made in understanding the psychopathology of addiction. These advances have identified changes in neural pathways that evolve following chronic substance use. Substance-induced alterations in brain functioning have both physiological (tolerance and dependence) and behavioral consequences, such as craving and the inability to control the impulse to use drugs despite adverse consequences—the defining characteristic of addiction. Neuroimaging technologies have been used to study the brain and the reinforcing and addictive properties of substances. In a parallel effort, genetic risk factors have been identified that predispose individuals to addictive disorders. Understanding that addiction has a fundamental biological component helps explain the difficulty that many people have in achieving and maintaining abstinence without pharmacological treatment. On the basis of this medical model of addiction, several medications have been developed to assist in normalizing the brain chemistry disrupted by chronic substance use or aid in the avoidance of substance use. By providing this support, new medications allow addicted individuals to focus on their psychosocial treatment and work a program of recovery.

This chapter first presents the basics of brain function, including the neurotransmitters and pathways involved in substance abuse. This understanding provides the foundation for the subsequent presentation of medications used to treat addictive disorders. This chapter focuses on medications approved by the U.S. Food and Drug Administration (FDA) for alcohol dependence and opioid dependence with an overview of promising new developments for stimulant and cannabis dependence. (Carroll & Kiluk, Chapter 12, this volume) in this book talks more specifically about integrating psychotherapy with pharmacotherapy.

Brain Basics

Neurons and the Brain

Microscopically, the brain is composed of a collection of cells, or *neurons*, that signal one another both chemically and electrically. Electrical signals are used to communicate within cells, and chemical signals are used to communicate between cells. Most neurons have a characteristic structure that consists of a globular *cell body* with numerous long, spindly projections coming off the central cell body (Figure 11.1). These projections are used in the process of signaling between neurons and receive communications from their sometimes-distant cell bodies. The *axon* of a signaling cell projects to the *dendrite* of the receiving cell, and the two projections come into close proximity with one another but do not touch. This coming together of the axon of the signaling cell and the dendrite of the receiving cell is the *synapse*, and the space between the two projections is the *synaptic cleft* (Figure 11.2). Cells are either *presynaptic* or *postsynaptic* to indicate the location

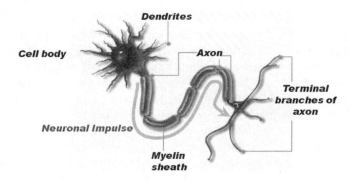

FIGURE 11.1. Structure of a neuron. Both axons and dendrites project from the central cell body. Electrical impulses travel down the axon, which is insulated by the myelin sheath, to the terminal branches of the axon. Adapted from the National Institutes of Health Image Bank.

of the cell relative to the signaling process being studied. The presynaptic cell is the cell that is sending the message; the postsynaptic cell is the cell that is receiving the message. When a neuron fires electrically, or *depolarizes*, a message is carried from one part of a cell to its projections. Neuronal firing causes the release of chemical *neurotransmitters* (e.g., dopamine) into the synapse that carry signals across the synaptic cleft from one neuron to another (Figure 11.2). At rest, neurotransmitters are stored in *vesicles* at the terminal ends of the axon of the presynaptic cell. When the cells depolarize, the vesicles fuse with the cell membrane, and a neurotransmitter is released from the presynaptic cell into the synaptic cleft. The neurotransmitter then diffuses out across the small space of the synaptic cleft to contact the postsynaptic cell membrane. *Receptors* on the postsynaptic cell membrane are proteins that await the arrival of specific neurotransmitters, much like a lock awaiting a specific key. The binding of the neurotransmitter to the receptor then activates that receptor, which in turn transmits a signal into the postsynaptic cell. Many receptors and neurotransmitter systems have been implicated in the neurobiology of substance abuse, including dopamine, serotonin, norepinephrine, glutamate, gamma-aminobutyric acid (GABA), acetylcholine, the endogenous opiate system, and the cannabinoid system (Kandel, Schwartz, & Jessell, 2000).

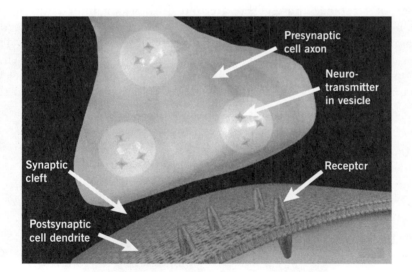

FIGURE 11.2. Structure of a synapse. Cells signal one another via synapses. In response to an electrical impulse, neurotransmitters are released from vesicles in the presynaptic cell axon. The neurotransmitters diffuse across the synaptic cleft to bind to receptors on the postsynaptic cell membrane. Adapted from the National Institutes of Health Image Bank.

Neuroanatomy Basics

On a larger scale, the brain is composed of the brainstem, the basal ganglia, and the cortex (Figure 11.3), as well as the many thousands of connections, or *tracts*, between these structures (Nolte, 2009). The brainstem is the most interior and primitive area of the brain. Several anatomical areas in the brainstem are thought to be involved in the pathogenesis of addictive behaviors, including the *ventral tegmental area (VTA), substantia nigra (SN)*, and *dorsal raphe nucleus (DRN)*. The area between the brainstem and the cortex is the basal ganglia and is made up of distinct areas, many of which are involved in the development and persistence of addiction. These include the *nucleus accumbens (NAc), bed nucleus of the stria terminalis (BNST)*, and *amygdala*. The outermost and most evolutionarily advanced anatomical area of the brain is the cortex, which communicates to the rest of the brain via the *thalamus*. Several cortical areas are implicated in the pathogenesis of drug-taking behaviors, including the *anterior cingulate cortex, dorsolateral prefrontal cortex, orbitofrontal cortex, insular cortex*, and *hippocampus* (Figure 11.4).

Neuroanatomy of Substance Abuse

The neurotransmitter dopamine is particularly important in the neurobiology of substance abuse. There are four distinct dopamine pathways in the brain: the mesolimbic pathway, the mesocortical pathway, the nigrostriatal pathway, and the tuberoinfundibular pathway (Figure 11.4). The first dopamine pathway in the brain is the *mesolimbic pathway*, which is composed of cells in the ventral tegmental area that project to the nucleus accumbens. It was originally thought that the release of dopamine in the

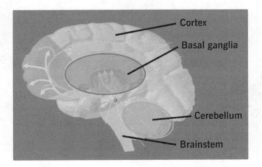

FIGURE 11.3. Major anatomical divisions of the brain. The brainstem is at the base of the brain. The basal ganglia are located on top of the brainstem. The cortex is the outermost structure, and the cerebellum sits off the back of the brain. Adapted from the National Institutes of Health Image Bank.

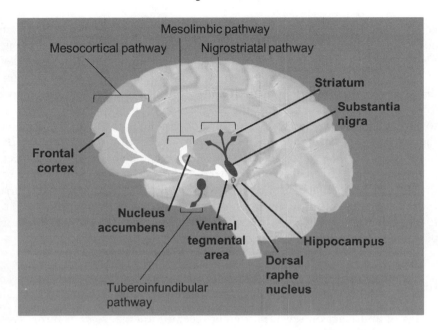

FIGURE 11.4. Brain areas involved in the neurobiology of addiction. Labeled in bold are the frontal cortex, nucleus accumbens, ventral tegmental area, dorsal raphe nucleus, hippocampus, substantia nigra, and striatum. Also represented are the four dopamine pathways in the brain: the mesolimbic pathway (white), the mesocortical pathway (white), the nigrostriatal pathway (gray), and the tuberoinfundibular pathway (gray). Adapted from the National Institutes of Health Image Bank.

nucleus accumbens was the neurobiological substrate that accounted for the experience of pleasure. However, further study suggested that the brain mechanisms underlying substance abuse were more complicated than first hypothesized. Dopamine cells of the mesolimbic pathway also project to a variety of other subcortical structures, including the amygdala, bed nucleus of the stria terminalis (BNST), lateral septal area, and lateral hypothalamus, which are also involved in the pathogenesis of substance abuse.

The second dopamine pathway in the brain is the *mesocortical pathway*, which consists of cells in the ventral tegmental area whose projections extend to cerebral cortical structures, especially the frontal lobes. This pathway is important for cognitive function, motivation, and emotional responses. It includes several cerebral cortical structures believed to have an important role in the addictive process, such as the dorsolateral prefrontal cortex (Dagher, Owen, Boecker, & Brooks, 1999), the orbitofrontal cortex (Elliott, Dolan, & Frith, 2000; Kringelbach, 2005), and the anterior cingulate (Allman, Hakeem, Erwin, Nimchinsky, & Hof, 2001; Bush, Luu,

& Posner, 2000). This neural system may contribute to the development of addiction in several ways. The prefrontal cortex is important in allowing people to control impulsive behavior. Hence, disruptions or abnormalities in this area of the brain may lead to increased impulsivity and subsequent drug use. In addition, the impaired ability of this circuit to inhibit behaviors may be involved in craving, the progression of drug use from impulsive to compulsive use and relapse. The third dopamine pathway in the brain is the *nigrostriatal pathway*, which consists of a collection of dopamine cells in the substantia nigra (adjacent to the ventral tegmental area) that project to the striatum. This pathway is involved in the production of movement in the normal brain (Nicola, Surmeier, & Malenka, 2000) and can account for the motor effects of some drugs of abuse (Gardner & Ashby, 2000). The fourth dopamine pathway is the *tuberoinfundibular pathway* and does not play a significant role in substance abuse.

Reward and Drug Taking

Drugs of abuse act on several different receptor and neurotransmitter systems (Gardner, 1997). However, the activation of dopamine-rich cells in the ventral tegmental area and the subsequent release of dopamine in the nucleus accumbens is particularly important because it is associated with reward. This biochemical phenomenon is observed with both natural pleasurable stimuli (e.g., food and sex) and a variety of drugs of abuse (e.g., alcohol, amphetamine, caffeine, cocaine, marijuana, nicotine, opiods, and phencyclidine) (Adinoff, 2004).

Drugs are classified by the response caused in a cell after they bind to their respective receptors. An *agonist* is a drug that stimulates (turns on) a response in a cell after binding to a receptor. An *antagonist* is a drug that blocks (turns off) the response caused by the agonist. A *partial agonist* is a drug that binds to and activates a receptor to a lesser degree when compared to a full agonist. Stimulant drugs such as cocaine (Ritz, Lamb, Goldberg, & Kuhar, 1987) and amphetamine (Bunney & Aghajanian, 1978) work to directly increase the concentration of dopamine in the nucleus accumbens by binding to proteins on the presynaptic membrane of the dopamine cell itself, but many other drugs of abuse work indirectly to increase dopamine in the nucleus accumbens. Some substances of abuse bind to receptors and cause downstream changes inside the cell that indirectly increase dopamine in the nucleus accumbens. For instance, tetrahydrocannabinol (THC, the active ingredient in marijuana) binds to and activates cannabinoid receptors throughout the brain. Opiods (i.e., heroin and morphine) bind to and activate opiod receptors in the ventral tegmental area, nucleus accumbens, and amygdala. Caffeine binds to and inactivates adenosine A2 receptors in the striatum. Alcohol and benzodiazepines increase activity of the GABA receptor. Alcohol also decreases functioning of the N-methyl-D-aspartate (NMDA) glutamate receptor. Phencyclidine (PCP) binds to the NMDA receptor and blocks ion movement through the channel in the protein. Nicotine binds to and activates nicotinic acetylcholine receptors. Each brain receptor that binds with an abused substance has a corresponding endogenous compound that is the natural key to unlock the activity of that receptor. For example, the endogenous endorphins and enkephalins bind to the opioid receptors, acetylcholine binds to the nicotinic receptor, and anandamide binds to the cannabinoid receptors. Many of the receptor and neurotransmitter systems serve as targets for existing and developing pharmacological treatment strategies for substance abusers.

However, dopamine increases alone do not fully explain the highly complex phenomenon of substance abuse, which has biological, developmental, social, learned, and psychological components. What makes a drug addictive is not directly proportionate to its primary site of action. There are two models that attempt to explain this complex relationship. In the *opponent processes* model, a drug of abuse produces euphoria (positive affective state) when acutely administered and dysphoria (negative affective state) when access to the drug is prevented. The withdrawal dysphoria is associated with decreased dopamine levels in the nucleus accumbens (Jentsch, Olausson, De La Garza, & Taylor, 2002) and may augment the transition from substance use to compulsive substance abuse (Koob & Le Moal, 2005). Substance-abusing individuals also exhibit drug-seeking behaviors at the expense of natural rewards. In the *incentive salience* model, addictive behavior is thought to form by associative learning that enhances the incentive salience (or importance) of drug-related cues in relation to natural rewards. This leaves the individual with a long-term vulnerability to relapse (Kalivas & Volkow, 2005). With continued drug use, there is a shift in how the brain imparts relative importance to different stimuli, from long-term reinforcers (e.g., healthy relationships, successful occupations) to short-term reinforcers associated with substance use. There is also thought to be behavioral sensitization, with repeated exposures to a drug of abuse, in which the impulsive liking of a drug for pure hedonic value is replaced by a more compulsive wanting of the drug with concomitant loss of control over inhibitory behaviors (Robinson & Berridge, 2000). In this way, the teaching of Alcoholics Anonymous (AA) to avoid people, places, and things associated with use is supported by neurobiological research, as these conditioned cues cause an activation of certain brain structures that lead a substance user to crave drugs of abuse.

The process of addiction itself has been conceptualized in three stages: binge, withdrawal, and craving. Each stage has been mapped onto particular anatomical areas in the brain (Koob & Volkow, 2010). In the *binge* stage, the ventral tegmental area and the nucleus accumbens (or ventral striatum) mediates the acute reinforcing effects of drugs of abuse. The transition from impulsive use to compulsive abuse is associated with a shift in activity from the ventral striatum to the dorsal striatum and orbitofrontal cortex. *Withdrawal* from drugs of abuse results from a period of acute abstinence after a prolonged period of consistent use and is associated with observable brain changes. It is associated with decreased dopamine activation in the nucleus accumbens and is mediated by the amygdala. *Craving* describes an intense desire to use a substance and can be triggered by use of a small amount of the drug itself (Self & Nestler, 1998) or by cues that are associated with drug use (Jentsch et al., 2002). The effects of craving are thought to be mediated by a wider network consisting of the orbitofrontal cortex, dorsal striatum, prefrontal cortex, amygdala, hippocampus, and insula. The consolidation of memories that leads to craving is likely mediated by the neurotransmitter glutamate and involves the amygdala and hippocampus as well as cortical regions such as the orbitofrontal cortex and the anterior cingulate cortex. Also associated with substance abuse and relapse is a decreased ability to inhibit certain behaviors (e.g., drug use), which is mediated by the cingulate cortex, the dorsolateral prefrontal cortex, and the inferior frontal cortices. Because of the loss of these higher brain functions, there is an emergence of behaviors associated with shorter term, immediate reward (Goldstein & Volkow, 2002). The inability to inhibit behaviors, often a risk factor for the development of substance abuse, also becomes increasingly impaired. Thus, there appears to be a lack of willpower in the ability to further resist substance use and relapse (Adinoff et al., 2007). The changes that occur in the brain as a result of substance abuse are complex; many do not return to predrug use levels even after prolonged abstinence. While some of the detailed neurobiological changes are still to be elucidated, it is clear there are dramatic shifts in brain functioning that result from substance abuse. Table 11.1 summarizes the areas of the brain that are involved in addictive behavior.

Medications for Substance Abuse

This section discusses the current pharmacological treatment options for the major classes of abused drugs. (The integrations of pharmacology and psychotherapy are discussed in Chapter 12.) These include medications approved by the FDA for alcohol and opioid addiction, as well as promising medications for the treatment of cocaine, methamphetamine, and cannabis addiction. Medications are presented in sections organized by specific drugs of abuse. For each medication, background information as well as clinically relevant considerations are included that should be of benefit to substance abuse treatment providers.

TABLE 11.1. Brain Areas Involved in Addiction

Amygdala	• Subcortical structure • Consolidation of emotional memories (Paton, Belova, Morrison, & Salzman, 2006) • Fear conditioning (LeDoux, 2003)
Anterior cingulate cortex	• Cortical structure • Modulation of emotional responses, impulsivity (Bush et al., 2000) • Error detection, problem solving (Allman et al., 2001)
Bed nucleus of the stria terminalis (BNST)	• Subcortical structure • Major output pathway of the amygdala (Choi et al., 2007) • Reactions to fearful stimuli (Fox et al., 2010) and stress (Somerville, Whalen, & Kelley, 2010)
Dorsal raphe nucleus (DRN)	• Midbrain structure • Location of serotonin cell bodies that project widely throughout the brain (O'Hearn & Molliver, 1984) • Regulates arousal and vigilance (Abrams et al., 2005) • Modulates activity of the ventral tegmental area (Yoshimoto & McBride, 1992)
Dorsolateral prefrontal cortex (DLPFC)	• Cortical structure • Planning, sequencing, and cognitive control (Dagher et al., 1999)
Hippocampus	• Primitive cortex • Long-term memory (Canales, 2010) and spatial navigation (Sharma, Rakoczy, & Brown-Borg, 2010)
Insular cortex	• Cortical structure • Processing negative emotional experience (Critchley, Wiens, Rotshtein, Ohman, & Dolan, 2004) and pain (Baliki, Geha, & Apkarian, 2009) • Integrating information from multiple sensory modalities (Taylor, Seminowicz, & Davis, 2009)
Nucleus accumbens (NAc)	• Subcortical structure, part of the ventral striatum • Regulation of reward (Willuhn, Wanat, Clark, & Phillips, 2010) • Response to fear (Schwienbacher, Fendt, Richardson, & Schnitzler, 2004) • Response to novelty (Legault & Wise, 2001)
Orbitofrontal cortex (OFC)	• Cortical structure • Decision making (Kringelbach, 2005) and impulsivity in novel situations (Elliott et al., 2000)
Striatum	• Subcortical structure, composed of caudate and putamen • Regulation of motor activity (Voorn, Vanderschuren, Groenewegen, Robbins, & Pennartz, 2004)

(cont.)

TABLE 11.1. *(cont.)*

Substantia nigra (SN)	• Midbrain structure • Location of dopamine cell bodies that are the origin of the nigrostriatal dopamine circuit • Regulation of movement (Nicola et al., 2000)
Thalamus	• Between cerebral cortex and midbrain • Relay area for information into and out of the cerebral cortex (Jones, 2007)
Ventral tegmental area (VTA)	• Midbrain structure • Location of dopamine cell bodies that are the origin of the mesolimbic and mesocortical dopamine circuits • Drug and natural reward circuitry (Alcaro, Huber, & Panksepp, 2007)

Alcohol Dependence

Naltrexone

Naltrexone is an opioid receptor antagonist that is approved by the FDA for treatment of alcohol dependence in an oral formulation and an intramuscular, sustained-release formulation. It is also approved for the treatment of opioid dependence (see "Opioids").

History. Naltrexone was originally developed as a treatment for heroin dependence in the 1960s. In 1994, after several studies demonstrated its efficacy in treating alcohol-dependent individuals (O'Malley et al., 1992; Volpicelli, Alterman, Hayashida, & O'Brien, 1992), naltrexone was approved by the FDA for the treatment of alcohol dependence. In 2006, the FDA approved the sustained-release formulation, which is given by monthly intramuscular injection. This format may benefit patients with difficulties adhering to medication.

Pharmacology. Naltrexone appears to disrupt the rewarding and reinforcing effects of alcohol through its effects on the opioid receptor and, subsequently, dopamine release. In animal models, naltrexone administration decreases dopamine release, thereby attenuating reinforcement from alcohol (Benjamin, Grant, & Pohorecky, 1993). Naltrexone may also interfere with the transmission of reward signals by blocking stimulation of the opioid receptors by endogenous opioid compounds (endorphins, enkephalins, and dynorphins) (Morris, Hopwood, Whelan, Gardiner, & Drummond, 2001). Consistent with the postulated mechanism of decreasing the reward associated with alcohol, naltrexone decreases heavy drinking more than it increases abstinence (Pettinati et al., 2006).

Evidence and Research. The COMBINE (Combined Pharmacotherapies and Behavioral Interventions Study) trial evaluated the comparative efficacy of naltrexone, acamprosate, and behavioral interventions for treatment of opioid addiction. Naltrexone was found to be highly effective in decreasing drinking in treated subjects (Anton et al., 2006). A meta-analysis (a study that combines the results of multiple smaller studies to increase the statistical strength) of 24 naltrexone trials found that naltrexone decreased the risk of relapse in short-term treatment (up to 12 weeks), relative to placebo. Longer treatment courses (12 weeks or longer) resulted primarily in improvements in time to first drink and craving (Srisurapanont & Jarusuraisin, 2005). A review of 29 studies similarly found that most studies demonstrated decreased heavy or excessive drinking outcomes, rather than improved abstinence rates, with naltrexone versus placebo (Pettinati et al., 2006). A study of the sustained-release formulation of naltrexone (Vivitrol) demonstrated both its safety and efficacy in reducing the number of heavy drinking days (Kranzler, Modesto-Lowe, & Nuwayser, 1998).

Formulation and Dosing. Naltrexone hydrochloride (ReVia and Depade) is available in 50-mg tablets and is taken orally. Dosing typically begins with 25 mg (half-tablet) daily for up to 1 week with a subsequent increase to a maintenance dose of 50 mg daily. Most studies have tested the efficacy of the 50-mg dose, so there is limited data assessing the efficacy of the higher dose (100 mg) that is frequently prescribed. The sustained-release formulation (Vivitrol) comes in a 380-mg solution that is administered by intramuscular injection once every 4 weeks by a trained clinician.

Side Effects. The most common side effects are nausea, headache, dizziness, nervousness, fatigue, insomnia, vomiting, anxiety, and somnolence.

Contraindications and Safety. The main concerns when prescribing naltrexone are inducing opioid withdrawal in patients who have been using opioids and hepatotoxicity (see "Opioid Dependence").

Pregnancy. All medications approved by the FDA are assigned a Pregnancy Category classification based on evidence of risk to the fetuses of pregnant women. Data come from animal and/or human studies. All FDA-approved medications in this chapter are classified as Pregnancy Category C. This indicates that animal studies have demonstrated adverse effects on the fetus, but there are no adequate human studies to assess the risk in human fetuses. For this category, the potential benefits may justify use in pregnant women following a thorough informed consent discussion.

Acamprosate

Acamprosate is a relatively new medication that is FDA-approved for the treatment of alcohol dependence, specifically for maintenance of abstinence from alcohol use.

History. Acamprosate was originally developed in Europe and has been in use there since the 1980s for alcohol dependence treatment. It was approved in the United States by the FDA in 2004.

Pharmacology. Acamprosate helps normalize glutamate neurotransmitter systems altered by chronic alcohol consumption (Mason & Heyser, 2010). Acamprosate, a structural analogue of the inhibitory neurotransmitter GABA, may attenuate alcohol withdrawal symptoms by depressing the neuronal hyperexcitable state associated with withdrawal. The primary mechanism appears to be suppression of the excitatory glutamate neurotransmitter system (Wilde & Wagstaff, 1997). Normalization of glutamate neurotransmission may account for its reported ability to decrease cravings and subsequent alcohol intake. Craving can be conceptualized as the anticipation of the delivery of a positive reinforcing effect (e.g., pleasant intoxication symptoms) or conversely, the removal of a negative reinforcing effect (e.g., unpleasant withdrawal symptoms). By diminishing withdrawal symptoms through inhibition of the excitatory glutamate system acamprosate may reduce craving and thereby increase abstinence from alcohol (Littleton, 1995).

Evidence and Research. A meta-analysis of 33 trials demonstrated that acamprosate was safe and well tolerated, increased abstinence and compliance with treatment, and decreased relapses to alcohol (Bouza, Angeles, Munoz, & Amate, 2004). The COMBINE study (described in the naltrexone section), however, found acamprosate to be no more effective than placebo (Anton et al., 2006).

Formulation and Dosing. Acamprosate (Campral) is available in 333-mg oral tablets. Typical dosing is 666 mg three times daily for an approximate daily total of 2 grams. It should not be used for patients who are actively drinking as it is approved for the maintenance of abstinence from alcohol and not for decreasing alcohol intake. It can be safely given to patients with liver disease because it is eliminated from the body mostly by the kidneys.

Side Effects. Acamprosate tends to be well tolerated without serious side effects. The most common side effects include diarrhea, nausea, flatulence, and headaches.

Contraindications and Safety. Acamprosate should be lowered to 333 mg three times daily in patients with mild to moderate renal impairment and should not be given to those with severe impairment. Studies have also shown a significant but small increase in suicidal and depressive symptoms versus placebo (1.4% vs. 0.5% in studies lasting 6 months or less, and 2.4% vs. 0.8% in yearlong studies).

Pregnancy. Acamprosate is classified as a Pregnancy Class C medication by the FDA (see "Alcohol Dependence").

Disulfiram

Disulfiram is the oldest FDA-approved medication for treatment of alcohol dependence.

History. Disulfiram has been used since the 19th century in the production of rubber. An American physician working at a chemical plant in 1949 discovered its potential use in treating alcoholism. He had observed workers exposed to disulfiram becoming sober due to adverse physical reactions they had after subsequently drinking alcohol. Ten years later, scientists in Denmark studying disulfiram as a treatment for parasitic infections observed the same phenomenon in staff exposed to disulfiram who subsequently consumed alcohol (Suh, Pettinati, Kampman, & O'Brien, 2006). This led to investigations into its potential for the treatment of alcohol dependence and its eventual approval by the FDA over 50 years ago.

Pharmacology. The body normally metabolizes alcohol in a three-step process. Alcohol is first converted (using the enzyme alcohol dehydrogenase) to the toxic intermediate compound acetaldehyde. Acetaldehyde dehydrogenase then converts acetaldehyde into acetic acid, which is further converted to water and carbon dioxide. Disulfiram blocks the action of acetaldehyde dehydrogenase, preventing the conversion of acetaldehyde into acetic acid. This means that a person taking disulfiram who then consumes alcohol will experience a buildup of toxic acetaldehyde, which manifests as unpleasant physiological symptoms, including facial flushing, headache, diaphoresis, tachycardia, nausea, vomiting, palpitation, and hyperventilation (Petersen, 1992). These symptoms typically emerge within 20 minutes of alcohol intake and can last for up to several hours. More dangerous symptoms include convulsions, cardiovascular collapse, respiratory depression, arrhythmias, and myocardial infarction (Suh et al., 2006).

Patients taking disulfiram must avoid even small amounts of alcohol, as consumption of even small quantities can lead to severe symptoms. Conceptually, disulfiram therapy works as a form of operant learning with the unpleasant physiological reaction serving as a negative reinforcer, thereby increasing abstinent behavior.

Evidence and Research. While some studies have demonstrated the ability of disulfiram treatment to help alcohol-dependent patients reduce their alcohol consumption (Laaksonen, Koski-Jannes, Salaspuro, Ahtinen, & Alho, 2008), a review of 24 studies revealed a surprising lack of evidence supporting the use of disulfiram (Hughes & Cook, 1997). In the early 1980s, for example, a highly influential trial showed no evidence that treatment with disulfiram improved abstinence rates or time to first drink. However, the results were clearly affected by the low treatment adherence rates (around 20%) associated with disulfiram therapy (Fuller et al., 1986). Because disulfiram does not help with cravings, patients can simply stop taking disulfiram on days when the urge to drink becomes overwhelming. Disulfiram administered in a supervised setting may be more successful in a subset of the alcohol-dependent population with longer histories of alcohol dependence (Diehl et al., 2010).

Formulation and Dosing. Disulfiram (Antabuse) is available in 250-mg and 500-mg oral tablets. The typical daily dose is 250 mg daily, with a range of 125 mg to 500 mg (the maximum approved daily dose). Disulfiram should not be started if alcohol has been consumed within the previous 12 hours.

Side Effects. Common side effects in abstinent patients include mild headache, skin rash, acne, drowsiness, fatigue, impotence, and a metallic taste in the mouth. Infrequently, disulfiram-induced hepatotoxicity can progress to liver failure, even in those without a prior history of liver problems. Hepatotoxicity risk peaks after 60 days of treatment and is usually reversible if disulfiram is stopped before the development of liver failure (Barth & Malcolm, 2010).

Contraindications and Safety. Disulfiram is contraindicated in patients with a history of severe cardiac or liver problems and those with previous allergic reactions to the medication.

Pregnancy. Disulfiram is classified as a Pregnancy Class C medication by the FDA (see "Alcohol dependence").

Other Medications

While this section has exclusively focused on medications that are FDA-approved for the treatment of alcoholism, others have also been shown to be of benefit. Baclofen, a $GABA_B$ receptor agonist, may be of particular benefit in alcohol-dependent subjects with impaired liver functioning (Addolorato et al., 2007). Ondansetron, a 5-HT$_3$ antagonist, is particularly effective in those with an early onset of alcohol problems (Johnson et al., 2000). A multisite trial has also shown topiramate, which has actions at the GABA$_A$ and glutamate receptors, to be useful in the treatment of alcohol-dependence (Johnson et al., 2007).

Opioid Dependence: Antagonist Medications

Naltrexone

Naltrexone is an opioid receptor antagonist approved by the FDA for the treatment of both alcohol and opioid addiction.

History. In response to the rising drug experimentation and abuse of the 1960s, the Special Action Office for Drug Abuse Prevention (SAODAP) was created in 1971. The following year, Congress passed the Drug Abuse Office and Treatment Act which included, among its various provisions, a mandate to increase research funding for development of nonaddictive antagonist medications for heroin addiction (Julius, 1979). From this research, several compounds showed promise; EN-1639A (naltrexone) had the ideal characteristics for an outpatient medication for the treatment of opioid addiction. Naltrexone was made by modifying naloxone, a short-acting, intravenously delivered opioid antagonist that is used to treat opioid overdose. These modifications improved naltrexone's absorption when administered orally and significantly increased its duration of action (Resnick, Volavka, Freedman, & Thomas, 1974). In 1983, naltrexone was approved by the FDA for opioid addiction treatment in an oral tablet that is dosed daily. In 2010, the FDA approved a sustained-release, monthly intramuscular injectable formulation for the same indication.

Pharmacology. Naltrexone is a nonaddictive opioid receptor antagonist that competitively blocks the opioid receptor, preventing opioids from binding and subsequently blocking the euphoria and reinforcing effects of opioids (Coviello, Cornish, Lynch, Alterman, & O'Brien, 2010). By blocking the opioid-induced high, naltrexone presumably decreases or extinguishes opioid use (Rawson, Glazer, Callahan, & Liberman, 1979). Although naltrexone may help also reduce opioid cravings (Judson, Carney, & Goldstein, 1981), many patients have reported a minimal effect on craving.

Evidence and Research. The Heroin Antagonist and Learning Therapy (HALT) Project compared oral naltrexone therapy and behavioral treatments in opioid-addicted subjects and found that oral naltrexone, either with or without behavioral treatments, was highly effective in extinguishing opioid-taking behaviors (Rawson et al., 1979). It has recently been reported that sustained-release naltrexone increases abstinence and treatment retention while reducing cravings and relapse risk (Gastfriend, 2011).

Formulation and Dosing, Side Effects, and Pregnancy. See "Alcohol dependence."

Contraindications and Safety. Naltrexone may inadvertently induce opioid withdrawal in patients who are actively using or have recently used opioids. Therefore, patients should only start on naltrexone after at least a week of abstinence. With longer acting opioids that are slow to be eliminated from the body, like methadone, the risk is even higher. Avoiding iatrogenic (physician-caused) withdrawal is especially important for patients who are contemplating treatment with the injectable, sustained-release formulation of naltrexone. In these patients, a persistent withdrawal state could emerge if sustained-release naltrexone is administered too early. The easiest way to assess risk of naltrexone-induced opioid withdrawal is by performing a challenge test. A patient is given a small dose of naloxone intravenously or naltrexone orally and observed for about half an hour for the emergence of any withdrawal symptoms. Absence of any withdrawal symptoms indicates that the patient is a good candidate to initiate naltrexone treatment.

Due to the risk of hepatotoxicity, naltrexone is contraindicated in patients with acute hepatitis or liver failure. Caution should be exercised in prescribing to patients with a history of current or past liver disease. As naltrexone and its main metabolite are primarily excreted in the urine, caution is also recommended when prescribing to patients with renal insufficiency.

Special Considerations: Treatment Adherence. Similar to the use of disulfiram for alcohol (see "Disulfiram"), the lack of patient adherence limits the efficacy of naltrexone. This may be due to naltrexone's general lack of efficacy at decreasing opioid craving, that is, patients taking naltrexone orally may not take their daily dose if they think they are going to use opioids in the near future. Thus, like disulfiram, oral naltrexone is widely believed to mostly benefit a subset of psychosocially stable and highly motivated patients, such as opioid-dependent healthcare professionals (van der Brink, Goppel, & von Ree, 2003). The sustained release formulation may be of additional benefit, as it is effective for a period of 4 weeks following a single intramuscular injection. Thus, patients do not have the option of suddenly discontinuing naltrexone when they want to return to using opioids. The injectable form of naltrexone increases treatment retention in opioid-addicted individuals (Comer et al., 2006). The improvement in retaining patients in substance abuse treatment is important as it sets the stage for other treatment interventions to be utilized, especially psychosocial and behavioral therapies (See Carroll & Kiluk, Chapter 12, this volume).

Opioid Dependence: Agonist Medications

Agonist medications stimulate the opioid receptor either completely (full agonists) or incompletely (partial agonists). The degree of agonism, or stimulation, of the receptor largely determines its physiological effects and clinical usefulness in treating opioid-addicted patients. Agonist therapy is generally considered to be most effective as a maintenance treatment rather than for only detoxification or short-term use.

Methadone

Methadone is a synthetic *full opioid agonist* that has been approved by the FDA for over 40 years. It is approved for maintenance treatment of opioid addiction, detoxification of opioid withdrawal symptoms, and for the treatment of severe pain.

History. German scientists originally developed methadone as a synthetic opioid in 1939 under the trade name Amidon. Following the end of World War II, the Allied nations took control over Germany's patents and research records. This led to the introduction of methadone to the U.S. market in 1947. Originally approved for its analgesic and cough-suppressing properties, it was not until the 1960s that methadone was investigated for treating opioid addiction.

Groundbreaking studies in the 1960s demonstrated that methadone maintenance treatment in heroin-dependent patients prevented withdrawal, did not produce euphoric effects like heroin, helped attenuate cravings, and enabled addicted patients to resume productive lives (Kreek, 2000). Methadone received approval for a new FDA indication of opioid addiction in the early 1970s. Strict regulations from several pieces of legislation in that decade, including the 1973 Methadone Control Act, established strict controls that highly regulated the dispensing of methadone to addicted patients in special opioid treatment programs. The Substance Abuse and Mental Health Services Administration certifies these methadone clinics, and they are registered with the Drug Enforcement Administration (DEA). The often-burdensome regulations have persisted to the present day.

Pharmacology. Methadone is an opioid medication with a long duration and slow onset of action. It is a full agonist at the opioid receptor (Kristensen, Christensen, & Christup, 1994). Stimulation of the opioid receptor is predominantly responsible for both the therapeutic and adverse effects of methadone, including analgesia, physical dependence, respiratory depression, constipation, pupillary constriction, and euphoria. The primary use of methadone in opioid-addicted patients is to reduce cravings in abstinent patients without producing the intense euphoric effects of heroin. In this way, methadone is utilized as a maintenance medication to keep addicted patients from abusing opioids.

Methadone is administered orally and has a slower onset of action than intravenously administered heroin. As a consequence, it lacks an intense euphoric effect. In addition, a *cross-tolerance* develops between heroin (as well as other opioids) and methadone after chronic opioid use (Dumas & Pollack, 2008). "Cross tolerance" refers to the phenomenon whereby persistent use of an opioid agonist (e.g., heroin) results in physiological tolerance to many of the effects (including euphoria) of other members of the medication class (e.g., other opioids). For instance, a cross-tolerance occurs between all opioids including heroin, methadone, morphine, oxycodone, and hydrocodone.

Methadone also exhibits antagonism at the NMDA glutamate receptor (Ebert, Andersen, & Krogsgaard-Larsen, 1995). These properties may contribute to the ability of methadone to reduce cravings in opioid-addicted patients (Preston, Umbricht, & Epstein, 2000), as NMDA stimulation has been implicated in the development and evolution of various abstinence-related phenomenon, including cravings, withdrawal, and affective changes (Bisaga & Popik, 2000).

Research and Evidence. A large study showed a decrease in illicit opioid use with medium and high doses of methadone (up to 50 mg and 100 mg daily, respectively) as measured by negative urine drug screens and treatment adherence, with better success rates at higher doses (Strain, Bigelow, Liebson, & Stitzer, 1999). Additionally, a study of over 800 opioid-addicted individuals in methadone treatment demonstrated a lower rate of mortality among those who had continued in methadone maintenance versus those who had dropped out of or who had left treatment. This includes a remarkable 20% lower risk of death from unnatural causes, primarily heroin overdose (Fugelstad, Stenbacka, Leifman, Nylander, & Thiblin, 2007). Methadone also improves medical and social problems associated with the abuse of opioids. A meta-analysis investigating the effect of methadone on illicit opioid use, HIV risk behaviors, and drug-related criminal behavior revealed improvements in all three outcomes (Marsch, 1998).

Formulation and Dosing. Methadone (Dolophine) is available in 5- and 10-mg tablets and a cherry-flavored solution (Methadose) containing 10 mg of methadone per milliliter. Methadone tablets can be prescribed by physicians outside of methadone clinics for severe pain without any of the strict federal regulations, while Methadose is used exclusively for treatment of opioid addiction, and only in certified and registered methadone clinics. Methadone is generally started at 20–30 mg for the initial dose with another 5 or 10 mg dose several hours later if the patient is still experiencing significant withdrawal symptoms. The maximum cumulative dose on the first day is 40 mg. Subsequent titration of methadone dose for maintenance therapy should be done gradually and cautiously due to its long duration of action and risk of overdose and death from respiratory depression if increased too rapidly. This risk is amplified in patients who may be concomitantly using central nervous system depressants such as alcohol or benzodiazepines. Typical effective daily maintenance doses are between 80 and 120 mg. Daily doses under 60 mg are less effective and may lead to poorer treatment retention rates than doses above 80 mg (Caplehorn & Bell, 1991). Some patients may require twice daily dosing of methadone due to break-through cravings from increased metabolism. These rapid metabolizers often need higher total daily doses as well (Adinoff, 2008).

Side Effects. Common side effects include constipation, nausea, vomiting, dizziness, drowsiness, dry mouth, headache, sweating, itching, lightheadedness, and weakness.

Safety and Contraindications. The foremost safety consideration is overdose with resultant respiratory depression and death. This is primarily a concern due to methadone's slow onset of action and slow elimination from the body, leading to an accumulation and overdose symptoms that may present in a delayed fashion. Methadone has also been associated with rare cases of serious cardiac arrhythmias (QT interval prolongation and torsade de pointes), typically with high doses administered multiple times daily (Krantz, Kutinsky, Robertson, & Mehler, 2003).

Pregnancy. Methadone is classified as a Pregnancy Class C medication by the FDA.

Buprenorphine

Buprenorphine is approved by the FDA for the treatment of opioid addiction. It works similarly to methadone but differs in its *partial* stimulation of the opioid receptor (Figure 11.5). In addition, practitioners are able to prescribe buprenorphine in outpatient office-based settings (that do not require DEA approval, as is required for methadone maintenance treatment).

History. Buprenorphine was developed in the United Kingdom and marketed as an analgesic medication beginning in 1978. The Drug Addiction Treatment Act of 2000 in the United States allowed opioid addiction treatment with certain opioid agonist medications to occur in an outpatient setting (rather than just methadone clinics). There were no medications that fit under the law until the FDA approved buprenorphine in 2002. Physicians are required to receive additional training to prescribe outpatient buprenorphine for addiction.

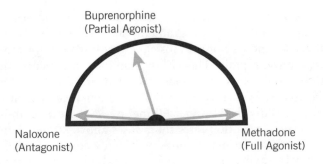

FIGURE 11.5. Pharmacology of therapeutic opiates. Compounds stimulate opiod receptors to different degrees. Methadone, a full agonist, activates opiod receptors to the highest degree. Naltrexone, an antagonist, turns the receptor completely off. Buprenorphine is a partial agonist and activates the receptor partially but not to the degree of a full agonist.

Pharmacology. Buprenorphine is an opioid with partial agonism of the opioid receptor. It is the partial agonism at the opioid receptor that is responsible for much of its unique clinical properties as a treatment for opioid addiction. As a partial agonist, buprenorphine incompletely stimulates the opioid receptor. This results in buprenorphine's ability to prevent or attenuate opioid withdrawal symptoms and cravings in abstinent opioid-addicted patients. At the same time, buprenorphine does not cause the highly reinforcing euphoric effects that full agonists (i.e., heroin or methadone) can cause, thus reducing the abuse potential (Jasinski, Pevnick, & Griffith, 1978). There is also a ceiling effect in its subjective effects on mood. That is, there is a plateauing of buprenorphine's subjective effects even with higher doses. The partial agonism at the opioid receptor and the ceiling effect are also thought to be responsible for the lower risk of respiratory depression and death in overdose compared with full agonist opioids (Robinson, 2002), demonstrating buprenorphine's strong safety profile and appropriateness for outpatient, office-based treatment (Walsh, Preston, Stitzer, Cone, & Bigelow, 1994). Buprenorphine has a relatively gradual onset of action and a long duration of action, which weakens the addictive potential and allows for dosing on a daily or even every-other-day schedule.

Research and Evidence. A large, multicenter study of outpatients revealed a dramatic improvement in the percentage of negative urine drug screens as well as decreased craving compared to placebo in the subjects treated with buprenorphine. In fact, the clinical trial ended early so that the patients receiving placebo could start taking buprenorphine (Fudala et al., 2003). A slow-release, subcutaneously implantable formulation of buprenorphine that provides a steady amount of buprenorphine to the circulation for 6 months has been shown in early studies to increase negative urine drug screens, decrease cravings, and increase treatment retention by twofold over standard daily sublingual buprenorphine therapy (Ling et al., 2010). The extended-release formulation, not yet available for clinical use, may be especially useful in patients for whom treatment adherence has been an issue.

Formulation and Dosing. Buprenorphine comes in a tablet and in a film, both designed to disintegrate when placed under the tongue (sublingual). The tablet is available with buprenorphine only (Subutex) or in a combination (Suboxone) of buprenorphine and naloxone, the opioid receptor-blocking medication. The film is only available in the combination form. Subutex comes in 2-mg and 8-mg tablets. Suboxone has a 4:1 buprenorphine: naloxone ratio and is available in a 2-mg buprenorphine/0.5-mg naloxone tablet/film and an 8-mg buprenorphine/2-mg naloxone tablet/film. Naloxone helps prevent the intravenous injection of solubilized Suboxone tablets (see "Special Considerations: Diversion and Abuse" below).

Side Effects. Common side effects include drowsiness, dizziness, constipation, nausea, vomiting, diarrhea, abdominal discomfort, headache, sweating, weakness, flushing, and insomnia.

Safety and Contraindications. Buprenorphine is generally considered to be a safe medication for opioid addiction treatment due to its favorable side effect profile and the ceiling effect described above. Although there have been reports of deaths associated with buprenorphine, these primarily occur when buprenorphine tablets are ground up, solubilized, and intravenously injected. This is particularly dangerous when buprenorphine is injected concomitantly with benzodiazepines (Tracqui, Kintz, & Ludes, 1998). Therefore, caution should be exercised when prescribing buprenorphine to patients who are using central nervous system depressants such as benzodiazepines or alcohol.

When transitioning patients from methadone maintenance to buprenorphine it is important to avoid inducing acute withdrawal from methadone by starting buprenorphine too early. This is due to the precipitated withdrawal phenomenon that can occur when methadone's full agonist activity at the opioid receptor is blocked by buprenorphine's partial agonist activity, leading to a net decrease in opioid receptor stimulation. Patients on methadone maintenance should have their dose gradually tapered (due to methadone's slow excretion from the body) and buprenorphine should be started after the onset of some mild withdrawal symptoms have emerged, as this would indicate that methadone is no longer occupying most of the opioid receptors (Breen et al., 2003).

Pregnancy. Buprenorphine is classified as a Pregnancy Class C medication by the FDA.

Special Considerations: Opioid Agonist Therapy

Controversy

Since the early days of methadone maintenance therapy there has been controversy surrounding the use of opioid agonists for the treatment of opioid addiction (Brown, Jansen, & Bass, 1974). Critics have argued that maintenance therapy with either methadone or buprenorphine constitutes a substitution of one addiction for another. Thus, the argument is that addiction is never actually treated or cured; it is just transferred to a different addicting drug. However, agonist therapy now is considered not only a legitimate treatment for opioid addiction, but also one of the most effective treatments available. It enables patients to improve and recover their psychosocial functioning, health, and overall quality of life, as well as avoid many of the maladaptive behavioral patterns associated with opioid addiction. While a physical dependence remains, the primary symptoms of addiction (loss of control, compulsive use, and continued use despite adverse consequences) are subdued or completely ameliorated.

Medication Selection

Due to the stigma of using agonist medications, some patients and providers may be unwilling to consider methadone or buprenorphine as a treatment option. For these patients, naltrexone may be an appropriate choice, particularly the injectable, sustained-release version, in conjunction with psychosocial interventions. For those patients who are able and willing to take methadone or buprenorphine, the choice between the two for maintenance therapy often depends on individual characteristics and previous treatment experiences. Both medications are effective when used for short-term detoxification of acute withdrawal symptoms and for long-term maintenance therapy (Ahmadi, 2003; Bickel et al., 1988; Stimmel, Goldberg, Rotkopf, & Cohen, 1977). However, patients with more severe opioid addiction with strong cravings may do better with methadone treatment due to methadone's full agonist activity at the opioid receptor. In addition, the more highly structured environment of the methadone clinic may be beneficial to these patients. Similarly, methadone treatment may be indicated for individuals who have failed office-based buprenorphine treatment. On the other hand, patients with more stable psychosocial situations (e.g., housing, employment) may do well with buprenorphine on an outpatient basis, which has the added benefit of avoiding the stigma associated with methadone clinics.

Diversion and Abuse

As discussed previously, methadone is dispensed in a highly regulated fashion in special methadone clinics with direct observation of dosing by clinic staff. Thus, diversion and misuse is primarily a concern in patients allowed take-home doses of methadone for unsupervised administration. Rates of methadone diversion via intravenous injection in Australia revealed that more highly regulated methadone clinics (like those in the United States) had dramatically lower rates of diversion than less regulated ones. Rates of diversion were under 5% in the more highly regulated clinics versus over 60% at clinics that provided take-home doses (Ritter & Di Natale, 2005).

Given that buprenorphine is more often dosed in less regulated settings compared to methadone, there has been heightened concern of the potential for diversion and abuse. Even though buprenorphine tablets taken sublingually have not been shown to result in euphoric effects, ground up and intravenously administered buprenorphine has been theorized to increase its positive reinforcing effects enough to significantly increase its abuse potential (Sung & Conry, 2006). Buprenorphine abuse has been observed in Europe and other regions where buprenorphine is frequently prescribed without naloxone. Consequently, a formulation containing buprenorphine and the opioid receptor antagonist naloxone was released in the United States as Suboxone. The rationale for including naloxone is based on the theorized ability of naloxone to block the effects of buprenorphine and/or cause unpleasant withdrawal symptoms when the medication is injected intravenously, thus decreasing its abuse liability. Some 80% of intravenous heroin abusers reported having a bad experience when injecting solubilized Suboxone but not with buprenorphine alone (Alho, Sinclair, Vuori, & Holopainen, 2007). Because of naloxone's poor sublingual absorption, it typically is not absorbed when Suboxone tablets are taken sublingually. Little diversion of the combined buprenorphine and naloxone exists, which is the form used widely in most of the United States. When diversion does occur, it is primarily used by addicted patients for the self-medication of withdrawal symptoms rather than for intoxication or euphoria (Mitchell et al., 2009). In fact, opioid-addicted subjects were less likely to report subjective reinforcing effects from buprenorphine combined with naloxone (taken sublingually as directed) than from buprenorphine alone or from heroin (Comer et al., 2010).

Pregnancy

Pregnant women who are addicted to opioids comprise a high-risk population. Opioid abuse during pregnancy increases the risk of obstetrical and medical complications for both the mother and the fetus. Bringing women into substance abuse treatment improves both maternal and fetal outcomes (Kaltenbach & Berghella, 1998). Detoxification from opioids while pregnant is widely discouraged due to concerns of risk to the fetus caused by *in utero* opioid withdrawal. In addition, the risk of relapse in pregnant women is exceedingly high even if detoxification is successful. Thus, methadone maintenance has been widely considered the treatment of choice for opioid-addicted women during pregnancy (Kandall, Doberczak, Jantunen, & Stein, 1999).

One of the frequent consequences in neonates born of methadone maintained women is neonatal abstinence syndrome (NAS). This is an opioid-withdrawal syndrome in the newborns due to their development of physical dependence on methadone during gestation. NAS usually requires care in a neonatal intensive care unit for several days or more and detoxification with opioids (such as morphine drops). NAS is associated with developmental delay in the first year of life, but children tend to reach normative levels of functioning by age 2 (McCance-Katz, 1991).

Buprenorphine is both safe and effective in pregnant women (Johnson, Jones, & Fischer, 2003). In fact, neonates of buprenorphine-treated women, relative to those women treated with methadone, have almost half the incidence of NAS and require less morphine for fewer days for the treatment of NAS. They also have shorter hospital stays than methadone-treated women (Jones et al., 2010; Kakko, Heilig, & Sarman, 2008).

Adolescents

Abuse of opioids, especially pain medications like hydrocodone and oxycodone, has been an increasingly common problem in the adolescent population; an epidemiological survey of 12th-grade students in the United States found that opioid pain medication abuse was the second most frequently abused substance after marijuana (Compton & Volkow, 2006). Treatment for this patient population has typically involved buprenorphine rather than methadone, largely due to the highly regulated and controlled nature of methadone clinics. Under the Panini State Methadone Maintenance Treatment Guidelines of 1992, methadone maintenance in the United States is only allowed in adolescents after they have failed at least two attempts of detoxification or rehabilitation treatment (Simkin & Grenoble, 2010). Adolescents treated with buprenorphine for withdrawal, relative to those treated with clonidine, have fewer withdrawal symptoms, more negative urine drug screens, decreased HIV-risk behavior, and are more likely to remain in treatment (Marsch et al., 2005). Opioid-addicted adolescents undergoing a 12-week maintenance period on buprenorphine, compared to a 2-week detoxification period, resulted in decreased overall opioid use, intravenous substance administration, and use of other drugs (Woody et al., 2008). These studies support the use of maintenance buprenorphine treatment in adolescents.

Prescription Opioid Addiction

Abuse and addiction to prescription opioids has become increasingly problematic over the past decade for not just adolescents, but the general population as well. In treatment with buprenorphine in an outpatient-based setting, prescription opioid-addicted individuals treated with buprenorphine
tended to stay in treatment longer and have more opioid-negative urine
drug screens than those who were not on maintenance therapy. Buprenorphine may be a good option for this population (Moore et al., 2007).

Stimulant Dependence

Although there are currently no FDA-approved medications for the treatment of stimulant addiction, numerous medications have been investigated
for their potential utility in treating individuals addicted to cocaine or
methamphetamine. Current research in stimulant addiction has focused
on the dopamine, GABA, glutamate, and serotonin systems as well as
immunological therapies (Ross & Peselow, 2009). Studies of antiepileptics
(carbamazepine, phenytoin), dopamine agonists (bromocriptine), amanta-
dine, antidepressants (fluoxetine, desipramine, imipramine, bupropion),
and naltrexone were reviewed in 2002 and none were considered effective
in treating cocaine addiction (Silva de Lima, de Oliveira Soares, Reisser,
& Farrell, 2002). Disulfiram, the cocaine vaccine, modafinil, vigabatrin,
D-cycloserine, and topiramate have shown promise for the development of
cocaine addiction treatments (Kampman, 2010; Price et al., 2009). Incon-
clusive findings have been reported on the efficacy of various other medications, including risperidone, imipramine, and amlodipine in the treatment of methamphetamine addiction (Meredith, Jaffe, Ang-Lee, & Saxon,
2005). Some of the more promising medications will be reviewed.

Disulfiram

Disulfiram has shown promise in treating cocaine addiction separately or
in conjunction with coexisting alcohol dependence (Carroll et al., 2004).
Individuals with alcohol and cocaine addiction who are taking disulfiram,
in combination with naltrexone or alone, were more likely to be abstinent
from both cocaine and alcohol compared to those taking a placebo (Pettinati
et al., 2008). However, a Cochrane systematic review of disulfiram studies
did not find clear evidence of its efficacy for treatment of cocaine addiction
(Pani et al., 2010). Disulfiram may attenuate the reinforcing euphoric properties of cocaine (Baker, Jatlow, & McCance-Katz, 2007), decrease craving, and increase the dysphoric effects of cocaine (Haile, Kosten, & Kosten,
2009). In addition to blocking the enzyme acetaldehyde dehydrogenase (see
"Alcohol"), disulfiram also blocks the enzyme dopamine beta-hydroxylase.

This enzyme converts dopamine to norepinephrine. Treatment with disulfiram then leads to increased dopamine levels, which may be responsible for its beneficial effects in the treatment of cocaine addiction (Petrakis et al., 2000).

Cocaine Vaccine

Another promising treatment for cocaine addiction is the development of a vaccine that stimulates production of antibodies directed against cocaine. These anticocaine antibodies bind to cocaine molecules and make the antibody–cocaine complex too large to cross the blood–brain barrier. Binding cocaine with antibodies makes cocaine unable to affect brain reward pathways and limits its other damaging physiological effects throughout the body (Sofuoglu & Kosten, 2006). Cocaine vaccines are currently being developed and one has now progressed to clinical trials (Kinsey, Kosten, & Orson, 2010). The safety of this vaccine and its ability to effectively stimulate cocaine-directed antibodies has been established (Kosten et al., 2002). The vaccine has also been shown to decrease cocaine self-administration in animal models of addiction (Fox et al., 1996) as well as to attenuate the euphoric effects of cocaine and decrease cocaine use in individuals addicted to cocaine (Martell, Mitchell, Poling, Gonsai, & Kosten, 2005; Martell et al., 2009).

Modafinil

Modafinil (Provigil) is a nonstimulant medication approved by the FDA for the treatment of the sleep disorder narcolepsy. Modafinil is believed to modulate the dopamine, GABA, and glutamate systems among others, and has been shown in some studies to reduce cocaine cravings and increase abstinence rates (Martinez-Raga, Knecht, & Cepeda, 2008).

Bupropion

Bupropion is a norepinephrine and dopamine reuptake-inhibiting medication that is FDA-approved for the treatment of major depression and nicotine dependence. It has been demonstrated to decrease subjective reinforcing effects and cue-induced cravings in methamphetamine-addicted individuals (Newton, De La Garza, Kalechstein, Tziortzis, & Jacobsen, 2009). Bupropion, in conjunction with behavioral therapies, was reported to increase abstinence in patients with low to moderate degrees of methamphetamine addiction (Elkashef et al., 2006). In other studies, however, bupropion was no more effective than placebo in reducing methamphetamine use (Shoptaw et al., 2008).

Modafinil

Modafinil, in addition to its potential for cocaine addiction treatment, has also been studied for the treatment of methamphetamine addiction. Although no differences were found between modafinil and placebo in abstinence rates, cravings, or severity of dependence in methamphetamine-addicted subjects, medication-adherent subjects did provide more negative urine drug screens (Shearer et al., 2009).

Cannabis Dependence

There are no FDA-approved medications for the treatment of cannabis addiction. Various medications have been studied, including tetrahydrocannabinol (THC), nefazodone, bupropion, divalproex, and naltrexone. Most of these have not been shown to be effective in treating cannabis addiction with the exception of THC, the active ingredient in cannabis, which has shown some promise (Budney, Roffman, Stephens, & Walker, 2007).

Conclusion and Future Directions

The past two decades have seen dramatic advances in the pharmacological treatment of substance use disorders. As described in this chapter, the use of oral naltrexone for alcohol dependence, the new formulation of extended-release naltrexone for both alcohol and opioid dependence, acamprosate for alcohol dependence, and buprenorphine for opioid withdrawal and maintenance have all greatly benefitted treatment outcomes in addicted individuals. Nevertheless, medications for addiction treatment remain significantly underutilized. Concerns regarding cost, differing philosophical approaches to treatment, availability, and the absence of the resources necessary for prescribing and dispensing medication have limited the use of these pharmacological approaches. Fortunately, the situation is gradually improving as the benefits of pharmacological intervention in this patient population have become increasingly evident. Physician involvement in addiction treatment has become more widespread and some medications (e.g., opioid agonists) have become more accessible.

An additional factor in the enhanced use of medications for substance abuse is the heightened awareness of the benefits that accrue from combining pharmacotherapy with psychosocial treatments and support groups. Substance abuse is a chronic disease, and medications for any chronic disease, of course, are not a panacea. Limited success is expected in a substance-abusing individual with medications alone in the absence of other behavioral interventions, in much the same way as one would expect limited success from cardiac rehabilitation in a patient who persists in smoking. Medications, behavioral treatments, and support groups all potentiate each other's beneficial effects in the treatment of substance abuse when used in combination. Thus, maximizing treatment outcomes requires rigorous attention to all aspects of recovery.

Despite impressive advances in pharmacological treatments, there are some noteworthy disappointments. To date, there are no FDA-approved medications for the treatment of cocaine, amphetamine, or cannabis dependence and none appear to be on the near horizon. This is not for lack of trying. Several medications have proven successful in decreasing stimulant use in both animal studies and open label trials (when the individual knows what pill he or she is taking) only to later show disappointing outcomes in a "gold standard" double-blind, placebo-controlled clinical trial. In the face of this disappointment, however, dramatic progress has been made in understanding the neurobiology underlying the development and persistence of addictive disorders. Although the translation from the laboratory to the clinical setting is difficult, these achievements are certain to yield concrete benefits over time.

Advances in our understanding of the neurobiology of substance abuse may require a more sophisticated assessment of the addicted individual. Some medications may be more effective for those with specific genetic backgrounds. For instance, alcohol-dependent patients with a variant of the opioid receptor (OPRM1) are far more responsive to naltrexone than those with a different OPRM1 gene (Anton et al., 2008; Oslin et al., 2003). In addition, brain scans may identify a specific neural circuit or receptor configuration that is particularly responsive to a specific medication or even a combination of medications. Although similar claims have been made since genetic testing and brain-imaging techniques have become available, the ease of obtaining a full-gene analysis and the stunning improvements in measuring brain functioning suggest that these promises are closer to fruition. At this time, however, there is no scientific evidence supporting the use of brain imaging to either diagnose or advise treatment approaches for substance abuse (Adinoff & Devous, 2010; Leuchter, 2009).

An important caveat to this optimism is warranted, however. Many medications used to treat addictive disorders lack sufficient (or any!) evidence that they are, in fact, beneficial. Surprisingly, many of the medications commonly used to treat cocaine and amphetamine have even been shown to be ineffective. The dangers inherent in this approach include inducing unrealistic expectations from the patient and the treatment team as well as exposing a patient to potential side effects from a medication that offers little likelihood of benefit. Furthermore, these medications may be quite expensive yet yield no benefit except to the company claiming a presumed cure for addiction. Recent examples of expensive treatments without scientific support include Prometa (a combination of hydroxyzine [an antihistamine], flumazenil [a benzodiazepine antagonist], and gabapentin) for alcohol, cocaine, or opioid addiction and rapid detoxification for opioid withdrawal (Collins, Kleber, Whittington, & Heitler, 2005; Pfab, Pfab, Hirtl, & Zilker, 1999). When the time comes that we can prescribe safe and effective medications specific to a person's own genetic and biologic profile, an additional benefit will likely be evident. This medicalization of substance use disorders will clearly demonstrate the inherent neurobiological basis of substance abuse and will significantly diminish the social stigma commonly associated with this disease.

References

Abrams, J. K., Johnson, P. L., Hay-Schmidt, A., Mikkelsen, J. D., Shekhar, A., & Lowry, C. A. (2005). Serotonergic systems associated with arousal and vigilance behaviors following administration of anxiogenic drugs. *Neuroscience, 133*(4), 983–997.

Addolorato, G., Leggio, L., Ferrulli, A., Cardone, S., Vonghia, L., & Mirijello, A. (2007). Effectiveness and safety of baclofen for maintenance of alcohol abstinence in alcohol-dependent patients with liver cirrhosis: Randomised, double-blind controlled study. *Lancet, 370*(9603), 1915–1922.

Adinoff, B. (2004). Neurobiologic processes in drug reward and addiction. *Harvard Review of Psychiatry, 12*(6), 305–320.

Adinoff, B. (2008). Divided doses for methadone maintenance. *American Journal of Psychiatry, 165*(3), 303–305.

Adinoff, B., & Devous, M. (2010). Scientifically unfounded claims in diagnosing and treating patients. *American Journal of Psychiatry, 167*(5), 598.

Adinoff, B., Rilling, L. M., Williams, M. J., Schreffler, E., Schepis, T. S., & Rosvall, T. (2007). Impulsivity, neural deficits, and the addictions: The "oops" factor in relapse. *Journal of Addictive Diseases, 26*(Suppl. 1), 25–39.

Ahmadi, J. (2003). Methadone versus buprenorphine maintenance for the treatment of heroin-dependent outpatients. *Journal of Substance Abuse Treatment, 24*(3), 217–220.

Alcaro, A., Huber, R., & Panksepp, J. (2007). Behavioral functions of the mesolimbic dopaminergic system: An affective neuroethological perspective. *Brain Research Reviews, 56*(2), 283–321.

Alho, H., Sinclair, D., Vuori, E., & Holopainen, A. (2007). Abuse liability of buprenorphine-naloxone tablets in untreated IV drug users. *Drug and Alcohol Dependence, 88*(1), 75–78.

Allman, J. M., Hakeem, A., Erwin, J. M., Nimchinsky, E., & Hof, P. (2001). The anterior cingulate cortex: The evolution of an interface between emotion and cognition. *Annals of the New York Academy of Sciences, 935*, 107–117.

Anton, R. F., O'Malley, S. S., Ciraulo, D. A., Cisler, R. A., Couper, D., & Donovan, D. M. (2006). Combined pharmacotherapies and behavioral interventions for alcohol dependence: The COMBINE study: A randomized controlled trial. *JAMA: Journal of the American Medical Association, 295*(17), 2003–2017.

Anton, R. F., Oroszi, G., O'Malley, S., Couper, D., Swift, R., & Pettinati, H. (2008).

An evaluation of mu-opioid receptor (OPRM1) as a predictor of naltrexone response in the treatment of alcohol dependence: Results from the Combined Pharmacotherapies and Behavioral Interventions for Alcohol Dependence (COMBINE) study. *Archives of General Psychiatry, 65*(2), 135–144.

Baker, J. R., Jatlow, P., & McCance-Katz, E. F. (2007). Disulfiram effects on responses to intravenous cocaine administration. *Drug and Alcohol Dependence, 87*(2–3), 202–209.

Baliki, M. N., Geha, P. Y., & Apkarian, A. V. (2009). Parsing pain perception between nociceptive representation and magnitude estimation. *Journal of Neurophysiology, 101*(2), 875–887.

Barth, K. S., & Malcolm, R. J. (2010). Disulfiram: An old therapeutic with new applications. *CNS and Neurological Disorders—Drug Targets, 9*(1), 5–12.

Benjamin, D., Grant, E. R., & Pohorecky, L. A. (1993). Naltrexone reverses ethanol-induced dopamine release in the nucleus accumbens in awake, freely moving rats. *Brain Research, 621*(1), 137–140.

Bickel, W. K., Stitzer, M. L., Bigelow, G. E., Liebson, I. A., Jasinski, D. R., & Johnson, R. E. (1988). A clinical trial of buprenorphine: Comparison with methadone in the detoxification of heroin addicts. *Clinical Pharmacology and Therapeutics, 43*(1), 72–78.

Bisaga, A., & Popik, P. (2000). In search of a new pharmacological treatment for drug and alcohol addiction: N-methyl-D-aspartate (NMDA) antagonists. *Drug and Alcohol Dependence, 59*(1), 1–15.

Bouza, C., Angeles, M., Munoz, A., & Amate, J. M. (2004). Efficacy and safety of naltrexone and acamprosate in the treatment of alcohol dependence: A systematic review. *Addiction, 99*(7), 811–828.

Breen, C. L., Harris, S. J., Lintzeris, N., Mattick, R. P., Hawken, L., Bell, J. (2003). Cessation of methadone maintenance treatment using buprenorphine: Transfer from methadone to buprenorphine and subsequent buprenorphine reductions. *Drug and Alcohol Dependence, 71*(1), 49–55.

Brown, B. S., Jansen, D. R., & Bass, U. F. 3rd. (1974). Staff attitudes and conflict regarding the use of methadone in the treatment of heroin addiction. *American Journal of Psychiatry, 131*(2), 215–219.

Budney, A. J., Roffman, R., Stephens, R. S., & Walker, D. (2007). Marijuana dependence and its treatment. *Addiction Science and Clinical Practice, 4*(1), 4–16.

Bunney, B. S., & Aghajanian, G. K. (1978). d-Amphetamine-induced depression of central dopamine neurons: Evidence for mediation by both autoreceptors and a striato–nigral feedback pathway. *Naunyn Schmiedebergs Archives of Pharmacology, 304*(3), 255–261.

Bush, G., Luu, P., & Posner, M. I. (2000). Cognitive and emotional influences in anterior cingulate cortex. *Trends in Cognitive Sciences, 4*(6), 215–222.

Canales, J. J. (2010). Comparative neuroscience of stimulant-induced memory dysfunction: Role for neurogenesis in the adult hippocampus. *Behavioural Pharmacology, 21*(5–6), 379–393.

Caplehorn, J. R., & Bell, J. (1991). Methadone dosage and retention of patients in maintenance treatment. *Medical Journal of Australia, 154*(3), 195–199.

Carroll, K. M., Fenton, L. R., Ball, S. A., Nich, C., Frankforter, T. L., & Shi, J. (2004). Efficacy of disulfiram and cognitive behavior therapy in cocaine-dependent outpatients: A randomized placebo-controlled trial. *Archives of General Psychiatry, 61*(3), 264–272.

Choi, D. C., Furay, A. R., Evanson, N. K., Ostrander, M. M., Ulrich-Lai, Y. M., & Herman, J. P. (2007). Bed nucleus of the stria terminalis subregions differentially regulate hypothalamic–pituitary–adrenal axis activity: Implications for the integration of limbic inputs. *Journal of Neuroscience, 27*(8), 2025–2034.

Collins, E. D., Kleber, H. D., Whittington, R. A., & Heitler, N. E. (2005). Anesthesia-assisted vs. buprenorphine- or clonidine-assisted heroin detoxification and naltrexone induction. *JAMA: Journal of the American Medical Association, 294*(8), 903–913.

Comer, S. D., Sullivan, M. A., Vosburg, S. K., Manubay, J., Amass, L., & Cooper, Z. D. (2010). Abuse liability of intravenous buprenorphine/naloxone and buprenorphine alone in buprenorphine-maintained intravenous heroin abusers. *Addiction, 105*(4), 709–718.

Comer, S. D., Sullivan, M. A., Yu, E., Rothenberg, J. L., Kleber, H. D., & Kampman, K. (2006). Injectable, sustained-release naltrexone for the treatment of opioid dependence: A randomized, placebo-controlled trial. *Archives of General Psychiatry, 63*(2), 210–218.

Compton, W. M., & Volkow, N. D. (2006). Major increases in opioid analgesic abuse in the United States: Concerns and strategies. *Drug and Alcohol Dependence, 81*(2), 103–107.

Coviello, D. M., Cornish, J. W., Lynch, K. G., Alterman, A. I., & O'Brien, C. P. (2010). A randomized trial of oral naltrexone for treating opioid-dependent offenders. *American Journal on Addictions, 19*(5), 422–432.

Critchley, H. D., Wiens, S., Rotshtein, P., Ohman, A., & Dolan, R. J. (2004). Neural systems supporting interoceptive awareness. *Nature Neuroscience, 7*(2), 189–195.

Dagher, A., Owen, A. M., Boecker, H., & Brooks, D. J. (1999). Mapping the network for planning: A correlational PET activation study with the Tower of London task. *Brain, 122*(Pt. 10), 1973–1987.

Diehl, A., Ulmer, L., Mutschler, J., Herre, H., Krumm, B., & Croissant, B. (2010). Why is disulfiram superior to acamprosate in the routine clinical setting?: A retrospective long-term study in 353 alcohol-dependent patients. *Alcohol and Alcoholism, 45*(3), 271–277.

Dumas, E. O., & Pollack, G. M. (2008). Opioid tolerance development: A pharmacokinetic/pharmacodynamic perspective. *AAPS Journal, 10*(4), 537–551.

Ebert, B., Andersen, S., & Krogsgaard-Larsen, P. (1995). Ketobemidone, methadone and pethidine are non-competitive N-methyl-D-aspartate (NMDA) antagonists in the rat cortex and spinal cord. *Neuroscience Letters, 187*(3), 165–168.

Elkashef, A., Fudala, P. J., Gorgon, L., Li, S. H., Kahn, R., & Chiang, N. (2006). Double-blind, placebo-controlled trial of selegiline transdermal system (STS) for the treatment of cocaine dependence. *Drug and Alcohol Dependence, 85*(3), 191–197.

Elliott, R., Dolan, R. J., & Frith, C. D. (2000). Dissociable functions in the medial and lateral orbitofrontal cortex: Evidence from human neuroimaging studies. *Cerebral Cortex, 10*(3), 308–317.

Fox, A. S., Shelton, S. E., Oakes, T. R., Converse, A. K., Davidson, R. J., & Kalin,

N. H. (2010). Orbitofrontal cortex lesions alter anxiety-related activity in the primate bed nucleus of stria terminalis. *Journal of Neuroscience, 30*(20), 7023–7027.

Fox, B. S., Kantak, K. M., Edwards, M. A., Black, K. M., Bollinger, B. K., & Botka, A. J. (1996). Efficacy of a therapeutic cocaine vaccine in rodent models. *Nature Medicine, 2*(10), 1129–1132.

Fudala, P. J., Bridge, T. P., Herbert, S., Williford, W. O., Chiang, C. N., & Jones, K. (2003). Office-based treatment of opiate addiction with a sublingual-tablet formulation of buprenorphine and naloxone. *New England Journal of Medicine, 349*(10), 949–958.

Fugelstad, A., Stenbacka, M., Leifman, A., Nylander, M., & Thiblin, I. (2007). Methadone maintenance treatment: The balance between life-saving treatment and fatal poisonings. *Addiction, 102*(3), 406–412.

Fuller, R. K., Branchey, L., Brightwell, D. R., Derman, R. M., Emrick, C. D., & Iber, F. L. (1986). Disulfiram treatment of alcoholism. A Veterans Administration cooperative study. *JAMA: Journal of the American Medical Association, 256*(11), 1449–1455.

Gardner, E. L. (1997). Brain reward mechanisms. In P. R. J. H. Lowinson, R. B. Millman, & J. G. Langrod (Eds.), *Substance abuse: A comprehensive textbook* (pp. 51–85). Baltimore: Williams & Wilkins.

Gardner, E. L., & Ashby, C. R. Jr. (2000). Heterogeneity of the mesotelencephalic dopamine fibers: Physiology and pharmacology. *Neuroscience Biobehavioral Reviews, 24*(1), 115–118.

Gastfriend, D. R. (2011). Intramuscular extended-release naltrexone: Current evidence. *Annals of the New York Academy of Science, 1216*(1), 144–166.

Goldstein, R. Z., & Volkow, N. D. (2002). Drug addiction and its underlying neurobiological basis: Neuroimaging evidence for the involvement of the frontal cortex. *American Journal of Psychiatry, 159*(10), 1642–1652.

Haile, C. N., Kosten, T. R., & Kosten, T. A. (2009). Pharmacogenetic treatments for drug addiction: Cocaine, amphetamine and methamphetamine. *American Journal of Drug and Alcohol Abuse, 35*(3), 161–177.

Hughes, J. C., & Cook, C. C. (1997). The efficacy of disulfiram: A review of outcome studies. *Addiction, 92*(4), 381–395.

Jasinski, D. R., Pevnick, J. S., & Griffith, J. D. (1978). Human pharmacology and abuse potential of the analgesic buprenorphine: A potential agent for treating narcotic addiction. *Archives of General Psychiatry, 35*(4), 501–516.

Jentsch, J. D., Olausson, P., De La Garza, R., & Taylor, J. R. (2002). Impairments of reversal learning and response perseveration after repeated, intermittent cocaine administrations to monkeys. *Neuropsychopharmacology, 26*(2), 183–190.

Johnson, B. A., Roache, J. D., Javors, M. A., DiClemente, C. C., Cloninger, C. R., & Prihoda, T. J. (2000). Ondansetron for reduction of drinking among biologically predisposed alcoholic patients: A randomized controlled trial. *JAMA: Journal of the American Medical Association, 284*(8), 963–971.

Johnson, B. A., Rosenthal, N., Capece, J. A., Wiegand, F., Mao, L., Beyers, K. (2007). Topiramate for treating alcohol dependence: A randomized controlled trial. *JAMA: Journal of the American Medical Association, 298*(14), 1641–1651.

Johnson, R. E., Jones, H. E., & Fischer, G. (2003). Use of buprenorphine in pregnancy: Patient management and effects on the neonate. *Drug and Alcohol Dependence, 70*(Suppl. 2), S87–S101.

Jones, E. G. (2007). *The thalamus* (2nd ed.). New York: Cambridge University Press.

Jones, H. E., Kaltenbach, K., Heil, S. H., Stine, S. M., Coyle, M. G., & Arria, A. M. (2010). Neonatal abstinence syndrome after methadone or buprenorphine exposure. *New England Journal of Medicine, 363*(24), 2320–2331.

Judson, B. A., Carney, T. M., & Goldstein, A. (1981). Naltrexone treatment of heroin addiction: Efficacy and safety in a double-blind dosage comparison. *Drug and Alcohol Dependence, 7*(4), 325–346.

Julius, D. A. (1979). Research and development of naltrexone: A new narcotic antagonist. *American Journal of Psychiatry, 136*(6), 782–786.

Kakko, J., Heilig, M., & Sarman, I. (2008). Buprenorphine and methadone treatment of opiate dependence during pregnancy: Comparison of fetal growth and neonatal outcomes in two consecutive case series. *Drug and Alcohol Dependence, 96*(1–2), 69–78.

Kalivas, P. W., & Volkow, N. D. (2005). The neural basis of addiction: A pathology of motivation and choice. *American Journal of Psychiatry, 162*(8), 1403–1413.

Kaltenbach, K., & Berghella, V. (1998). Opiod dependence during pregnancy: Effects and management. *Obstetrics and Gynecology Clinics of North America, 25*(1), 139–151.

Kampman, K. M. (2010). What's new in the treatment of cocaine addiction? *Current Psychiatry Reports, 12*(5), 441–447.

Kandall, S. R., Doberczak, T. M., Jantunen, M., & Stein, J. (1999). The methadone-maintained pregnancy. *Clinics in Perinatology, 26*(1), 173–183.

Kandel, E. R., Schwartz, J. H., & Jessell, T. M. (2000). *Principles of neural science* (4th ed.). New York: McGraw-Hill, Health Professions Division.

Kinsey, B. M., Kosten, T. R., & Orson, F. M. (2010). Anti-cocaine vaccine development. *Expert Review of Vaccines, 9*(9), 1109–1114.

Koob, G. F., & Le Moal, M. (2005). Plasticity of reward neurocircuitry and the "dark side" of drug addiction. *Nature Neuroscience, 8*(11), 1442–1444.

Koob, G. F., & Volkow, N. D. (2010). Neurocircuitry of addiction. *Neuropsychopharmacology, 35*(1), 217–238.

Kosten, T. R., Rosen, M., Bond, J., Settles, M., Roberts, J. S., & Shields, J. (2002). Human therapeutic cocaine vaccine: Safety and immunogenicity. *Vaccine, 20*(7–8), 1196–1204.

Krantz, M. J., Kutinsky, I. B., Robertson, A. D., & Mehler, P. S. (2003). Dose-related effects of methadone on QT prolongation in a series of patients with torsade de pointes. *Pharmacotherapy, 23*(6), 802–805.

Kranzler, H. R., Modesto-Lowe, V., & Nuwayser, E. S. (1998). Sustained-release naltrexone for alcoholism treatment: A preliminary study. *Alcoholism: Clinical and Experimental Research, 22*(5), 1074–1079.

Kreek, M. J. (2000). Methadone-related opioid agonist pharmacotherapy for heroin addiction: History, recent molecular and neurochemical research and future in mainstream medicine. *Annals of the New York Academy of Science, 909*, 186–216.

Kringelbach, M. L. (2005). The human orbitofrontal cortex: Linking reward to hedonic experience. *Nature Reviews of Neuroscience, 6*(9), 691–702.

Kristensen, K., Christensen, C. B., & Christup, L. L. (1994). The mu1, mu2, delta, kappa opioid receptor binding profiles on methadone stereoisomers and morphine. *Life Sciences, 56*(2), 45–50.

Laaksonen, E., Koski-Jannes, A., Salaspuro, M., Ahtinen, H., & Alho, H. (2008). A randomized, multicentre, open-label, comparative trial of disulfiram, naltrexone and acamprosate in the treatment of alcohol dependence. *Alcohol and Alcoholism, 43*(1), 53–61.

LeDoux, J. (2003). The emotional brain, fear, and the amygdala. *Cellular and Molecular Neurobiology, 23*(4–5), 727–738.

Legault, M., & Wise, R. A. (2001). Novelty-evoked elevations of nucleus accumbens dopamine: Dependence on impulse flow from the ventral subiculum and glutamatergic neurotransmission in the ventral tegmental area. *European Journal of Neuroscience, 13*(4), 819–828.

Leuchter, A. F. (2009). Book review: *Healing the hardware of the soul*, by Daniel Amen. *American Journal of Psychiatry, 166*, 625.

Ling, W., Casadonte, P., Bigelow, G., Kampman, K. M., Patkar, A., & Bailey, G. L. (2010). Buprenorphine implants for treatment of opioid dependence: A randomized controlled trial. *JAMA: Journal of the American Medical Association, 304*(14), 1576–1583.

Littleton, J. (1995). Acamprosate in alcohol dependence: How does it work? *Addiction, 90*(9), 1179–1188.

Marsch, L. A. (1998). The efficacy of methadone maintenance interventions in reducing illicit opiate use, HIV risk behavior and criminality: A meta-analysis. *Addiction, 93*(4), 515–532.

Marsch, L. A., Bickel, W. K., Badger, G. J., Stothart, M. E., Quesnel, K. J., & Stanger, C. (2005). Comparison of pharmacological treatments for opioid-dependent adolescents: A randomized controlled trial. *Archives of General Psychiatry, 62*(10), 1157–1164.

Martell, B. A., Mitchell, E., Poling, J., Gonsai, K., & Kosten, T. R. (2005). Vaccine pharmacotherapy for the treatment of cocaine dependence. *Biological Psychiatry, 58*(2), 158–164.

Martell, B. A., Orson, F. M., Poling, J., Mitchell, E., Rossen, R. D., & Gardner, T. (2009). Cocaine vaccine for the treatment of cocaine dependence in methadone-maintained patients: A randomized, double-blind, placebo-controlled efficacy trial. *Archives of General Psychiatry, 66*(10), 1116–1123.

Martinez-Raga, J., Knecht, C., & Cepeda, S. (2008). Modafinil: A useful medication for cocaine addiction?: Review of the evidence from neuropharmacological, experimental and clinical studies. *Current Drug Abuse Reviews, 1*(2), 213–221.

Mason, B. J., & Heyser, C. J. (2010). Acamprosate: A prototypic neuromodulator in the treatment of alcohol dependence. *CNS and Neurological Disorders: Drug Targets, 9*(1), 23–32.

McCance-Katz, E. F. (1991). The consequences of maternal substance abuse for the child exposed in utero. *Psychosomatics, 32*(3), 268–274.

Meredith, C. W., Jaffe, C., Ang-Lee, K., & Saxon, A. J. (2005). Implications of chronic methamphetamine use: A literature review. *Harvard Review of Psychiatry, 13*(3), 141–154.

Mitchell, S. G., Kelly, S. M., Brown, B. S., Reisinger, H. S., Peterson, J. A., Ruhf, A., et al. (2009). Uses of diverted methadone and buprenorphine by opioid-addicted individuals in Baltimore, Maryland. *American Journal on Addictions, 18*(5), 346–355.

Moore, B. A., Fiellin, D. A., Barry, D. T., Sullivan, L. E., Chawarski, M. C., & O'Connor, P. G. (2007). Primary care office-based buprenorphine treatment: Comparison of heroin and prescription opioid dependent patients. *Journal of General Internal Medicine, 22*(4), 527–530.

Morris, P. L., Hopwood, M., Whelan, G., Gardiner, J., & Drummond, E. (2001). Naltrexone for alcohol dependence: A randomized controlled trial. *Addiction, 96*(11), 1565–1573.

Newton, T. F., De La Garza, R., Kalechstein, A. D., Tziortzis, D., & Jacobsen, C. A. (2009). Theories of addiction: Methamphetamine users' explanations for continuing drug use and relapse. *American Journal on Addiction, 18*(4), 294–300.

Nicola, S. M., Surmeier, J., & Malenka, R. C. (2000). Dopaminergic modulation of neuronal excitability in the striatum and nucleus accumbens. *Annual Review of Neuroscience, 23*, 185–215.

Nolte, J. (2009). *The human brain: An introduction to its functional anatomy* (6th ed.). Philadelphia: Mosby/Elsevier.

O'Hearn, E., & Molliver, M. E. (1984). Organization of raphe-cortical projections in rat: A quantitative retrograde study. *Brain Research Bulletin, 13*(6), 709–726.

O'Malley, S. S., Jaffe, A. J., Chang, G., Schottenfeld, R. S., Meyer, R. E., & Rounsaville, B. (1992). Naltrexone and coping skills therapy for alcohol dependence: A controlled study. *Archives of General Psychiatry, 49*(11), 881–887.

Oslin, D. W., Berrettini, W., Kranzler, H. R., Pettinati, H., Gelernter, J., & Volpicelli, J. R. (2003). A functional polymorphism of the mu-opioid receptor gene is associated with naltrexone response in alcohol-dependent patients. *Neuropsychopharmacology, 28*(8), 1546–1552.

Pani, P. P., Trogu, E., Vacca, R., Amato, L., Vecchi, S., & Davoli, M. (2010). Disulfiram for the treatment of cocaine dependence. *Cochrane Database of Systematic Reviews* (1), CD007024.

Paton, J. J., Belova, M. A., Morrison, S. E., & Salzman, C. D. (2006). The primate amygdala represents the positive and negative value of visual stimuli during learning. *Nature, 439*(7078), 865–870.

Petersen, E. N. (1992). The pharmacology and toxicology of disulfiram and its metabolites. *Acta Psychiatrica Scandinavica, 369*(Suppl.), 7–13.

Petrakis, I. L., Carroll, K. M., Nich, C., Gordon, L. T., McCance-Katz, E. F., & Frankforter, T. (2000). Disulfiram treatment for cocaine dependence in methadone-maintained opioid addicts. *Addiction, 95*(2), 219–228.

Pettinati, H. M., Kampman, K. M., Lynch, K. G., Xie, H., Dackis, C., & Rabinowitz, A. R. (2008). A double blind, placebo-controlled trial that combines disulfiram and naltrexone for treating co-occurring cocaine and alcohol dependence. *Addictive Behaviors, 33*(5), 651–667.

Pettinati, H. M., O'Brien, C. P., Rabinowitz, A. R., Wortman, S. P., Oslin, D. W., & Kampman, K. M. (2006). The status of naltrexone in the treatment of alcohol dependence: Specific effects on heavy drinking. *Journal of Clinical Psychopharmacology, 26*(6), 610–625.

Pfab, R., Pfab, R., Hirtl, C., & Zilker, T. (1999). Opiate detoxification under anesthesia: No apparent benefit but suppression of thyroid hormones and risk of pulmonary and renal failure. *Clinical Toxicology, 37*(1), 43–50.

Preston, K. L., Umbricht, A., & Epstein, D. H. (2000). Methadone dose increase and abstinence reinforcement for treatment of continued heroin use during methadone maintenance. *Archives of General Psychiatry, 57*(4), 395–404.

Price, K. L., McRae-Clark, A. L., Saladin, M. E., Maria, M. M., DeSantis, S. M., & Back, S. E. (2009). D-cycloserine and cocaine cue reactivity: Preliminary findings. *American Journal of Drug and Alcohol Abuse, 35*(6), 434–438.

Rawson, R. A., Glazer, M., Callahan, E. J., & Liberman, R. P. (1979). Naltrexone and behavior therapy for heroin addiction. *NIDA Research Monographs, 25*, 26–43.

Resnick, R. B., Volavka, J., Freedman, A. M., & Thomas, M. (1974). Studies of EN-1639A (naltrexone): A new narcotic antagonist. *American Journal of Psychiatry, 131*(6), 646–650.

Ritter, A., & Di Natale, R. (2005). The relationship between take-away methadone policies and methadone diversion. *Drug and Alcohol Reviews, 24*(4), 347–352.

Ritz, M. C., Lamb, R. J., Goldberg, S. R., & Kuhar, M. J. (1987). Cocaine receptors on dopamine transporters are related to self-administration of cocaine. *Science, 237*(4819), 1219–1223.

Robinson, S. E. (2002). Buprenorphine: An analgesic with an expanding role in the treatment of opioid addiction. *CNS Drug Reviews, 8*(4), 377–390.

Robinson, T. E., & Berridge, K. C. (2000). The psychology and neurobiology of addiction: An incentive-sensitization view. *Addiction, 95*(Suppl. 2), S91–S117.

Ross, S., & Peselow, E. (2009). Pharmacotherapy of addictive disorders. *Clinical Neuropharmacology, 32*(5), 277–289.

Schwienbacher, I., Fendt, M., Richardson, R., & Schnitzler, H. U. (2004). Temporary inactivation of the nucleus accumbens disrupts acquisition and expression of fear-potentiated startle in rats. *Brain Research, 1027*(1–2), 87–93.

Self, D. W., & Nestler, E. J. (1998). Relapse to drug-seeking: Neural and molecular mechanisms. *Drug and Alcohol Dependence, 51*(1–2), 49–60.

Sharma, S., Rakoczy, S., & Brown-Borg, H. (2010). Assessment of spatial memory in mice. *Life Sciences, 87*(17–18), 521–536.

Shearer, J., Darke, S., Rodgers, C., Slade, T., van Beek, I., & Lewis, J. (2009). A double-blind, placebo-controlled trial of modafinil (200 mg/day) for methamphetamine dependence. *Addiction, 104*(2), 224–233.

Shoptaw, S., Heinzerling, K. G., Rotheram-Fuller, E., Steward, T., Wang, J., & Swanson, A. N. (2008). Randomized, placebo-controlled trial of bupropion for the treatment of methamphetamine dependence. *Drug and Alcohol Dependence, 96*(3), 222–232.

Silva de Lima, M., de Oliveira Soares, B. G., Reisser, A. A., & Farrell, M. (2002).

Pharmacological treatment of cocaine dependence: A systematic review. *Addiction, 97*(8), 931–949.

Simkin, D. R., & Grenoble, S. (2010). Pharmacotherapies for adolescent substance use disorders. *Child and Adolescent Psychiatry Clinics of North America, 19*(3), 591–608.

Sofuoglu, M., & Kosten, T. R. (2006). Emerging pharmacological strategies in the fight against cocaine addiction. *Expert Opinion on Emerging Drugs, 11*(1), 91–98.

Somerville, L. H., Whalen, P. J., & Kelley, W. M. (2010). Human bed nucleus of the stria terminalis indexes hypervigilant threat monitoring. *Biological Psychiatry, 68*(5), 416–424.

Srisurapanont, M., & Jarusuraisin, N. (2005). Naltrexone for the treatment of alcoholism: A meta-analysis of randomized controlled trials. *International Journal of Neuropsychopharmacology, 8*(2), 267–280.

Stimmel, B., Goldberg, J., Rotkopf, E., & Cohen, M. (1977). Ability to remain abstinent after methadone detoxification: A six-year study. *JAMA: Journal of the American Medical Association, 237*(12), 1216–1220.

Strain, E. C., Bigelow, G. E., Liebson, I. A., & Stitzer, M. L. (1999). Moderate- vs high-dose methadone in the treatment of opioid dependence: A randomized trial. *JAMA: Journal of the American Medical Association, 281*(11), 1000–1005.

Suh, J. J., Pettinati, H. M., Kampman, K. M., & O'Brien, C. P. (2006). The status of disulfiram: A half of a century later. *Journal of Clinical Psychopharmacology, 26*(3), 290–302.

Sung, S., & Conry, J. M. (2006). Role of buprenorphine in the management of heroin addiction. *Annals of Pharmacotherapy, 40*(3), 501–505.

Taylor, K. S., Seminowicz, D. A., & Davis, K. D. (2009). Two systems of resting state connectivity between the insula and cingulate cortex. *Human Brain Mapping, 30*(9), 2731–2745.

Tracqui, A., Kintz, P., & Ludes, B. (1998). Buprenorphine-related deaths among drug addicts in France: A report on 20 fatalities. *Journal of Analytical Toxicology, 22*(6), 430–434.

van der Brink, W. A., Goppel, M. B., & van Ree, J. M. C. (2003). Management of opioid dependence. *Current Opinion in Psychiatry, 16*(3), 297–304.

Volpicelli, J. R., Alterman, A. I., Hayashida, M., & O'Brien, C. P. (1992). Naltrexone in the treatment of alcohol dependence. *Archives of General Psychiatry, 49*(11), 876–880.

Voorn, P., Vanderschuren, L. J., Groenewegen, H. J., Robbins, T. W., & Pennartz, C. M. (2004). Putting a spin on the dorsal–ventral divide of the striatum. *Trends in Neurosciences, 27*(8), 468–474.

Walsh, S. L., Preston, K. L., Stitzer, M. L., Cone, E. J., & Bigelow, G. E. (1994). Clinical pharmacology of buprenorphine: ceiling effects at high doses. *Clinical Pharmacology and Therapeutics, 55*(5), 569–580.

Wilde, M. I., & Wagstaff, A. J. (1997). Acamprosate: A review of its pharmacology and clinical potential in the management of alcohol dependence after detoxification. *Drugs, 53*(6), 1038–1053.

Willuhn, I., Wanat, M. J., Clark, J. J., & Phillips, P. E. (2010). Dopamine signaling in the nucleus accumbens of animals self-administering drugs of abuse. *Current Topics in Behavioral Neuroscience, 3,* 29–71.

Woody, G. E., Poole, S. A., Subramaniam, G., Dugosh, K., Bogenschutz, M., & Abbott, P. (2008). Extended vs short-term buprenorphine-naloxone for treatment of opioid-addicted youth: A randomized trial. *JAMA: Journal of the American Medical Association, 300*(17), 2003–2011.

Yoshimoto, K., & McBride, W. J. (1992). Regulation of nucleus accumbens dopamine release by the dorsal raphe nucleus in the rat. *Neurochemical Research, 17*(5), 401–407.

Chapter 12

Integrating Psychotherapy and Pharmacotherapy in Substance Abuse Treatment

Kathleen M. Carroll
Brian D. Kiluk

Although this book focuses mainly on psychotherapeutic approaches commonly used in the treatment of substance abuse, medications also play a vital role in treatment. This chapter (1) describes differences in the roles and functions of psychotherapy and pharmacotherapy in the treatment system; (2) discusses the potential advantages of the two forms of treatment alone and in combination; and (3) concentrates on the pharmacological treatment of alcohol and opioid dependence (the only classes of substance dependence for which effective and approved pharmacotherapies exist), with an emphasis on describing how outcomes can be enhanced and extended through combining them with psychotherapy. Although this chapter covers many of the same medications presented in Chapter 11, this chapter is more concerned with the practical integration of pharmacotherapy and psychotherapy. It should be noted that in this chapter "psychotherapy" is used as a general term for several types of psychosocial treatment, including individual and group counseling, psychotherapy, and behavior therapy.

The Roles of Psychotherapy and Pharmacotherapy

The Roles of Psychotherapy

Most psychotherapies for substance abuse and dependence address common issues, despite often wide differences in theory, technique, and strategies. Although approaches vary in the degree to which emphasis is placed on these common tasks, some attention to these issues is likely to be involved in any successful treatment (Rounsaville, Carroll, & Back, 2004). The following is a brief description of areas typically addressed through psychotherapy.

Setting the Resolve to Stop

It is rare to encounter a substance-abusing person who seeks treatment without some degree of ambivalence regarding cessation of drug use. Even at the time of treatment seeking, which usually occurs only after substance-related problems have become severe, substance abusers usually can identify many ways in which they want or feel the need for drugs and have difficulty developing a clear picture of what life without drugs might be like (Rounsaville et al., 2004). Moreover, given the substantial external pressures that may prompt treatment, many patients remain highly ambivalent about treatment itself. Roughly 25–50% of individuals receiving substance abuse treatment report some form of formal pressure to do so (Perron & Bright, 2008), and thus the associated resistance/ambivalence must be addressed if the patient is to experience him- or herself as an active participant in treatment. Although some evidence suggests that individuals mandated to substance abuse treatment have similar treatment outcomes to those non-mandated (see Klag, O'Callaghan, & Creed, 2005), internal motivation is still an important focus of psychotherapy. Treatments based on principles of motivational psychology, such as motivational interviewing (Miller & Rollnick, 2002), concentrate on strategies intended to bolster the patient's own motivational resources. However, most behavioral treatments include some exploration of what the patient stands to lose or gain through continued substance use as a means to enhance motivation for treatment and abstinence.

Teaching Coping Skills

Social learning theory posits that substance abuse may represent a means of coping with difficult situations, positive and negative affect, invitations by peers to use substances, and so on. By the time substance use is severe enough for treatment, use of substances may represent the individual's single, overgeneralized means of coping with a variety of situations, settings, and states. If stable abstinence is to be achieved, treatment must help the patient to recognize the high-risk situations in which he or she is most likely to use substances and to develop other, more effective means of coping with them. Although cognitive-behavioral approaches concentrate almost exclusively on skills training as a means of preventing relapse to substance use (e.g., Carroll, 1998; Marlatt & Donovan, 2005; Monti, Kadden, Rohsenhow, Cooney, & Abrams, 2002), most treatment approaches touch on the relationship between high-risk situations and substance use to some extent. The format for teaching skills to manage high-risk situations varies widely, from group discussion/instruction to rehearsal through role plays, imaginal exposure, or emotional induction. The past decade has seen an increase in the use of computer technology as a format for teaching/rehearsing coping skills; virtual reality has been used to induce craving for more effective coping rehearsal (e.g., Saladin, Brady, Graap, & Rothbaum, 2006), and several new computer-assisted therapies have been developed that incorporate coping skills training (e.g., Carroll et al., 2008; Riper et al., 2007). In addition to teaching skills for avoiding or coping with high-risk situations, skills training may target how to repair relationship difficulties, increase use of social support, effectively communicate, or regulate emotion.

Changing Reinforcement Contingencies

By the time treatment is sought, many substance abusers spend the preponderance of their time acquiring, using, and recovering from substance use to the exclusion of other endeavors. The abuser may be estranged from family and friends and may have few social contacts who do not use alcohol/drugs. If the patient is still working, employment often becomes no more than a means of acquiring money to buy drugs; the fulfilling or challenging aspects of work have faded away. Few other activities, such as hobbies, athletics, or involvement with community or church groups, can stand up to the demands of substance dependence. Typically, the rewards available in daily life are narrowed progressively to those derived from substance use, and other diversions may be neither available nor perceived as enjoyable. When substance use is stopped, its absence may leave the patient with the need to fill the time that had been spent using drugs and to find rewards that can substitute for those derived from drug use. Thus, most behavioral treatments encourage patients to identify and develop fulfilling alternatives to substance use, as exemplified by the community reinforcement approach (CRA; Azrin, 1976) or contingency management (Budney & Higgins, 1998), both of which stress the development of alternate reinforcers for substance use.

Fostering Management of Painful Affect

The most commonly cited reasons for relapse are powerful negative affects (Marlatt & Donovan, 2005). Some have suggested that fluctuation in negative affect and failure of affect regulation is a critical dynamic underlying the development of compulsive drug use (Baker, Piper, McCarthy, Majeskie, & Fiore, 2004). Moreover, many substance abusers have difficulty recognizing and articulating their affect states (Keller, Carroll, Nich, & Rounsaville, 1995; Taylor, Parker, & Bagby, 1990). Thus, an important common task in substance abuse treatment is to help patients develop ways of coping with powerful dysphoric affects and to learn to recognize and identify the probable cause of these feelings (Rounsaville et al., 2004). Again, virtually all forms of psychotherapy for substance abuse include techniques for coping with strong affect.

Improving Interpersonal Functioning and Enhancing Social Supports

Social support networks are an important protective factor against relapse (Dobkin, De Civita, Paraherakis, & Gill, 2002; Longabaugh, Beattie, Noel, Stout, & Malloy, 1993). Typical issues presented by drug abusers are damage to relationships when using drugs was the principal priority, failure to achieve satisfactory relationships even prior to having initiated drug use, and inability to identify friends or intimates who are not themselves drug users (Rounsaville et al., 2004). The focus on building and maintaining a network of social supports for abstinence is a central part of treatments such as family therapy (McCrady & Epstein, 1995), 12-step approaches (Nowinski & Baker, 2003), interpersonal therapy (Rounsaville, Gawin, & Kleber, 1985), and network therapy (Galanter, 1993).

Fostering Compliance with Pharmacotherapy

Treatment compliance is often difficult among substance abusers (so much so that abusers are typically excluded from clinical trials of treatments for other disorders). Thus, when pharmacotherapies are used in the treatment of substance abuse, it is not surprising that high rates of noncompliance are seen. So, one major role for behavioral treatments is to foster compliance with pharmacotherapy (Carroll, 1997a). Strategies include, for example, regular monitoring of medication compliance through pill counts or medication serum levels; encouragement of patient self-monitoring (e.g., through medication logs or diaries); clear communication between patient and staff about the study medication; contracting with patients for adherence; directly reinforcing adherence through incentives or rewards; providing telephone or written reminders about appointments or taking medication;

preparing and educating patients about the disorder and its treatment; and the provision of extensive support and encouragement by the patient's family (see O'Donohue & Levensky, 2006).

It should be noted, however, that some traditional treatment approaches have a long-standing opposition to the use of pharmacological approaches in the treatment of substance use disorders. While many traditional programs and self-help groups have become more accepting of pharmacotherapies, clinicians may find it helpful to prepare a patient for the reaction he or she may encounter in such groups, reiterate the rationale and expected benefits of the medication, and point out the difference between drugs of abuse and prescribed pharmacotherapies.

The Roles of Pharmacotherapy

The target symptoms addressed and the roles typically played by pharmacotherapy differ from those of behavioral treatments in their course of action, time to effect, target symptoms, and durability of benefits (Elkin, Pilkonis, Docherty, & Sotsky, 1988a, 1988b). In general, pharmacotherapies have a much more narrow application than do most behavioral treatments. That is, most behavioral therapies are applicable across a range of treatment settings (e.g., inpatient, outpatient, residential), modalities (e.g., group, individual, family), and populations. For example, 12-step, cognitive-behavioral, contingency management, or motivational enhancement approaches have been used, with only minor modifications, regardless of whether the patient is an opiate, alcohol, cocaine, or marijuana user. In contrast, most pharmacotherapies are applicable only to a single class of substance use and exert their effects over a narrow band of symptoms. For example, methadone produces cross-tolerance for opioids but has little effect on concurrent cocaine abuse; disulfiram produces nausea after alcohol ingestion but not after ingestion of other substances. However, recently a few exceptions have been identified. Naltrexone, which was initially used to treat opiate addiction, has also been found to be effective at treating alcohol dependence (see Bouza, Angeles, Munoz, & Amate, 2004). Also disulfiram, which has been used for more than 50 years as a treatment for alcohol dependence, has demonstrated effectiveness at treating non-alcoholic cocaine-dependent patients (Carroll et al., 2004).

Common roles and indications for pharmacotherapy in the treatment of substance use disorders include the following (Rounsaville et al., 2004):

Detoxification

For those classes of substances that produce substantial physical withdrawal syndromes (e.g., alcohol, opioids, sedative–hypnotics), medications are often needed to control the dangerous or distressing symptoms associated with withdrawal. Benzodiazepines remain the standard of care for managing symptoms of alcohol withdrawal, including seizures and delirium tremens (see Mayo-Smith, 2009). Due to the potential abuse and other complications associated with benzodiazepines, there has been some recent interest and promising evidence for the use of anticonvulsants at treating alcohol withdrawal symptoms, but further investigations are needed (Barrons & Roberts, 2009; Myrick et al., 2009). Agents such as methadone, clonidine, naltrexone, and buprenorphine are most often used for the management of opioid withdrawal (see Tetrault & O'Connor, 2009). However, there are differences in the use of these medications during the withdrawal phase. For instance, methadone and buprenorphine, which are long-acting opioid substitutions, are designed to lessen the severity of the withdrawal symptoms by tapering the dosage over several days or weeks, whereas naltrexone is designed to accelerate withdrawal symptoms producing a more rapid detoxification period that can then be managed with clonidine, buprenorphine, or sedatives over a shorter duration. Due to the intensity of the intervention, only clinicians who are experienced with the use of rapid detoxification procedures should try this and other "ultrarapid" detoxifications (Kosten & O'Connor, 2003; Stine & Kosten, 2009a). In the past, the role of behavioral treatments during detoxification was considered extremely limited due to the level of discomfort, agitation, and confusion the patient may experience, particularly in the short term. However, a review of studies suggested that psychotherapy was effective in increasing retention and abstinence in the course of longer term outpatient detoxification protocols (Amato et al., 2008a).

Stabilization and Maintenance

A widely used example of the use of a medication for long-term stabilization of drug users is methadone maintenance for opioid dependence, a treatment strategy that involves the daily administration of a long-acting opioid (methadone) as a substitute for the illicit use of short-acting opioids (typically heroin). Other examples include buprenorphine for opioid dependence and nicotine replacement therapies for smoking (not reviewed here). These maintenance-type therapies permit the patient to function normally without experiencing withdrawal symptoms, cravings, or side effects. A large body of research supports the use of maintenance therapies for opioid dependence; these will be reviewed in detail in the section on specific pharmacotherapies. Briefly, one of the benefits of maintenance therapies, such as methadone and buprenorphine, is their effect on treatment retention. For instance, they may provide the opportunity to evaluate and treat other problems that often coexist with opioid dependence (e.g., medical, legal, and occupational problems) or provide a level of stabilization that permits the inception of psychotherapy and other aspects of treatment (see Martin, Zweben, & Payte, 2009; Mattick, Breen, Kimber, & Davoli, 2009; Mattick, Kimber, Breen, & Davoli, 2008).

Antagonist and Other Behaviorally Oriented Pharmacotherapies

Another pharmacological strategy is the use of *antagonist treatment*, that is, the use of medications that block the effects of specific drugs. An example of this approach is naltrexone, an effective, long-acting opioid antagonist. Naltrexone is nonaddicting, does not have the reinforcing properties of opioids, has few side effects and, most important, effectively blocks the effects of opioids (Stine & Kosten, 2009b). Therefore, naltrexone treatment represents a potent behavioral strategy: as opioid ingestion will not be reinforced while the patient is taking naltrexone, unreinforced opioid use allows extinction of relationships between conditioned drug cues and drug use. For example, a naltrexone-maintained patient, anticipating that opioid use will not result in desired drug effects, may be more likely to learn to live in a world full of drug cues and high-risk situations without resorting to drug use. However, as discussed later, medication compliance issues have significantly affected the usefulness of oral naltrexone for opioid dependence.

Treatment of Coexisting Disorders

An important role of pharmacotherapy in the treatment of substance use disorders is as a treatment for coexisting psychiatric syndromes that may precede or play a role in substance dependence. The frequent co-occurrence of other mental disorders, particularly affective and anxiety disorders, with substance use disorders is well documented in a variety of populations and settings (Kessler et al., 1994; Regier et al., 1990). Given that psychiatric disorders often precede development of substance use disorders, several researchers and clinicians have hypothesized that individuals with primary psychiatric disorders may be attempting to self-medicate their psychiatric symptoms with drugs and alcohol (e.g., Markou, Kosten, & Koob, 1998). Thus, effective pharmacological treatment of the underlying psychiatric disorder may improve not only the psychiatric disorder but also the perceived need for and therefore the use of illicit drugs (Rosenthal & Westreich, 1999). Examples of this type of approach include the use of antidepressant treatment for depressed abusers of alcohol (Cornelius et al., 1997), opioids (Nunes, Quitkin, Brady, & Stewart, 1991), and cocaine (Margolin, Avants, & Kosten, 1995). Pharmacological treatment of psychiatric disorders in substance users is not an explicit focus of this chapter; below we review only those medications that target substance use directly.

Combining Behavioral and Pharmacological Treatments

Enormous progress has been made in the development of effective pharmacotherapies for several substance use disorders. (See Table 12.1 for a brief overview.) However, there are three important considerations that need to be addressed before discussing specific pharmacotherapies.

First, nonpharmacological, behavioral treatments constitute the bulk of substance abuse treatment in the United States. Numerous studies point to the benefits of purely psychosocial or behavioral approaches for many substance use disorders (Hubbard, Craddock, Flynn, Anderson, & Etheridge, 1997; Higgins, 1999; McLellan & McKay, 1998). In most cases, pharmacotherapies (other than those used for detoxification or treatment of comorbid disorders) are typically seen as adjunctive strategies, to be used when behavioral treatment alone has been demonstrated to be insufficient for a particular individual.

Second, there are no effective pharmacotherapies for most types of illicit drug use. Classes of drug use for which no robustly effective pharmacotherapies have been found include cocaine, marijuana, hallucinogens, methamphetamine, inhalants, phencyclidine, and sedatives/hypnotics/anxiolytics. Although major advances have been made in identifying physiological mechanisms of action for many of these substances, and although in a few cases (such as marijuana) specific receptors have been identified that should accelerate progress in identifying pharmacological treatments, psychotherapies remain the sole available treatment for these classes of drug dependence.

Third, there is general consensus that even for the most potent pharmacotherapies for drug use, purely pharmacological approaches are insufficient for most substance abusers; the best outcomes are seen for combined treatments. Pharmacotherapeutic treatments that are delivered alone, without psychotherapeutic support, are usually insufficient to promote stable abstinence in drug abusers. As described above, most pharmacotherapies are relatively narrow in their actions; they may help to detoxify, stabilize, or treat coexisting disorders, but are rarely considered "complete treatments" by themselves. Furthermore, because few patients will persist in or comply with a purely pharmacotherapeutic approach, pharmacotherapies delivered alone, without any supportive or compliance-enhancing elements, are usually not considered feasible.

Even where pharmacotherapy is the primary treatment approach (as in the case of methadone maintenance), some form of psychosocial treatment is used to provide at least a minimal supportive structure within which pharmacotherapeutic treatment can be conducted effectively. Furthermore, it is widely recognized that drug effects can be enhanced or diminished by the context in which the drug is delivered. That is, a drug administered in the context of a supportive clinician–patient relationship, with clear

TABLE 12.1. Summary of Indicated Pharmacotherapy for Various Drugs of Abuse

Drug of abuse	Pharmacotherapy	Effect
Alcohol	Disulfiram	Deterrent to drinking; produces aversive physiological reaction when combined with alcohol.
	Naltrexone (oral and extended-release injectable)	Reduces craving for alcohol; limits heavy drinking episodes
	Acamprosate	Reduces alcohol withdrawal symptoms and craving for alcohol.[a]
Opioids	Methadone	Prevents onset of opioid withdrawal; reduces craving; blocks euphoric effects of opioids.
	LAAM[b]	Prevents onset of opioid withdrawal.
	Buprenorphine	Prevents onset of opioid withdrawal; blocks euphoric effect of opioids.
	Naltrexone (oral and extended-release injectable)	Blocks euphoric effect of opioids; potentially reduces cravings.
Cocaine	Disulfiram[c]	Reduces reinforcing effects of cocaine.
Marijuana	None	
Amphetamines	None	
Sedatives/Anxiolytics	None	
Other	None	

[a]Mechanism of action has not been identified.
[b]No longer clinically available in United States.
[c]Some evidence of effectiveness but not yet approved for treatment of cocaine dependence.

expectations of possible drug benefits and side effects, close monitoring of drug compliance, and encouragement for abstinence, is more likely to be effective than a drug delivered without such elements. Even with primarily pharmacotherapeutic treatments, a psychotherapeutic component is almost always included to foster patients' retention in treatment and compliance with pharmacotherapy and to address the numerous comorbid psychosocial problems that occur among individuals with substance use disorders (Carroll, Kosten, & Rounsaville, 2004; Rounsaville et al., 2004).

Pharmacological Treatments

Pharmacotherapy of Alcohol Dependence

Disulfiram

The most commonly used pharmacological adjunct for the treatment of alcohol dependence is disulfiram, or Antabuse. Disulfiram interferes with the normal metabolism of alcohol, which results in an accumulation of acetaldehyde. Drinking following ingestion of disulfiram results in an intense physiological reaction, characterized by flushing, rapid or irregular heartbeat, dizziness, nausea, and headache (Fuller, 1989). Thus, disulfiram treatment is intended to work as a deterrent to drinking.

Despite the sustained popularity and widespread use of disulfiram, there have been few placebo-controlled clinical trials, and empirical support for its effectiveness has been mixed (Garbutt, West, Carey, Lohr, & Crews, 1999). Most studies on disulfiram treatment did not use control groups, and participants were often not blinded to the treatment groups because of (1) researchers' desire to assess the psychological threat of adverse reactions and (2) the problem of unmasking the blind through disulfiram's side effects (Suh, Pettinati, Kampman, & O'Brien, 2006). One of the most cited disulfiram trials that included a "blinded" group reported that disulfiram was no more effective than inactive doses of disulfiram or no medication in terms of abstinence, time to first drink, unemployment, or social stability (Fuller et al., 1986). However, for subjects who did drink, disulfiram treatment was associated with significantly fewer total drinking days. Moreover, rates of compliance with disulfiram in the study were low (20% of all subjects were judged by the authors as adherent to the medication regimen), although complete abstinence rates were high (43%) among compliant subjects. This study illustrates several important limitations of disulfiram: (1) compliance is a major problem and (2) many patients are unwilling to take disulfiram. In Fuller et al. (1986), 62% of those eligible for the study refused to participate.

One approach to address the poor compliance with disulfiram treatment is through subcutaneous implantation, a technique first introduced in 1968 (Kellan & Wesolkowski, 1968). Although initially considered a promising approach to circumvent adherence problems, the effectiveness of disulfiram implants remains questionable (Suh et al., 2006). Reasons proposed for the lack of efficacy are (1) an inadequate amount of disulfiram released/absorbed through implantation (Hughes & Cook, 1997), and (2) the psychological effect of disulfiram is potentially more powerful than the pharmacological effect (Johnsen & Morland, 1991).

A review of disulfiram research trials suggested that it is more effective when compliance is monitored (Brewer, Meyers, & Johnson, 2000). Thus, several studies have evaluated the effectiveness of psychotherapy as a strategy to improve retention and compliance with disulfiram. One of the most effective strategies may be disulfiram contracts, where the patient's spouse or significant other agrees to observe the patient take disulfiram each day and reward the patient (through praise) for compliance (O'Farrell & Bayog, 1986). Adding behavioral marital therapy with a disulfiram contract produces greater adherence, better drinking outcomes, higher marital satisfaction, and less domestic violence (O'Farrell, Choquette, Cutter, Brown, & McCourt, 1993; O'Farrell, Choquette, & Cutter, 1998). Azrin, Sisson, Meyers, and Godley (1982) reported positive and durable results from a randomized clinical trial comparing unmonitored disulfiram to disulfiram contracts, where disulfiram ingestion was monitored by the patient's spouse or administered as part of a multifaceted behavioral program, the community reinforcement approach (CRA). CRA was developed by Hunt and Azrin (1973) as a broad-spectrum approach (incorporating skills training, behavioral family therapy, and job-finding training) that also includes a disulfiram component. At 6-month follow-up, the traditionally treated group reported over 50% drinking days, while the group that received CRA was almost completely abstinent. This example illustrates how psychotherapy can be integrated with pharmacotherapy to produce better outcomes than either treatment alone.

Naltrexone

A major development in the treatment of alcohol dependence was the U.S. Food and Drug Administration's (FDA's) approval of naltrexone in 1994. The application of naltrexone, a mu-opioid antagonist, to the treatment of alcoholism derived from findings that indicated naltrexone reduced alcohol consumption in animals (Volpicelli, Davis, & Olgin, 1986) and alcohol craving and use in humans (Volpicelli, O'Brien, Alterman, & Hayashida, 1990). Although many randomized clinical trials have shown naltrexone to be more effective than placebo in reducing alcohol use and craving (e.g., O'Malley et al., 1992), recent reviews suggest naltrexone's primary effect is a reduction in relapse to heavy drinking, as opposed to increasing abstinence rates (Bouza et al., 2004; Srisurapanont & Jarusuraisin, 2005).

However, as with disulfiram, naltrexone's beneficial effects appear limited to the subgroup of patients who are compliant with the daily dosing regimen (Volpicelli et al., 1997). Yet compliance is relatively rare. A recent analysis of data from a commercial, community-based claims database of 1,138 patients with alcohol-related disorders who received a prescription for oral naltrexone revealed that only 14% were considered compliant (defined as having filled prescriptions for ≥80% of the 6-month treatment period), and a majority (52%) filled only a single prescription for the medication (Kranzler, Stephenson, Montejano, Wang, & Gastfriend, 2008). This underscores the importance of delivering naltrexone in conjunction with a behavioral approach that addresses compliance.

Thus, it is not surprising that naltrexone's effects have been found to differ somewhat with the nature of the behavioral treatment with which it is delivered. For example, Anton and colleagues (1999) reported high rates of retention, compliance, and significant effects of naltrexone in a randomized trial comparing naltrexone and placebo among abstinent alcoholics who received cognitive-behavioral therapy (CBT). Yet Krystal, Cramer, Krol, Kirk, and Rosenheck (2001) found no differences in outcome in a randomized trial comparing naltrexone and placebo among alcohol-dependent patients who received a 12-step-oriented therapy. Additionally, several trials have reported the combination of naltrexone with a cognitive-behavioral approach that emphasized coping skills/relapse prevention were more successful at reducing heavy drinking and multiple relapses for those who did drink, compared to therapy approaches that emphasized complete abstinence (Heinala et al., 2001; O'Malley et al., 1992), or motivational enhancement (Anton et al., 2005). However, in the context of a primary care clinic, there were no differences in naltrexone's effectiveness when combined with either medical management or weekly CBT (O'Malley et al., 2003).

Another approach to addressing compliance with naltrexone is through an extended-release injectable formulation (XR-NTX; Vivitrol), which was approved by the FDA in 2006 for the treatment of alcohol dependence. These once-monthly injections, in combination with psychosocial support, have been effective at reducing heavy drinking days, with less potential for hepatoxicity compared to oral naltrexone (Garbutt et al., 2005; Kranzler, Wesson, & Billot, 2004). However, injectable naltrexone appears to have greater effects in individuals who are able to abstain from alcohol prior to initiation of treatment; patients who had a 7-day period of abstinence prior to their first injection had an 80% reduction in heavy drinking rates, compared with active drinkers who had a 21% reduction (Garbutt et al., 2005). In fact, a subsequent analysis of this data revealed that patients with at least 4 days of alcohol abstinence prior to initiation of XR-NTX displayed significantly longer initial abstinence (i.e., time to first drink), and fewer drinking days per month, than those receiving placebo

(O'Malley, Garbutt, Gastfriend, Dong, & Kranzler, 2007). Thus, although the extended-release naltrexone appears to be effective at reducing heavy drinking days compared to placebo, the treatment effects are considerably increased for patients who can attain a brief period of abstinence prior to treatment initiation.

Acamprosate

Acamprosate, or calcium acetylhomotaurinate, has a molecular structure similar to several endogenous amino acids. Although its mechanism of action is not entirely clear, its main interaction is with the glutamatergic system (Al Quatari, Bouchenafa, & Littleton, 1998). There is some evidence to suggest that acamprosate works by reducing alcohol withdrawal symptoms (Spanagel, Putzke, Stefferl, Schöbitz, & Zieglgänsberger, 1996), as well as by reducing craving (Littleton, 1995) and the rewarding effects of alcohol (McGeehan & Olive, 2003). It was approved by the FDA in 2004, in conjunction with psychosocial treatment, for the maintenance of abstinence from alcohol, and appears to have no abuse potential and a benign side effect profile. Several large multicenter studies indicated that acamprosate was equally effective no matter what type of psychosocial treatment it was combined with, and some have suggested it can be used with little additional psychosocial treatment outside of medical management (Weiss & Kueppenbender, 2006). Two meta-analyses have confirmed the efficacy of acamprosate in maintaining abstinence in alcohol-dependent patients (Bouza et al., 2004; Srisurapanont & Jarusuraisin, 2005), and a recent review of 24 randomized clinical trials with nearly 7,000 participants concluded that acamprosate, combined with psychosocial intervention, was effective at reducing the risk of drinking after detoxification and increasing the number of days abstinent compared to placebo (Rosner et al., 2010). The authors noted a wide variability in the type of psychosocial treatments used in these studies, so the most effective combination approach remains unclear. However, much of the evidence in this review was from studies conducted in Europe; two recent U.S. studies did not support acamprosate's efficacy (Anton et al., 2006; Mason, Goodman, Chabac, & Lehert, 2006). Differences in study design and sample characteristics may account for this discrepancy, yet the usefulness of acamprosate in the United States is uncertain.

Combining Pharmacotherapies

The combination of naltrexone and acamprosate has been examined in conjunction with psychosocial treatment for alcohol dependence in two studies. One, a 12-week clinical trial conducted in Germany with 160 detoxified alcohol-dependent patients, all receiving weekly cognitive-behavioral group therapy, found that the combination of naltrexone and acamprosate was significantly better than acamprosate alone, but not naltrexone alone, in delaying time to first relapse (Kiefer et al., 2003). The other, Project COM-BINE (Anton et al., 2006), was one of the largest multisite randomized clinical trials for examining pharmacotherapies for alcohol dependence in the United States. This study of 1,383 recently alcohol-abstinent volunteers compared the efficacy of naltrexone and acamprosate, alone or in combination, in the context of brief medical management with or without a more intensive combined behavioral intervention (CBI) that integrated cognitive-behavioral and motivational enhancement therapy. Results demonstrated that patients receiving medical management with naltrexone, CBI, or both fared better on drinking outcomes, whereas acamprosate did not demonstrate efficacy with or without CBI. These findings remained consistent, although somewhat diminished, up to 1 year after treatment was discontinued (Donovan et al., 2008).

The combination of naltrexone and disulfiram for the treatment of alcohol dependence has also been evaluated in patients with various comorbid psychiatric disorders. The evidence suggests the combination of these two pharmacotherapies is no more effective than either medication alone at reducing drinking (Petrakis et al., 2005; Petrakis, Nich, & Ralevski, 2006; Petrakis et al., 2007).

Pharmacotherapy of Opioid Dependence

Methadone Maintenance

The inception of methadone maintenance treatment revolutionized the treatment of opioid addiction. It displayed the previously unseen ability to keep addicts in treatment and to reduce their illicit opioid use, outcomes with which nonpharmacological treatments had fared comparatively poorly (O'Malley, Anderson, & Lazare, 1972). Methadone prevents the onset of opioid withdrawal for approximately 24 hours (depending on individual metabolism), and is thought to provide a satiating effect for the user without producing an opioid "high." Beyond its ability to retain opioid addicts in treatment and help control opioid use, methadone maintenance reduces the risk of HIV infection through reducing intravenous drug use (Sees et al., 2000; Ball, Lange, Myers, & Friedman, 1988), increases adherence to antiretroviral therapy for those infected with HIV (Roux et al., 2008; Uhlmann et al., 2010), and provides the opportunity to evaluate and treat concurrent disorders, including medical, family, and psychiatric problems (Lowinson et al., 2004). A recent review of 11 randomized clinical trials evaluating the effectiveness of methadone maintenance compared to placebo or other nonpharmacological therapy concluded that methadone is able to retain patients in treatment longer and to reduce illicit opioid use better than drug-free alternative treatments (Mattick et al., 2009). In this review the authors noted no statistically significant reduction in criminal activity and mortality, yet there is considerable evidence from individual studies to suggest otherwise—patients receiving methadone maintenance show reduced criminal activity and mortality (Clausen, Anchersen, & Waal, 2008; Gibson et al., 2008; Lind, Chen, Weatherburn, & Mattick, 2005; Marsch, 1998; Sees et al., 2000).

While methadone is generally effective, there is a great deal of variability in the success across different maintenance programs. This is likely the result of variability in methadone dosing, with roughly one-third of methadone facilities providing doses below recommended levels in a recent survey (Pollack & D'Aunno, 2008), as well as variability in the provision and quality of psychosocial services (Corty & Ball, 1987). Additional problems with methadone maintenance treatment include illicit diversion of take-home methadone doses, difficulties with detoxification from methadone maintenance to a drug-free state, and the concurrent use of other substances, particularly alcohol, cocaine, and benzodiazepines among methadone-maintained subjects (Brands et al., 2008; Stine & Kosten, 2009b). A range of psychosocial treatments have been evaluated for their ability to address these drawbacks, as well as to enhance and extend the benefits of methadone maintenance. Later in this chapter, we review several types of behavioral approaches that have been identified as effective in enhancing and extending the benefits of methadone maintenance treatment. Despite the evidence of effectiveness, there are many barriers that limit the implementation and access to methadone maintenance treatments, such as limited patient and community acceptance of methadone as well as regulatory restrictions and the lack of availability in many areas of the country (Rounsaville & Kosten, 2000). Development of alternative maintenance agents, and especially agents that can be more readily administered with reduced clinic attendance and outside of traditional methadone maintenance settings, have addressed some of the problems associated with limited access to treatment.

Buprenorphine

Buprenorphine, a partial mu agonist and a kappa antagonist initially used for the management of acute pain, was introduced in the 1970s as a substitution agent for the treatment of opioid dependence due to its low physical dependence liability and minimal withdrawal symptoms (Jasinski, Pevnick, & Griffith, 1978). Because of its unique pharmacological properties, it has become an attractive alternative to methadone; ceiling effects at higher buprenorphine doses result in a lower risk of overdose, compared with methadone (Walsh, Preston, Stitzer, Cone, & Bigelow, 1994), and withdrawal symptoms following abrupt discontinuation of buprenorphine are relatively mild compared to heroin or methadone withdrawal (Kosten & O'Connor, 2003). However, due to concerns about the abuse liability and diversion risks, a sublingual tablet of buprenorphine combined with nalox-one (an opioid antagonist) was developed to limit abuse potential. When this sublingual tablet is taken as directed, buprenorphine exerts its partial agonist effects, but if diverted and injected, the naloxone exerts its opioid receptor antagonist effect and is aversive, negating the euphoric effects of the injected buprenorphine (Chiang & Hawks, 2003; Mendelson & Jones, 2003). The U.S. FDA approved buprenorphine and buprenorphine/nalox-one (Suboxone) in 2002 based on evidence of safety and effectiveness (e.g., Kosten, Schottenfeld, Ziedonis, & Falcioni, 1993; Ling, Wesson, Chara-vastra, & Klett, 1996). With the passage of the Drug Addiction Treatment Act of 2000 (DATA 2000), physicians with qualified training and certifica-tion were able to prescribe buprenorphine outside of traditional substance treatment programs, which may be preferable to some patients concerned with the stigma associated with methadone clinics. Several studies have supported the effectiveness of office-based buprenorphine treatment (Fiel-lin et al., 2006; Fiellin et al., 2002; Fudala et al., 2003). In a review of 24 randomized clinical trials examining the effectiveness of buprenorphine compared to methadone or placebo, the authors concluded that buprenor-phine is an effective intervention for use in the maintenance treatment of heroin dependence, but appears less effective than methadone at adequate dosages (Mattick et al., 2008).

Although generally effective, concerns with sublingual buprenor-phine treatment include diversion and nonmedical use (even with the buprenorphine–naloxone combination), as well as poor treatment adher-ence (Alho, Sinclair, Vuori, & Holopainen, 2007; Bell, Trinh, Butler, Ran-dall, & Rubin, 2009). To address these issues, an implantable formula-tion of buprenorphine has been developed, which delivers buprenorphine over 6 months with a constant and low-level release of the medication. Investigations are still ongoing, but results from a recent multicenter, placebo-controlled trial are promising for this treatment method (Ling et al., 2010).

L-Alpha-Acetylmethadol

L-Alpha-acetylmethadol (LAAM) gained U.S. FDA approval in 1993 as the first alternative to methadone as a maintenance treatment for opioid dependence. Although similar to methadone in terms of physical depen-dence (Fraser & Isbell, 1952), LAAM is much longer acting than meth-adone, and can suppress symptoms of opiate withdrawal for more than 72 hours (Walsh, Johnson, Cone, & Bigelow, 1998). Therefore, LAAM could be administered on a thrice-weekly dosing schedule, as opposed to methadone's daily dosing. This permitted reduced clinic attendance, eliminated the need for take-home bottles, and reduced dispensing costs. A 2002 review, which reported on 15 randomized clinical trials and three controlled prospective studies published up until 2000, concluded that LAAM appeared more effective than methadone at reducing heroin use, but there was not enough evidence to draw firm conclusions about its safety (Clark et al., 2002). In 2001, the FDA required a "black box" warning of potentially fatal heart arrhythmias, stating that LAAM should be used only for patients who failed treatment with other agents, and all those receiving LAAM should have baseline electrocardiogram screening and periodic monitoring. Although not widely used initially, the use of LAAM dropped sharply after these warnings appeared, and in 2003 the sole manufacturer of LAAM withdrew it from the world market despite similar cardiac complications reported with the use of methadone (Jaffe, 2007). LAAM is no longer clinically available as a maintenance therapy (although it remains FDA-approved), yet based on the research evidence and recent trials, many have recommended that LAAM's availability be reconsidered (Anglin, Conner, Annon, & Longshore, 2009; Jaffe, 2007; Wolstein et al., 2009).

Behavioral Treatments in the Context of Maintenance Therapies

Before describing specific approaches that have been effective in enhancing opioid maintenance therapies, the context for such approaches should be set by brief review of a study that authoritatively established the importance of psychosocial treatments in the context of a pharmacotherapy as potent as methadone. McLellan, Arndt, Metzger, Woody, and O'Brien (1993) randomly assigned 92 opiate-dependent individuals to a 24-week trial that included (1) methadone maintenance alone, without psychosocial services; (2) methadone maintenance with standard services, which included regular meetings with a counselor; or (3) enhanced methadone maintenance, which included regular counseling plus on-site medical/psychiatric, employment, and family therapy. Although some patients did reasonably well in the methadone-alone condition, 69% of this group had to be transferred out of the condition within 3 months of the study inception because their substance use did not improve or even worsened, or because they experienced significant medical or psychiatric problems that required a more intensive level of care. In terms of drug use and psychosocial outcomes, the best outcomes were seen in the enhanced methadone maintenance condition, with intermediate outcomes for the standard methadone services condition, and poorest outcomes for the methadone-alone condition. Although methadone maintenance treatment has powerful effects in terms of keeping addicts in treatment, a purely pharmacological approach will not be sufficient for the large majority of patients.

Contingency Management Approaches

Several studies have evaluated the use of contingency management to reduce illicit drug use among those who are maintained on methadone. In these studies, a reinforcer is provided to patients who demonstrate specified target behaviors such as providing drug-free urine specimens, accomplishing specific treatment goals, or attending treatment sessions. For example, methadone take-home privileges might be contingent on reduced drug use, an approach that capitalizes on an inexpensive reinforcer that is potentially available in all methadone maintenance programs. Stitzer and colleagues (e.g., Stitzer & Bigelow, 1978; Stitzer, Iguchi, & Felch, 1992) have done extensive work in evaluating methadone take-home privileges as a reward for decreased illicit drug use. In a series of well-controlled trials, this group of researchers has demonstrated (1) the relative benefits of positive over negative contingencies (Stitzer, Bickel, Bigelow, & Liebson, 1986); (2) the attractiveness of take-home privileges over other incentives available within methadone maintenance clinics (Stitzer & Bigelow, 1978); (3) the effectiveness of rewarding drug-free urines over other, more distal behaviors such as group attendance (Iguchi et al., 1996); and (4) the benefits of using take-home privileges contingent on drug-free urines over noncontingent take-home privileges (Stitzer et al., 1992).

Silverman and colleagues (Silverman, Higgins, et al., 1996; Silverman, Wong, et al., 1996), drawing on the compelling work of Steve Higgins and colleagues (see Budney & Higgins, 1998), have evaluated a voucher-based contingency management system to address concurrent illicit drug use (typically cocaine) among methadone-maintained opioid addicts. In this approach, abstinence, verified through drug-free urine screens, is reinforced through a voucher system where patients receive points redeemable for items consistent with a drug-free lifestyle (e.g., movie tickets, sporting goods). Patients never receive money directly. To encourage longer periods of abstinence, the value of the points increases with each successive clean urine specimen, and the value of the points is reset to the lowest amount when the patient produces a drug-positive urine screen. Silverman and colleagues (Silverman, Higgins, et al., 1996; Silverman, Wong, et al., 1996) demonstrated the efficacy of this approach in reducing illicit opioid and cocaine use, and a recent meta-analysis reported its efficacy across a range of substance-use disorders (Lussier, Heil, Mongeon, Badger, & Higgins, 2006).

There are some drawbacks of this approach: although contingency management appears quite promising in modifying previously intractable problems in methadone maintenance programs, particularly continued illicit drug use among clients, they have rarely been implemented in clinical practice. One major obstacle to the implementation of contingency management voucher approaches in regular clinical settings is their cost (up to $1,200 over 12 weeks). However, a creative, less expensive contingency management approach, developed by Nancy Petry and colleagues (see Petry & Martin, 2002; Petry, Martin, & Simcic, 2005) has demonstrated effectiveness comparable to the voucher-based approach (Petry, Alessi, Hanson, & Sierra, 2007), with favorable cost-effectiveness results (Sindelar, Olmstead, & Pierce, 2007). In this prize-based contingency management system, patients earn chances to draw from a "prize bowl" filled with slips of paper designated with either a value exchangeable for prizes or an encouraging message (e.g., "good job"). A typical prize bowl contains 250 slips of paper, with roughly half redeemable for a prize ranging from $1 to $100 (majority worth $1, with only one slip of paper worth $100). This procedure helps reduce overall cost by providing an intermittent schedule of tangible rewards, yet still maintains aspects of a fixed ratio schedule that escalates with increased target behaviors (i.e., patients earn more draws with each successive target behavior).

A drawback of contingency management separate from cost issues is that the positive effects diminish over time when the behavioral intervention is terminated (Silverman, Higgins, et al., 1996). In methadone maintenance treatment, this may suggest that specific reinforcers grow weaker with time and/or are replaced by other reinforcers. For example, for clients entering a methadone program from the street, contingency payments or dose increases may be highly motivating. On the other hand, for clients who have been stabilized and are working, other reinforcers, such as take-home doses or permission to omit counseling sessions, may be more attractive. While contingency management procedures may prove effective only over short periods of time, they may still be valuable in that they provide an interruption to illicit drug use (or other undesirable behaviors). This may serve as an opportunity for other interventions to take effect. For instance, given findings that the positive effects of CBT often appear later in treatment, several studies have examined the combination of contingency management procedures with CBT (Epstein, Hawkins, Covi, Umbricht, & Preston, 2003; Rawson et al., 2002).

Other Psychotherapies

Several studies have evaluated other forms of psychotherapy as strategies to enhance outcome from opioid maintenance therapies. The landmark study in this area was done by Woody et al. (1983) and was replicated in community settings by members of this group (Woody, McLellan, Luborsky, & O'Brien, 1995). While the original study is now more than 25 years old, it remains the most impressive demonstration of the benefits and role of psychotherapy in the context of methadone maintenance programs. This study not only demonstrated improvement in more outcome domains for those receiving professional psychotherapy in addition to methadone, but it also demonstrated differential response to psychotherapy as a function of patient characteristics. This may point to the best use of psychotherapy (relative to drug counseling) when resources are scarce: while methadone-maintained opiate addicts with lower levels of psychopathology tended to improve regardless of whether they received professional psychotherapy or drug counseling, those with higher levels of psychopathology tended to improve only if they received psychotherapy.

In addition to improving treatment adherence and psychopathology symptoms, psychotherapy approaches within maintenance treatments can also reduce substance use other than opioids, such as cocaine and benzodiazepines. Studies examining interventions other than contingency management within methadone maintenance treatment have reported positive findings for the community reinforcement approach (CRA) and relapse prevention (Abbott, Weller, Delaney, & Moore, 1998), and CBT (Rawson et al., 2002; Rosenblum et al., 1995). However, there appears to be little difference across interventions when combined with methadone maintenance, and several studies have suggested that the level of intensity of the psychosocial intervention does not impact outcome (Avants et al., 1999; Magura, Rosenblum, Fong, Villano, & Richman, 2002).

Despite some evidence of the effectiveness of adding psychosocial interventions to opioid agonist maintenance, there remains some controversy regarding their inclusion in standard pharmacological maintenance treatments. Twelve different psychosocial interventions, including contingency management, and three different pharmacological maintenance therapies (methadone, buprenorphine, LAAM) were considered in a recent review of 28 randomized trials (Amato et al., 2008b). The authors concluded that any psychosocial intervention combined with any pharmacological maintenance treatment was not superior to any pharmacological maintenance treatment alone at improving retention rates, reducing opiate use during treatment, or reducing depression and other psychiatric symptoms. Although there was a difference in favor of combining a psychosocial intervention with a pharmacological maintenance treatment at improving abstinence rates, the results of this review were surprising, given that a prior review indicated a positive effect of adding a psychosocial intervention to pharmacological maintenance (Amato, Davoli, Ferri, & Vecchi, 2004). It should be noted, however, that the standard pharmacological maintenance treatments included in these reviews did routinely offer counseling sessions, so even the control conditions typically included some ancillary psychosocial intervention. Therefore, caution is warranted when concluding that additional psychosocial interventions are not needed with pharmacological maintenance treatment.

Naltrexone/Antagonist Treatment

Opioid antagonist treatment (naltrexone) offers many advantages over methadone maintenance. It is nonaddicting and can be prescribed without concerns about diversion, has a benign side effect profile, and may be less costly, in terms of demands on professional and patient time, than the daily or near-daily clinic visits required for methadone maintenance (Rounsaville, 1995). Naltrexone blocks the subjective effects of heroin for 24–36 hours. It is easy to administer (typically one tablet per day), produces a relatively small number of side effects, and does not produce tolerance. Most important are behavioral aspects of the treatment, as unreinforced opiate use allows extinction of relationships between cues and drug use.

However, naltrexone has not, despite its many advantages, fulfilled its promise. Naltrexone treatment is currently limited to only a minority of opioid addicts, primarily because of low interest, difficulties associated with induction, and high dropout rates early in treatment (Fudala, Greenstein, & O'Brien, 2004). Naltrexone treatment has other disadvantages compared with methadone, including (1) discomfort associated with detoxification and protracted withdrawal symptoms, (2) lack of negative consequences for abrupt discontinuation, and (3) no reinforcement for ingestion. These may all lead to inconsistent compliance with treatment and high rates of attrition.

A recent review of randomized clinical trials reported that naltrexone was significantly better than control conditions at reducing the number of opioid-positive urines. However, this effect was only present in a subgroup with high retention rates (Johansson, Berglund, & Lindgren, 2006). Moreover, some of the most promising data included studies utilizing contingency management approaches for enhancing retention, suggesting the importance of including a targeted behavioral therapy in improving the utility of an otherwise marginally effective pharmacotherapy for the general population of opioid addicts.

Outside of including some form of psychotherapy to improve medication compliance, long-acting sustained release formulations of naltrexone (both injectable and implantable formulations) have been evaluated as alternatives to the poorly adhered-to oral form. Intramuscular injectable formulations (XR-NTX) deliver a concentration of naltrexone over the course of 4 weeks following a single injection. Although they are mostly used for the treatment of alcohol dependence, a recent randomized clinical trial indicated that monthly injectable naltrexone plus twice-weekly relapse prevention increased treatment retention and reduced opioid use compared to placebo (Comer et al., 2006). In 2010, following evidence of feasibility and safety, the FDA approved XR-NTX (Vivitrol) for prevention of relapse to opioid dependence in detoxified patients. The implantable formulation of naltrexone has also shown positive results in a randomized controlled trial compared to oral naltrexone (Hulse, Morris, Arnold-Reed, & Tait, 2009). This implantable formulation requires a minor surgical procedure to insert the implant, which provides a sustained-release of naltrexone over 2–3 months. This offers less frequent treatment visits, yet is potentially less acceptable than the injectable formulation due to the surgical procedure required. More investigations are needed before this sustained-release formulation is available in mainstream treatment facilities, yet the early evidence is promising. Nevertheless, psychosocial interventions remain important as an adjunct to naltrexone treatment, not only because of adherence issues, but also due to the prevalence of nonopioid use during treatment.

Pharmacotherapy of Cocaine Dependence

To date, there is no approved pharmacotherapy for cocaine dependence. Common targets for cocaine pharmacotherapies have been similar to those of other abused substances: agonists, antagonists, anticraving agents, and agents directed toward underlying or co-occurring conditions. More than 30 medications have been evaluated in clinical trials, and although a large number of agents have shown promise in open-label or pilot studies, none have consistently been more effective than placebo or behavioral treatment alone when evaluated in rigorous randomized, double-blind evaluations. Gorelick (2009) and Preti (2007) have provided excellent reviews of the pharmacotherapy literature, and recent Cochrane reviews of the latest clinical trials confirmed the lack of evidence for the use of psychostimulants (Castellas et al., 2010), anticonvulsants (Minozzi et al., 2008), antidepressants (Silva de Lima, Farrell, Lima Reisser, & Soares, 2003), and antipsychotics (Amato, Minozzi, Pani, & Davoli, 2007) for the treatment of cocaine dependence.

Although the clinical community awaits an approved pharmacotherapy for general populations of cocaine users, it is important to note that some medications do have a place in the treatment of cocaine dependence, particularly medications for treating co-occurring psychiatric or substance use disorders. These agents are often useful because many of the comorbid disorders that accompany cocaine dependence also play a role in perpetuating cocaine dependence (as in the case of individuals who are self-medicating psychiatric symptoms with cocaine). Thus, despite a lack of overall support for treating cocaine dependence, there are a number of effective pharmacotherapies for the many psychiatric disorders that frequently accompany cocaine dependence.

Another strategy involves the use of pharmacotherapies to target substance use disorders that frequently co-occur with cocaine dependence. For example, based on high rates of comorbid alcohol dependence among clinical populations of cocaine-dependent individuals (Brady, Sonne, Randall,

Adinoff, & Malcolm, 1995; Carroll, Rounsaville, & Bryant, 1993), disulfiram has been investigated as a viable treatment option. Initial randomized clinical trials in individuals with co-occurring cocaine and alcohol dependence suggested that disulfiram was associated with significantly better retention, longer periods of abstinence from cocaine and alcohol, and significantly fewer cocaine-positive urine specimens (Carroll, Nich, Ball, McCance, & Rounsaville, 1998; Carroll et al., 2000). Two subsequent randomized trials of cocaine-dependent individuals undergoing agonist therapies (e.g., methadone or buprenorphine) suggested that disulfiram was an effective approach for treating cocaine dependence without co-occurring alcohol dependence (George et al., 2000; Petrakis et al., 2000). And in the most promising evidence to date, our Yale group reported that disulfiram and CBT were effective at reducing cocaine use within a sample of 121 cocaine-dependent individuals at a general outpatient substance abuse treatment program (Carroll et al., 2004). This was the first randomized, placebo-controlled, clinical trial to demonstrate disulfiram's effectiveness in nonalcoholic cocaine-dependent outpatients. It also demonstrated that including CBT with disulfiram was more effective than interpersonal therapy (IPT) and disulfiram at reducing cocaine use during treatment. More large-scale controlled trials are needed before disulfiram can be implemented as a standard treatment for cocaine dependence, but the combination of disulfiram with psychosocial treatment appears to be a potentially useful approach.

Compared to trials evaluating pharmacological treatment of cocaine dependence, evaluations of behavioral therapies such as contingency management, CBT, and manualized twelve-step approaches have been much more effective (see Higgins, Heil, Rogers, & Chivers, 2008; Dutra et al., 2008). Because we currently lack an effective pharmacological platform for cocaine dependence (analogous to methadone maintenance or buprenorphine for the treatment of opioid dependence), behavioral therapies for cocaine-dependent individuals have focused on key outcomes such as retention and the inception and maintenance of abstinence, rather than placing initial emphasis on secondary psychosocial problems (e.g., family, psychological, legal problems).

Pharmacotherapy of Other Drugs of Abuse

As stated earlier, approved pharmacotherapies exist only for alcohol and opioid dependence. However, considerable effort has been made over the last few decades to identify effective medications for the treatment of other drugs of abuse, most notably cannabis and methamphetamine. Several medications have been investigated for signs of effectiveness at treating these drug-dependent populations. In general, the medications include those either: (1) known to be effective in the treatment of other drug use disorders, (2) known to alleviate symptoms of withdrawal from the drug of abuse, and/or (3) considered to target specific receptor function or potential mechanism of action. Despite some promising results, the evidence is mostly limited to laboratory models and small open-label trials (Elkashef et al., 2008; Vandrey & Haney, 2009). Medication development efforts are still in the early stages, and more controlled clinical trials are needed to support broad clinical use of these medications. Nevertheless, when enough evidence is compiled for a medication to receive approval to treat a drug of abuse, such as cannabis or methamphetamine, proper treatment will likely still include some form of behavioral or psychosocial intervention (i.e., psychotherapy) to both improve adherence and treat the aspects of addiction not addressed by pharmacotherapy (e.g., motivation, coping skills, intra- and interpersonal conflicts).

Conclusion

Even for those classes of substance abuse for which there are powerful and effective pharmacotherapies, the availability of methadone, buprenorphine, and Antabuse (e.g., disulfiram) have by no means cured substance abuse. These powerful agents tend to work primarily on the symptoms of substance abuse that are time-limited and autonomous, but have little impact on the enduring behavioral characteristics of substance use. Adherence is a universally important aspect of effective pharmacotherapy; however, even with the development of long-acting injectable formulations designed to limit problems with compliance, high rates of noncompliance and treatment dropout remain. Pharmacotherapies work only if substance abusers see the value of stopping substance use, but substance abusers have consistently found ways to circumvent these pharmacological interventions. It is unlikely that we will develop a pharmacological intervention that gives addicts the motivation to stop using drugs, helps them see the value in renouncing substance use, improves their ability to cope with the day-to-day frustrations in living, or provides alternatives to the reinforcements that illicit drugs provide. The bulk of the evidence suggests that pharmacotherapies can be very effective treatment adjuncts, but in most cases the effects of pharmacotherapies can be broadened, enhanced, and extended by the addition of psychotherapy (Carroll, Kosten, & Rounsaville, 2004).

Psychotherapy and pharmacotherapies work through different mechanisms, and address different problems. Neither is completely effective by itself. Because the evidence suggests that the two forms of treatment tend to work better together than apart, the best strategy is to match the needs of the patient using integrated treatments that consider biological, psychological, and social factors (Carroll, 1997b).

Acknowledgment

Support was provided by Grant Nos. P50-DA09241, K02-DA00248, U10-DA13038, and T32-DA007238 from the National Instutute on Drug Abuse.

References

Abbott, P. J., Weller, S. B., Delaney, H., & Moore, B. A. (1998). Community reinforcement approach in the treatment of opiate addiction. *American Journal of Substance Abuse Treatment, 24,* 17–30.

Al Quatari, M., Bouchenafa, O., & Littleton, J. (1998). Mechanisms of action of acamprosate, Part II: Ethanol dependence modifies effects of acamprosate on NMDA receptor binding in membranes from rat cerebral cortex. *Alcoholism: Clinical and Experimental Research, 22,* 810–814.

Alho, H., Sinclair, D., Vuori, E., & Holopainen, A. (2007). Abuse liability of buprenorphine-naloxone tablets in untreated IV drug users. *Drug and Alcohol Dependence, 88,* 75–78.

Amato, L., Minozzi, S., Davoli, M., Vecchi, S., Ferri, M., & Mayet, S. (2008a). Psychosocial and pharmacological treatments versus pharmacological treatments for opioid detoxification. *Cochrane Database of Systematic Reviews 2008, Issue 4,* CD005031.

Amato, L., Minozzi, S., Davoli, M., Vecchi, S., Ferri, M., & Mayet, S. (2008b). Psychosocial combined with agonist maintenance treatments versus agonist maintenance treatments alone for treatment of opioid dependence. *Cochrane Database of Systematic Reviews 2008, Issue 4.* CD004147.

Amato, L., Davoli, M., Ferri, M., & Vecchi, S. (2004). Psychosocial and pharmacological treatments versus pharmacological treatments for opioid abuse and dependence. *Cochrane Database of Systematic Reviews 2004, Issue 2,* CD004147.

Amato, L., Minozzi, S., Pani, P. P., & Davoli, M. (2007). Antipsychotic medications for cocaine dependence. *Cochrane Database of Systematic Reviews 2007, Issue 3,* CD006306.

Anglin, M. D., Conner, B. T., Annon, J. J., & Longshore, D. (2009). Longitudinal effects of LAAM and methadone maintenance on heroin addict behavior. *Journal of Behavioral Health Services Research, 36,* 267–282.

Anton, R. F., Moak, D. H., Latham, P., Waid, L. R., Myrick, H., Voronin, K., et al. (2005). Naltrexone combined with either cognitive behavioral or motivational enhancement therapy for alcohol dependence. *Journal of Clinical Psychopharmacology, 25,* 349–357.

Anton, R. F., Moak, D. H., Waid, L. R., Latham, P. K., Malcolm, R. J., & Dias, J. K. (1999). Naltrexone and cognitive behavioral therapy for the treatment of outpatient alcoholics: Results of a placebo-controlled trial. *American Journal of Psychiatry, 156,* 1758–1764.

Anton, R. F., O'Malley, S. S., Ciraulo, D. A., Cisler, R. A., Couper, D., Donovan, D. M., et al. (2006). Combined pharmacotherapies and behavioral interventions for alcohol dependence: The COMBINE study: A randomized controlled trial. *Journal of the American Medical Association, 295,* 2003–2017.

Avants, S. K., Margolin, A., Sindelar, J. L., Rounsaville, B. J., Shottenfeld, R., Stine, S., et al. (1999). Day treatment versus enhanced standard methadone services for opioid dependent patients: A comparison of clinical efficacy and cost. *American Journal of Psychiatry, 156,* 27–33.

Azrin, N. H. (1976). Improvements in the community-reinforcement approach to alcoholism. *Behaviour Research and Therapy, 14,* 39–348.

Azrin, N. H., Sisson, R. W., Meyers, R., & Godley, M. (1982). Alcoholism treatment by disulfiram and community reinforcement therapy. *Journal of Behavior Therapy and Experimental Psychiatry, 13,* 105–112.

Baker, T. B., Piper, M. E., McCarthy, D. E., Majeskie, M. R., & Fiore, M. C. (2004). Addiction motivation reformulated: An affective processing model of negative reinforcement. *Psychological Review, 111,* 33–51.

Ball, J. C, Lange, W. R., Myers, C. P., & Friedman, S. R. (1988). Reducing the risk of AIDS through methadone maintenance treatment. *Journal of Health and Social Behavior, 29,* 214–216.

Barrons, R., & Roberts, N. (2009). The role of carbamazepine and oxcarbazepine in alcohol withdrawal syndrome. *Journal of Clinical Pharmacy and Therapeutics, 35,* 153–167.

Bell, J., Trinh, L., Butler, B., Randall, D., & Rubin, G. (2009). Comparing treatment retention in treatment and mortality in people after initial entry to methadone and buprenorphine treatment. *Addiction, 104,* 1193–1200.

Bouza, C., Angeles, M., Munoz, A., & Amate, J. M. (2004). Efficacy and safety of naltrexone and acamprosate in the treatment of alcohol dependence. *Addiction, 99,* 811–828.

Brady, K. T., Sonne, E., Randall, C. L., Adinoff, B., & Malcolm, R. (1995). Features of cocaine dependence with concurrent alcohol use. *Drug and Alcohol Dependence, 39,* 69–71.

Brands, B., Blake, J., Marsch, D. C., Sproule, B., Jeyapalan, R., & Li, S. (2008). The impact of benzodiazepine use on methadone maintenance treatment outcomes. *Journal of Addictive Diseases, 27,* 37–48.

Brewer, C., Meyers, R. J., & Johnson, J. (2000). Does disulfiram help to prevent relapse in alcohol abuse? *CNS Drugs, 14,* 329–341.

Budney, A. J., & Higgins, S. T. (1998). *A community reinforcement plus vouchers approach: Treating cocaine addiction.* Rockville, MD: National Institute on Drug Abuse.

Carroll, K. M. (1997a). Manual guided psychosocial treatment: A new virtual requirement for pharmacotherapy trials? *Archives of General Psychiatry, 54,* 923–928.

Carroll, K. M. (1997b). Integrating psychotherapy and pharmacotherapy to improve drug abuse outcomes. *Journal of Addictive Behaviors, 22,* 233–245.

Carroll, K. M. (1998). *A cognitive-behavioral approach: Treating cocaine addiction* (NIH Publication No. 98–4308). Rockville, MD: National Institute on Drug Abuse.

Carroll, K. M., Ball, S. A., Martino, S., Nich, C., Babuscio, T. A., Nuro, K. F., et al. (2008). Computer-assisted delivery of cognitive-behavioral therapy for addiction: A randomized trial of CBT4CBT. *American Journal of Psychiatry, 165,* 881–888.

Carroll, K. M., Fenton, L. R., Ball, S. A., Nich, C., Frankforter, T. L., Shi, J., et al. (2004). Efficacy of disulfiram and cognitive behavior therapy in cocaine-dependent outpatients. *Archives of General Psychiatry, 61,* 264–272.

Carroll, K. M., Kosten, T. R., & Rounsaville, B. J. (2004). Choosing a behavioral therapy platform for pharmacotherapy for substance users. *Drug and Alcohol Dependence, 75,* 123–134.

Carroll, K. M., Nich, C., Ball, S. A., McCance, E., & Rounsaville, B. J. (1998). Treatment of cocaine and alcohol dependence with psychotherapy and disulfiram. *Addiction, 93,* 713–728.

Carroll, K. M., Nich, C., Ball, S. A., McCance-Katz, E. F., Frankforter, T., & Rounsaville, B. J. (2000). One year follow-up of disulfiram and psychotherapy for cocaine-alcohol abusers: Sustained effects of treatment. *Addiction, 95,* 1335–1349.

Carroll, K. M., Rounsaville, B. J., & Bryant, K. J. (1993). Alcoholism in treatment seeking cocaine abusers: Clinical and prognostic significance. *Journal of Studies on Alcohol, 54,* 199–208.

Castellas, X., Casas, M., Perez-Mana, C., Roncero, C., Vidal, X., & Capella, D. (2010). Efficacy of psychostimulant drugs for cocaine dependence. *Cochrane Database of Systematic Reviews 2010, Issue 2,* CD007380.

Chiang, C. N., & Hawks, R. L. (2003). Pharmacokinetics of the combination tablet of buprenorphine and naloxone. *Drug and Alcohol Dependence, 70,* S39–S47.

Clark, N. C., Lintzeris, N., Gijsbers, A., Whelan, G., Dunlop, A., Ritter, A., et al. (2002). LAAM maintenance vs. methadone maintenance for heroin dependence. *Cochrane Database of Systematic Reviews 2002, Issue 2,* CD002210.

Clausen, T., Anchersen, K., & Waal, H. (2008). Mortality prior to, during and after opioid maintenance treatment (OMT): A national prospective cross-registry study. *Drug and Alcohol Dependence, 94,* 151–157.

Comer, S. D., Sullivan, M. A., Yu, E., Rothenberg, J. L., Kleber, H. D., Kampman, K., et al. (2006). Injectable, sustained-release naltrexone for the treatment of opioid dependence. *Archives of General Psychiatry, 63,* 210–218.

Cornelius, J. R., Salloum, I. M., Ehler, J. G., Jarrett, P. J., Cornelius, M. D., Perel, J. M., et al. (1997). Fluoxetine in depressed alcoholics: A double-blind, placebo-controlled trial. *Archives of General Psychiatry, 54,* 700–705.

Corty, E., & Ball, J. C. (1987). Admissions to methadone maintenance: Comparisons between programs and implications for treatment. *Journal of Substance Abuse Treatment, 4,* 181–187.

Dobkin, P. L., De Civita, M., Paraherakis, A., & Gill, K. (2002). The role of functional support in treatment retention and outcomes among outpatient adult substance abusers. *Addiction, 97,* 347–356.

Donovan, D. M., Anton, R. F., Miller, W. R., Longabaugh, R., Hosking, J. D., & Youngblood, M. (2008). Combined pharmacotherapies and behavioral interventions for alcohol dependence (the COMBINE study): Examination of posttreatment drinking outcomes. *Journal of Studies on Alcohol and Drugs, 69,* 5–13.

Dutra, L., Stathopoulou, G., Basden, S. L., Leyro, T. M., Powers, M. B., & Otto, M. W. (2008). A meta-analytic review of psychosocial interventions for substance use disorders. *American Journal of Psychiatry, 165,* 179–187.

Elkashef, A., Vocci, F., Hanson, G., White, J., Wickes, W., & Tiihonen, J. (2008). Pharmacotherapy of methamphetamine addiction: An update. *Substance Abuse, 29*, 31–49.

Elkin, I., Pilkonis, P. A., Docherty, J. P., & Sotsky, S. M. (1988a). Conceptual and methodological issues in comparative studies of psychotherapy and pharmacotherapy: I. Active ingredients and mechanisms of change. *American Journal of Psychiatry, 145*, 909–917.

Elkin, I., Pilkonis, P. A., Docherty, J. P., & Sotsky, S. M. (1988b). Conceptual and methodological issues in comparative studies of psychotherapy and pharmacotherapy: II. Nature and timing of treatment effects. *American Journal of Psychiatry, 145*, 1070–1076.

Epstein, D. H., Hawkins, W. E., Covi, L., Umbricht, A., & Preston, K. L. (2003). Cognitive-behavioral therapy plus contingency management for cocaine use: Findings during treatment and across 12–month follow-up. *Psychology of Addictive Behaviors, 17*, 73–82.

Fiellin, D. A., Pantalon, M. V., Chawarski, M. C., Moore, B. A., Sullivan, L. E., O'Connor, P. G., et al. (2006). Counseling plus buprenorphine–naloxone therapy for opioid dependence. *New England Journal of Medicine, 355*, 365–374.

Fiellin, D. A., Pantalon, M. V., Pakes, J. P., O'Connor, P. G., Chawarski, M. C., & Shottenfeld, R. C. (2002). Treatment of heroin dependence with buprenorphine in primary care. *American Journal of Drug and Alcohol Abuse, 28*, 231–241.

Fraser, H. F., & Isbell, H. (1952). Actions and addiction liabilities of alpha acetylmethadols in man. *Journal of Pharmacology and Experimental Therapeutics, 105*, 458–465.

Fudala, P. J., Bridge, T. P., Herbert, S., Williford, W. O., Chiang, C. N., Jones, K., et al. (2003). Office-based treatment of opiate addiction with a sublingual-tablet formulation of buprenorphine and naloxone. *New England Journal of Medicine, 349*, 949–958.

Fudala, P. J., Greenstein, R. A., & O'Brien, C. P. (2004). Alternative pharmacotherapies for opioid addiction. In J. H. Lowinsohn, P. Ruiz, & R. B. Millman (Eds.), *Substance abuse: A comprehensive textbook* (4th ed., pp. 641–653). New York: Williams & Wilkins.

Fuller, R. K. (1989). Antidipsotropic medications. In W. R. Miller & R. K. Hester (Eds.), *Handbook of alcoholism treatment approaches: Effective alternatives* (pp. 117–127). New York: Pergamon Press.

Fuller, R. K., Branchey, L., Brightwell, D. R., Derman, R. M., Emrick, C. D., Iber, F. L., et al. (1986). Disulfiram treatment for alcoholism: A Veterans Administration cooperative study. *Journal of the American Medical Association, 256*, 1449–1455.

Galanter, M. (1993). *Network therapy for alcohol and drug abuse: A new approach in practice.* New York: Basic Books.

Garbutt, J. C., Kranzler, H. R., O'Malley, S. S., Gastfriend, D. R., Pettinati, H. M., Silverman, B. L., et al. (2005). Efficacy and tolerability of long-acting injectable naltrexone for alcohol dependence: A randomized controlled trial. *Journal of the American Medical Association, 293*, 1617–1625.

Garbutt, J. C., West, S. L., Carey, T. S., Lohr, K. N., & Crews, F. T. (1999).

Pharmacological treatment of alcohol dependence: A review of the evidence. *Journal of the American Medical Association, 281,* 1318–1325.

George, T. P., Pakes, J., Chawarski, M. C., Carroll, K. M., Kosten, T. R., & Schottenfeld, R. S. (2000). Disulfiram versus placebo for cocaine abuse in buprenorphine-maintained subjects: A preliminary trial. *Biological Psychiatry, 47,* 1080–1086.

Gibson, A., Degenhart, L., Mattick, R. P., Ali, R., White, J., & O'Brien, S. (2008). Exposure to opioid maintenance treatment reduces long-term mortality. *Addiction, 103,* 462–468.

Gorelick, D. A. (2009). Pharmacologic therapies for cocaine, methamphetamine, and other stimulant addiction. In R. K. Ries, D. A. Fiellin, S. C. Miller, & R. Saitz (Eds.), *Principles of addiction medicine* (4th ed., pp. 671–688). Philadelphia: Lippincott, Williams & Wilkins.

Heinala, P., Alho, H., Kiianmaa, K., Lonnqvist, J., Kuoppasalmi, K., & Sinclair, J. D. (2001). Targeted use of naltrexone without prior detoxification in the treatment of alcohol dependence: A factorial double-blind, placebo-controlled trial. *Journal of Clinical Psychopharmacology, 21,* 287–292.

Higgins, S. T. (1999). We've come a long way: Comments on cocaine treatment outcome research. *Archives of General Psychiatry, 56,* 516–518.

Higgins, S. T., Heil, S. H., Rogers, R. E., & Chivers, L. (2008). Cocaine. In S. T. Higgins, K. Silverman, & S. H. Heil (Eds.), *Contingency management in substance abuse treatment* (pp. 19–41). New York: Guilford Press.

Hubbard, R. L., Craddock, S. G., Flynn, P. M., Anderson, J., & Etheridge, R. M. (1997). Overview of 1–year follow-up outcomes in the Drug Abuse Treatment Outcome Study (DATOS). *Psychology of Addictive Behaviors, 11,* 261–278.

Hughes, J. C., & Cook, C. C. (1997). The efficacy of disulfiram: A review of outcome studies. *Addiction, 92,* 381–395.

Hulse, G. K., Morris, N., Arnold-Reed, D., & Tait, R. J. (2009). Improving clinical outcomes in treating heroin dependence: Randomized controlled trial of oral or implant naltrexone. *Archives of General Psychiatry, 66,* 1108–1115.

Hunt, G. M., & Azrin, N. H. (1973). A community-reinforcement approach to alcoholism. *Behavior Research and Therapy, 11,* 91–104.

Iguchi, M. Y., Lamb, R. J., Belding, M. A., Platt, J. J., Husband, S. D., & Morral, A. R. (1996). Contingent reinforcement of group participation versus abstinence in a methadone maintenance program. *Experimental and Clinical Psychopharmacology, 4,* 1–7.

Jaffe, J. H. (2007). Can LAAM, like Lazarus, come back from the dead? *Addiction, 102,* 1342–1343.

Jasinski, D. R., Pevnick, J. S., & Griffith, J. D. (1978). Human pharmacology and abuse potential of the analgesic buprenorphine: A potential agent for treatment of narcotic addictions. *Archives of General Psychiatry, 35,* 501–516.

Johansson, B. A., Berglund, M., & Lindgren, A. (2006). Efficacy of maintenance treatment with naltrexone for opioid dependence: A meta-analytical review. *Addiction, 101,* 491–503.

Johnsen, J., & Morland, J. (1991). Disulfiram implant: A double-blind placebo controlled follow-up on treatment outcome. *Alcoholism: Clinical and Experimental Research, 15,* 532–536.

Kellan, A. M., & Wesolkowski, J. M. (1968). Disulfiram implantation for alcoholism. *Lancet, 1*, 925–926.

Keller, D. S., Carroll, K. M., Nich, C., & Rounsaville, B. J. (1995). Differential treatment response in alexithymic cocaine abusers: Findings from a randomized clinical trial of psychotherapy and pharmacotherapy. *American Journal on Addictions, 4*, 234–244.

Kessler, R. C., McGonagle, K. A., Zhao, S., Nelson, C. B., Hughes, M., Eshlemen, S., et al. (1994). Lifetime and 12-month prevalence of DSM-III-R psychiatric disorders in the United States: Results from the National Comorbidity Survey. *Archives of General Psychiatry, 51*, 8–19.

Kiefer, F., Jahn, H., Tarnaske, T., Helwig, H., Briken, P., Holzbach, R., et al. (2003). Comparing and combining naltrexone and acamprosate in relapse prevention of alcoholism: A double-blind, placebo-controlled study. *Archives of General Psychiatry, 60*, 92–99.

Klag, S., O'Callaghan, F., & Creed, P. (2005). The use of legal coercion in the treatment of substance abusers: An overview and critical analysis of thirty years of research. *Substance Use and Misuse, 40*, 1777–1795.

Kosten, T. R., & O'Connor, P. G. (2003). Management of drug and alcohol withdrawal. *New England Journal of Medicine, 348*, 1786–1795.

Kosten, T. R., Schottenfeld, R., Ziedonis, D., & Falcioni, J. (1993). Buprenorphine versus methadone maintenance for opioid dependence. *Journal of Nervous and Mental Disease, 181*, 358–364.

Kranzler, H. R., Stephenson, J. J., Montejano, L., Wang, S., & Gastfriend, D. R. (2008). Persistence with oral naltrexone for alcohol treatment: Implications for health-care utilization. *Addiction, 103*, 1801–1808.

Kranzler, H. R., Wesson, D. R., & Billot, L. (2004). Naltrexone depot for treatment of alcohol dependence: A multicenter, randomized, placebo-controlled trial. *Alcoholism: Clinical and Experimental Research, 28*, 1051–1059.

Krystal, J. H., Cramer, J. A., Krol, W. F., Kirk, G. F., & Rosenheck, R. A. (2001). Naltrexone in the treatment of alcohol dependence. *New England Journal of Medicine, 345*, 1734–1739.

Lind, B., Chen, S., Weatherburn, D., & Mattick, R. (2005). The effectiveness of methadone maintenance treatment in controlling crime: An Australian aggregate level analysis. *Journal of Criminology, 45*, 201–211.

Ling, W., Casadonte, P., Bigelow, G., Kampman, K. M., Patkar, A., & Bailey, G. L. (2010). Buprenorphine implants for treatment of opioid dependence: A randomized controlled trial. *Journal of the American Medical Association, 304*, 1576–1583.

Ling, W., Wesson, D. R., Charavastra, C., & Klett, C. J. (1996). A controlled trial comparing buprenorphine and methadone maintenance in opioid dependence. *Archives of General Psychiatry, 53*, 401–407.

Littleton, J. (1995). Acamprosate in alcohol dependence: How does it work? *Addiction, 90*, 1179–1188.

Longabaugh, R., Beattie, M., Noel, R., Stout, R., & Malloy, P. (1993). The effect of social support on treatment outcome. *Journal of Studies on Alcohol, 54*, 465–478.

Lowinson, J. H., Marion, I., Joseph, H., Langrod, J., Salsitz, E. A., Payte, J. T., et al. (2004). Methadone maintenance. In J. H. Lowinson, P. Ruiz, R. B.

Millman, & J. G. Langrod (Eds.), *Substance abuse: A comprehensive text-book* (4th ed., pp. 616–633). Philadelphia: Lippincott, Williams & Wilkins.

Lussier, J. P., Heil, S. H., Mongeon, J. A., Badger, G. J., & Higgins, S. T. (2006). A meta-analysis of voucher based reinforcement therapy for substance use disorders. *Addiction, 101,* 192–203.

Magura, S., Rosenblum, A., Fong, C., Villano, C., & Richman, B. (2002). Treating cocaine-using methadone patients: Predictors of outcomes in a psychosocial clinical trial. *Substance Use and Misuse, 37,* 1927–1955.

Margolin, A., Avants, S. K., & Kosten, T. R. (1995). Mazindol for relapse prevention to cocaine abuse in methadone-maintained patients. *American Journal of Drug and Alcohol Abuse, 21,* 469–481.

Markou, A., Kosten, T. R., & Koob, G. F. (1998). Neurobiological similarities in depression and drug dependence: A self-medication hypothesis. *Neuropsychopharmacology, 18,* 135–174.

Marlatt, G. A., & Donovan, D. (Eds.). (2005). *Relapse prevention: Maintenance strategies in the treatment of addictive behaviors* (2nd ed.). New York: Guilford Press.

Marsch, L. (1998). The efficacy of methadone maintenance interventions in reducing illicit opiate use, HIV risk behavior and criminality: A meta-analysis. *Addiction, 93,* 515–532.

Martin, J., Zweben, J. E., & Payte, J. T. (2009). Opioid maintenance treatment. In R. K. Ries, D. A. Fiellin, S. C. Miller, & R. Saitz (Eds.), *Principles of addiction medicine* (4th ed., pp. 671–688). Philadelphia: Lippincott, Williams & Wilkins.

Mason, B. J., Goodman, A., Chabac, S., & Lehert, P. (2006). Effect of oral acamprosate on abstinence in patients with alcohol dependence in a double-blind, placebo-controlled trial: The role of patient motivation. *Journal of Psychiatric Research, 40,* 383–393.

Mattick, R. P., Breen, C., Kimber, J., & Davoli, M. (2009). Methadone maintenance therapy versus no opioid replacement therapy for opioid dependence. *Cochrane Database of Systematic Reviews 2009, Issue 3,* CD002209.

Mattick, R. P., Kimber, J., Breen, C., & Davoli, M. (2008). Buprenorphine maintenance versus placebo or methadone maintenance for opioid dependence. *Cochrane Database of Systematic Reviews 2008, Issue 2,* CD002207.

Mayo-Smith, M. F. (2009). Management of alcohol intoxication and withdrawal. In R. K. Ries, D. A. Fiellin, S. C. Miller, & R. Saitz (Eds.), *Principles of addiction medicine* (4th ed., pp. 559–572). Philadelphia: Lippincott, Williams & Wilkins.

McCrady, B. S., & Epstein, E. E. (1995). Marital therapy in the treatment of alcohol problems. In N. S. Jacobson & A. S. Gurman (Eds.), *Clinical handbook of couple therapy* (pp. 369–393). New York: Guilford Press.

McGeehan, A. J., & Olive, M. F. (2003). The anti-relapse compound acamprosate inhibits the development of a conditioned place preference to ethanol and cocaine but not morphine. *British Journal of Pharmacology, 138,* 9–12.

McLellan, A. T., Arndt, I. O., Metzger, D. S., Woody, G. E., & O'Brien, C. P. (1993). The effects of psychosocial services in substance abuse treatment. *Journal of the American Medical Association, 269,* 1953–1959.

McLellan, A. T., & McKay, J. R. (1998). The treatment of addiction: What can research offer practice? In S. Lamb, M. R. Greenlick, & D. McCarty (Eds.), *Bridging the gap between practice and research: Forging partnerships with community based drug and alcohol treatment* (pp. 147–185). Washington, DC: National Academy Press.

Mendelson, J., & Jones, R. T. (2003). Clinical and pharmacological evaluation of buprenorphine and naloxone combinations: Why the 4:1 ratio for treatment? *Drug and Alcohol Dependence, 70*(Suppl. 2), S29–S37.

Miller, W. R., & Rollnick, S. (2002). *Motivational interviewing, second edition: Preparing people for change.* New York: Guilford Press.

Minozzi, S., Amato, L., Davoli, M., Farrell, M., Lima Reisser, A., & Pani, P. P., et al. (2008). Anticonvulsants for cocaine dependence. *Cochrane Database of Systematic Reviews 2008, Issue 2,* CD006754.

Monti, P. M., Kadden, R. M., Rohsenhow, D. J., Cooney, N. L., & Abrams, D. B. (2002). *Treating alcohol dependence: A coping skills training guide* (2nd ed.). New York: Guilford Press.

Myrick, H., Malcolm, R., Randall, P. K., Boyle, E., Anton, R. F., Becker, H. C., et al. (2009). A double-blind trial of gabapentin versus lorazepam in the treatment of alcohol withdrawal. *Alcoholism: Clinical and Experimental Research, 33,* 1582–1588.

Nowinski, J., & Baker, S. (2003). *The twelve-step facilitation handbook: A systematic approach to recovery from alcoholism and addiction.* Center City, MN: Hazelden.

Nunes, E. V., Quitkin, F. M., Brady, R., & Stewart, J. W. (1991). Imipramine treatment of methadone maintenance patients with affective disorder and illicit drug use. *American Journal of Psychiatry, 148,* 667–669.

O'Donohue, W. T., & Levensky, E. R. (Eds.). (2006). *Promoting treatment adherence: A practical handbook for health care providers.* Thousand Oaks, CA: Sage.

O'Farrell, T. J., & Bayog, R. D. (1986). Antabuse contracts for married alcoholics and their spouses: A method to insure Antabuse taking and decrease conflict about alcohol. *Journal of Substance Abuse Treatment, 3,* 1–8.

O'Farrell, T. J., Choquette, K. A., & Cutter, H. S. (1998). Couples relapse prevention sessions after behavioral marital therapy for male alcoholics: Outcomes during the three years after starting treatment. *Journal of Studies on Alcohol, 59,* 357–370.

O'Farrell, T. J., Choquette, K. A., Cutter, H. S., Brown, E. D., & McCourt, W. F. (1993). Behavioral marital therapy with and without additional couples relapse prevention sessions for alcoholics and their wives. *Journal of Studies on Alcohol, 54,* 652–666.

O'Malley, J. E., Anderson, W. H., & Lazare, A. (1972). Failure of outpatient treatment of drug abuse, I: Heroin. *American Journal of Psychiatry, 128,* 865–868.

O'Malley, S. S., Garbutt, J. C., Gastfriend, D. R., Dong, Q., & Kranzler, H. R. (2007). Efficacy of extended-release naltrexone in alcohol-dependent patients who are abstinent before treatment. *Journal of Clinical Psychopharmacology, 27,* 507–512.

O'Malley, S. S., Jaffe, A. J., Chang, G., Schottenfeld, R. S., Meyer, R. E., & Rounsaville, B. J. (1992). Naltrexone and coping skills therapy for alcohol dependence: A controlled study. *Archives of General Psychiatry, 49*, 881–887.

O'Malley, S. S., Rounsaville, B. J., Farren, C., Namkoong, K., Wu, R., Robinson, J., et al. (2003). Initial and maintenance naltrexone treatment for alcohol dependence using primary care vs specialty care: A nested sequence of 3 randomized trials. *Archives of Internal Medicine, 163*, 1695–1704.

Perron, B. E., & Bright, C. L. (2008). The influence of legal coercion on dropout from substance abuse treatment: Results of a national survey. *Drug and Alcohol Dependence, 92*, 123–131.

Petrakis, I. L., Carroll, K. M., Gordon, L., Nich, C., McCance, E., Katz, E. F., et al. (2000). Disulfiram treatment for cocaine dependence in methadone maintained opioid addicts. *Addiction, 95*, 219–228.

Petrakis, I. L., Nich, C., & Ralevski, E. (2006). Psychotic spectrum disorders and alcohol abuse: A review of pharmacotherapeutic strategies and a report on the effectiveness of naltrexone and disulfiram. *Schizophrenia Bulletin, 32*, 644–654.

Petrakis, I. L., Poling, J., Levinson, C., Nich, C., Carroll, K. M., & Rounsaville, B. J. (2005). Naltrexone and disulfiram in patients with alcohol dependence and comorbid psychiatric disorders. *Biological Psychiatry, 57*, 1128–1137.

Petrakis, I. L., Ralevski, E., Nich, C., Levinson, C., Carroll, K. M., Poling, J., et al. (2007). Naltrexone and disulfiram in patients with alcohol dependence and current depression. *Journal of Clinical Psychopharmacology, 27*, 160–165.

Petry, N. M., Alessi, S. M., Hanson, T., & Sierra, S. (2007). Randomized trial of contingent prizes versus vouchers in cocaine-using methadone patients. *Journal of Consulting and Clinical Psychology, 75*, 983–991.

Petry, N. M., & Martin, B. (2002). Low-cost contingency management for treating cocaine and opioid abusing methadone patients. *Journal of Consulting and Clinical Psychology, 70*, 398–405.

Petry, N. M., Martin, B., & Simcic, F. (2005). Prize reinforcement contingency management for cocaine dependence: Integration with group therapy in a methadone clinic. *Journal of Consulting and Clinical Psychology, 73*, 354–359.

Pollack, H. A., & D'Aunno, T. (2008). Dosage patterns in methadone treatments: Results from a national survey, 1988–2005. *Health Services Research, 43*, 2143–2163.

Preti, A. (2007). New developments in the pharmacotherapy of cocaine abuse. *Addiction Biology, 12*, 133–151.

Rawson, R. A., Huber, A., McCann, M., Shoptaw, S., Farabee, D., Reiber, C., et al. (2002). A comparison of contingency management and cognitive-behavioral approaches during methadone maintenance treatment for cocaine dependence. *Archives of General Psychiatry, 59*, 817–824.

Regier, D. A., Farmer, M. E., Rae, D. S., Locke, B. Z., Keith, S. J., Judd, L. L., et al. (1990). Comorbidity of mental disorders with alcohol and other drug use. *Journal of the American Medical Association, 264*, 2511–2518.

Riper, H., Kramer, J., Smit, F., Conijn, B., Schippers, G., & Cuijpers, P. (2007). Web-based self-help for problem drinkers: A pragmatic randomized trial. *Addiction, 103*, 218–227.

Rosenblum, A., Magura, S., Foote, J., Palij, M., Handelsman, L., Lovejoy, M., et al. (1995). Treatment intensity and reduction in drug use for cocaine dependent methadone patients: A dose–response relationship. *Journal of Psychoactive Drugs, 27,* 151–159.

Rosenthal, R. N., & Westreich, L. (1999). Treatment of persons with dual diagnoses of substance use disorder and other psychological therapies. In B. S. McCrady & E. E. Epstein (Eds.), *Addictions: A comprehensive guidebook* (pp. 439–476). New York: Oxford University Press.

Rosner, S., Hackl-Herrwerth, A., Leucht, S., Lehert, P., Vecchi, S., & Soyka, M. (2010). Acamprosate for alcohol dependence. *Cochrane Database of Systematic Reviews 2010, Issue 9,* CD004322.

Rounsaville, B. J. (1995). Can psychotherapy rescue naltrexone treatment of opioid addiction? In L. S. Onken & J. D. Blaine (Eds.), *Potentiating the efficacy of medications: Integrating psychosocial therapies with pharmacotherapies in the treatment of drug dependence* (National Institute on Drug Abuse Research Monograph Series No. 105, pp. 37–52). Rockville, MD: National Institute on Drug Abuse.

Rounsaville, B. J., Carroll, K. M., & Back, S. (2004). Individual psychotherapy. In J. H. Lowinsohn, P. Ruiz, R. B. Millman, & J.G. Langrod (Eds.), *Substance abuse: A comprehensive textbook* (4th ed., pp. 653–667). Philadelphia: Lippincott, Williams & Wilkins.

Rounsaville, B. J., Gawin, F. H., & Kleber, H. D. (1985). Interpersonal psychotherapy adapted for ambulatory cocaine abusers. *American Journal of Drug and Alcohol Abuse, 11,* 171–191.

Rounsaville, B. J., & Kosten, T. R. (2000). Treatment for opioid dependence: Quality and access. *Journal of the American Medical Association, 283,* 1337–1339.

Roux, P., Carrieri, M. P., Villes, V., Dellamonica, P., Poizot-Martin, I., Ravaux, I., et al. (2008). The impact of methadone or buprenorphine treatment and ongoing injection on highly active antiretroviral therapy (HAART) adherence: Evidence from the MANIF2000 cohort study. *Addiction, 103,* 1828–1836.

Saladin, M. E., Brady, K. T., Graap, K. M., & Rothbaum, B. O. (2006). VR to evaluate craving and cue reactivity in cocaine dependent individuals. *Addictive Behaviors, 31,* 1881–1894.

Sees, K. L., Delucchi, K. L., Masson, C., Rosen, A., Clark, H. W., Robillard, H., et al. (2000). Methadone maintenance vs. 180–day psychosocially enriched detoxification for treatment of opioid dependence: A randomized controlled trial. *Journal of the American Medical Association, 283,* 1303–1310.

Silva de Lima, M., Farrell, M., Lima Reisser, A., & Soares, B. (2003). Antidepressants for cocaine dependence. *Cochrane Database of Systematic Reviews 2003, Issue 2,* CD002950.

Silverman, K., Higgins, S. T., Brooner, R. K., Montoya, I. D., Cone, E. J., Schuster, C. R., et al. (1996). Sustained cocaine abstinence in methadone maintenance patients through voucher-based reinforcement therapy. *Archives of General Psychiatry, 53,* 409–415.

Silverman K., Wong, C. J., Higgins, S. T., Brooner, R. K., Montoya, I. D., Contoreggi, C., et al. (1996). Increasing opiate abstinence through voucher-based reinforcement therapy. *Drug and Alcohol Dependence, 41,* 157–165.

Sindelar, J. L., Olmstead, T. A., & Pierce, J. M. (2007). Cost-effectiveness of prize-based contingency management in methadone maintenance programs. *Addiction, 102,* 1463–1471.

Spanagel, R., Putzke, J., Stefferl, A., Schobitz, B., & Zieglgansberger, W. (1996). Acamprosate and alcohol, II: Effects on alcohol withdrawal in the rat. *European Journal of Pharmacology, 305,* 45–50.

Srisurapanont, M., & Jarusuraisin, N. (2005). Naltrexone for the treatment of alcoholism: A meta-analysis of randomized controlled trials. *International Journal of Neuropsychopharmacology, 8,* 267–280.

Stine, S. M., & Kosten, T. R. (2009a). Ultra rapid opiate detoxification. In R. K. Ries, D. A. Fiellin, S. C. Miller, & R. Saitz (Eds.), *Principles of addiction medicine* (4th ed., pp. 604–606). Philadelphia: Lippincott, Williams & Wilkins.

Stine, S. M., & Kosten, T. R. (2009b). Pharmacologic intervention for opioid dependence. In R. K. Ries, D. A. Fiellin, S. C. Miller, & R. Saitz (Eds.), *Principles of addiction medicine* (4th ed., pp. 651–670). Philadelphia: Lippincott, Williams & Wilkins.

Stitzer, M. L., Bickel, W. K., Bigelow, G. E., & Liebson, I. A. (1986). Effect of methadone dose contingencies on urinalysis test results of polydrug-abusing methadone maintenance patients. *Drug and Alcohol Dependence, 18,* 341–348.

Stitzer, M. L., & Bigelow, G. E. (1978). Contingency management in a methadone maintenance program: Availability of reinforcers. *International Journal of the Addictions, 13,* 737–746.

Stitzer, M. L., Iguchi, M. Y., & Felch, L. J. (1992). Contingent take-home incentive: Effects on drug use of methadone maintenance patients. *Journal of Consulting and Clinical Psychology, 60,* 927–934.

Suh, J. J., Pettinati, H. M., Kampman, K. M., & O'Brien, C. P. (2006). The status of disulfiram: A half of a century later. *Journal of Clinical Psychopharmacology, 26,* 290–302.

Taylor, G. J., Parker, J. D., & Bagby, R. M. (1990). A preliminary investigation of alexithymia in men with psychoactive substance dependence. *American Journal of Psychiatry, 147,* 1228–1230.

Tetrault, J. M., & O'Connor, P. G. (2009). Management of opioid intoxication and withdrawal. In R. K. Ries, D. A. Fiellin, S. C. Miller, & R. Saitz (Eds.), *Principles of addiction medicine* (4th ed., pp. 589–603). Philadelphia: Lippincott, Williams & Wilkins.

Uhlmann, S., Milloy, M. J., Kerr, T., Zhang, R., Guillemi, S., Marsh, D., et al. (2010). Methadone maintenance therapy promotes initiation of antiretroviral therapy among injection drug users. *Addiction, 105,* 907–913.

Vandrey, R., & Haney, M. (2009). Pharmacotherapy for cannabis dependence: How close are we? *CNS Drugs, 23,* 543–553.

Volpicelli, J. R., Davis, M. A., & Olgin, J. E. (1986). Naltrexone blocks the postshock increase of ethanol consumption. *Life Sciences, 38,* 841–847.

Volpicelli, J. R., O'Brien, C. P., Alterman, A. I., & Hayashida, M. (1990). Naltrexone and the treatment of alcohol dependence. In L. D. Reid (Ed.), *Opioids, bulimia, and alcohol abuse and alcoholism* (pp. 195–214). New York: Springer-Verlag.

Volpicelli, J. R., Rhines, K. C., Rhines, J. S., Volpicelli, L. A., Alterman, A. I., &

O'Brien, C. P. (1997). Naltrexone and alcohol dependence: Role of subject compliance. *Archives of General Psychiatry, 54,* 737–742.

Walsh, S. L., Johnson, R. E., Cone, E. J., & Bigelow, G. E. (1998). Intravenous and oral l-alpha-acetylmethadol: Pharmacodynamics and pharmacokinetics in humans. *Journal of Pharmacology and Experimental Therapeutics, 285,* 71–82.

Walsh, S. L., Preston, K. L., Stitzer, M. L., Cone, E. J., & Bigelow, G. E. (1994). Clinical pharmacology of buprenorphine: Ceiling effects at high doses. *Clinical Pharmacology and Therapeutics, 55,* 569–580.

Weiss, R. D., & Kueppenbender, K. D. (2006). Combining psychosocial treatment with pharmacotherapy for alcohol dependence. *Journal of Clinical Psychopharmacology, 26*(Suppl. 1), S37–S42.

Wolstein, J., Gastpar, M., Finkbeiner, T., Heinrich, C., Heitkamp, R., Poehlke, T., et al. (2009). A randomized, open label trial comparing methadone and levo-alpha-acetylmethadol (LAAM) in maintenance of treatment of opioid addiction. *Pharmacopsychiatry, 42,* 1–8.

Woody, G. E., Luborsky, L., McLellan, A. T., O'Brien, C. P., Beck, A. T., Blaine, J., et al. (1983). Psychotherapy for opiate addicts: Does it help? *Archives of General Psychiatry, 40,* 639–645.

Woody, G. E., McLellan, A. T., Luborsky, L., & O'Brien, C. P. (1995). Psychotherapy in community methadone programs: A validation study. *American Journal of Psychiatry, 152,* 1302–1308.

Chapter 13

Addressing Substance Abuse in Primary Care Settings
Screening and Brief Intervention

Kristen L. Barry
Frederic C. Blow

Alcohol and drug abuse, including abuse of psychoactive prescription medications, are important and growing concerns in the United States. Because substance use is associated with a number of physical, mental, social, and legal consequences (Adrian & Barry, 2003; Barry et al., 2006; Booth, Kwiatkowski, & Chitwood, 2000; Center for Disease Control and Prevention [CDC], 2005; Chen, Scheier, & Kandel, 1995; Garrity et al., 2007; Grant, 1995; Johnson, Brems, & Burke, 2002; Kandel, Huang, & Davies, 2001; Vincent, Shoobridge, Ask, Allsop, & Ali, 1998), it is important to train health care personnel in primary clinical settings to recognize and treat these issues.

Healthy People 2000 guidelines (U.S. Department of Health and Human Services, 1990) first recommended increasing the proportion of physical and mental health providers who screen and provide advice for alcohol and drug problems. Indeed, practitioners across specialties, including primary and emergency care personnel, have a crucial role in identifying and treating at-risk and problem substance use. To assist in this task, brief screening and intervention techniques have been developed for use within the limited time constraints of most medical settings.

The First Step: Screening and Assessment

Alcohol

The National Institute on Alcoholism and Alcohol Abuse (2005b) defines moderate alcohol use as no more than seven drinks per week or up to one standard drink per day for most adult women and no more than 14 drinks per week or up to two standard drinks per day for most adult men. A standard drink is defined as 12 grams of alcohol (e.g., 12 ounces of beer, 5 ounces of wine, or 1.5 ounces of 80-proof distilled spirits). Drinking at these levels is generally not associated with health risks (U.S. Department of Health and Human Services & U.S. Department of Agriculture, 2005). For adults ages 65 years and older, the Center for Substance Abuse Treatment's Treatment Improvement Protocol (TIP) on older adults (Blow, 1998) recommends that both men and women consume no more than one standard drink per day (no more than seven standard drinks per week).

Certain people should not consume alcohol at all. These include women who are pregnant or trying to become pregnant, individuals taking certain over-the-counter or prescription drugs, those with medical conditions worsened by alcohol, individuals planning to drive a vehicle or engage in other activities requiring alertness, and those recovering from alcohol dependence.

The Alcohol Use Disorders Identification Test (AUDIT), developed by the World Health Organization (WHO; National Institute on Alcoholism and Alcohol Abuse, 2005b), is one brief screening tool for identifying individuals who are drinking at hazardous or harmful levels (Babor, Kranzler, & Lauerman, 1989; see also Barry & Fleming, 1993; Fiellin, Reid, & O'Connor, 2000; Fleming, Barry, & MacDonald, 1991; Schmidt, Barry, & Fleming, 1995). The AUDIT, which is well validated in adults under 65 years of age, assesses abuse by identifying physical and social problems of alcohol use with a 10-item questionnaire. A briefer version relating only to alcohol consumption is the AUDIT-C, composed of the first three items of the AUDIT (quantity, frequency, and binge).

Psychoactive Prescription Medications

The misuse of psychoactive prescription medications, defined as use in greater quantities or more often than prescribed, is a growing problem in the United States. The few screening instruments that have been tested and validated to determine misuse of psychoactive prescription medications generally have focused on chronic opioid use and/or patients seen in specialty clinics dealing with pain. One such screening instrument for detecting problems is the Pain Medication Questionnaire (PMQ). With 26 questions, the PMQ is one of the shorter instruments that can also be used in a self-report format (Adams et al., 2004). Each question is answered using a 5-point Likert-scale format ranging from "disagree" (0) to "agree" (4). Higher PMQ scores have been associated with a history of substance abuse, higher levels of psychosocial distress, and poorer functioning (Adams et al., 2004; Holmes et al., 2006). The PMQ may prove most useful in evaluating patients who are in, or plan to be in, a multidisciplinary pain clinic so that clinicians can maximize patient selection for such programs. The tool is also useful in gauging patients who are already taking opioids. However, in primary health care settings, a few screener questions may be useful in leading to the next steps if a more formal assessment is indicated.

Screening can take place at patient intake, during routine appointments, before prescribing medications (particularly those that interact with alcohol or other drugs), or in emergency departments (EDs). Likewise, screening can be effectively used with patients who may be pregnant or trying to conceive, with patients who have health conditions that may be affected by alcohol use, with patients with illnesses and problems that are not responding to treatment as expected, with adolescents and young adults, and with those who may be more likely to drink heavily.

Getting Started: Simple Screening Questions

Screening for problem substance use is a critical first step in identifying patients who may need further assessment and those who may be suitable candidates for brief interventions. Screening generally identifies at-risk and harmful substance use, while more extensive assessment measures the severity of and problems associated with use. The screening and assessment process should help determine if a patient's substance use is appropriate for brief intervention or warrants a different approach.

The following brief approaches to screening are adapted from the *Helping Patients Who Drink Too Much* (National Institute on Alcoholism and Alcohol Abuse, 2005b). Simple questions about heavy substance use days can be used during a clinical interview or before a patient is seen, followed up with further questions as indicated.

Alcohol

Prescreening Question
- "Do you drink beer, wine, or other alcoholic beverages?"

Follow-Up Questions
- "If yes, how many times in the [past year; past 3 months; past 6 months] have you had: five or more drinks in a day [for men under 65 years]/four or more drinks in a day [for women under 65 years]?"

- "On average, how many days per week do you drink alcoholic beverages? On a day when you drink alcohol, how many drinks do you have?"

Psychoactive Prescription Medications

Prescreening Questions

- "Do you use medications for pain, anxiety, or to help you sleep? If yes, what medications do you take?"
- "Do you sometimes use prescription drugs for sleep, pain, or anxiety in a way that is different than prescribed?"

Follow-Up Questions

- If yes, follow up with additional questions regarding which substances, frequency, and quantity of use.

Illegal Drugs

Prescreening Question

- "Do you use any drugs such as marijuana, cocaine, or other illegal drugs?"

Follow-Up Questions

- Any use of illegal drugs warrants asking follow-up questions regarding amounts and any consequences related to use, driving while high, and so on.

Brief Motivational Approaches to Change

A spectrum of prevention, intervention, and treatment approaches can be used across the range of alcohol and drug abuse patterns (see Figure 13.1). Brief motivational interventions (Miller & Rollnick, 2002) are designed to increase an individual's motivation to change. Brief interventions for alcohol and drug problems are time-limited, patient-centered approaches, focused on reducing or eliminating drinking and drug use. Brief interventions are characterized by few sessions (five or less, but often just one) or brief duration (a few minutes to an hour) (Barry, 1999). A large body of research shows the efficacy and effectiveness of brief interventions across treatment settings, populations, and provider types (Whitlock, Polen, Green, Orleans, & Klein, 2004). Brief interventions are designed to provide immediate attention to individuals at risk for further problems, to determine the

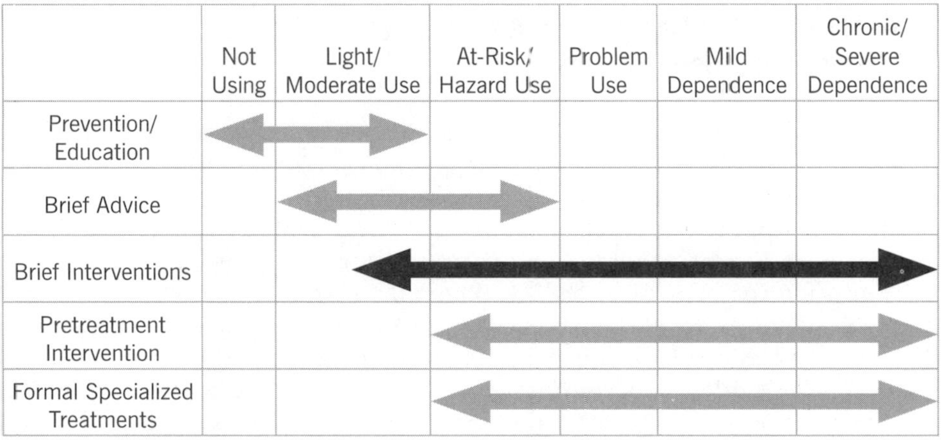

	Not Using	Light/ Moderate Use	At-Risk,' Hazard Use	Problem Use	Mild Dependence	Chronic/ Severe Dependence
Prevention/ Education	←——→					
Brief Advice		←————→				
Brief Interventions		←——————————————————→				
Pretreatment Intervention			←————————————→			
Formal Specialized Treatments			←————————————→			

FIGURE 13.1. Spectrum of interventions and target audience.

level of care needed to address substance use problems, and to prevent or minimize potential consequences.

Cognitive and social psychology provide the theoretical frameworks for brief motivational interventions, especially through the transtheoretical model of change (TTM; Prochaska & DiClemente, 1984). This model sees behavior change readiness as a progression through a series of stages: precontemplation, contemplation, preparation, action, and maintenance (Prochaska & DiClemente, 1992). *Precontemplation* is the stage at which there is no intention to change behavior in the foreseeable future. *Contemplation* is the stage in which people are aware that a problem exists and are seriously considering overcoming it but they have yet to commit to take action. *Preparation* is the stage in which individuals decide to take action soon. *Action* is the stage in which individuals actually modify some part of their behavior or environment to overcome their problem. Finally, *maintenance* is the stage in which people work to prevent relapse and maximize the gains they achieved in the action phase.

Brief motivational interventions are designed to aid individuals in moving through the stages of change. In motivational approaches, the practitioner uses open-ended questions to explore the positive and negative aspects of substance use. The practitioner also paraphrases key motivational points, reflecting back what the client has said. Additional tasks may include providing personalized feedback, helping to develop a plan for change, and anticipating the challenges in making changes and in maintaining changes. At the time of the intervention, the patient can be at any stage; he or she may or may not be ready to initiate changes in behavior. To assist with tracking progress, patients may be given personal workbooks to plan the elements needed for changing.

SBIRT Model of Comprehensive Care across the Spectrum of Substance Use Patterns

A comprehensive model for addressing alcohol and drug use in medical settings includes screening, brief intervention, and referral to treatment (SBIRT). *Screening* quickly assesses the severity of substance use and identifies the appropriate level of intervention/treatment. *Brief intervention* focuses on increasing insight and awareness regarding substance use and motivation for behavioral change. *Referral to treatment* provides access to specialty care for those who need more extensive treatment (Substance Abuse and Mental Health Services Administration, 2008; see Figure 13.2). SBIRT offers opportunities for early detection, focused motivational enhancement, and targeted encouragement to seek needed substance abuse treatment.

Brief Intervention Research

Alcohol

Primary Care Settings

Traditional approaches to alcohol and other drug problems have focused on long-term therapy. There is, however, increasing evidence that brief interventions delivered in health care settings can effectively reduce drinking,

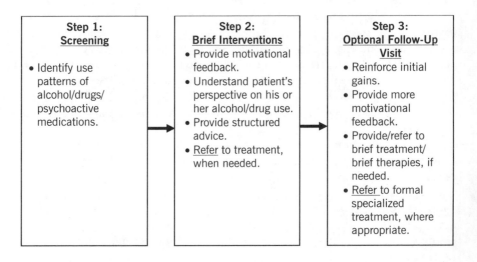

FIGURE 13.2. Conducting screening, brief intervention, and referral to treatment (SBIRT). Adapted from Substance Abuse and Mental Health Services Administration, Committee on Trauma Quick Guide (2007).

particularly for at-risk and problem users. There have been over 100 trials of brief intervention techniques over the past 25 years. Early studies in Europe and other countries demonstrated a significant (10–20%) reduction in drinking for brief intervention groups compared to control groups (Kristenson, Ohlin, Hulten-Nosslin, Trell, & Hood, 1983; Saunders, Aasland, Babor, DeLa Fuente & Grant, 1993; Wallace, Cutler, & Haines, 1988). Brief intervention trials then moved to the United States to primary care, emergency care, and specialty populations such as individuals with mental health disorders presenting to psychiatric emergency services (Barry et al., 2006; Milner, Barry, Blow, & Welsh, 2010).

The largest proportion of intervention studies have been conducted in primary care and emergency medicine settings targeting at-risk alcohol users, with fewer addressing illicit drug users who meet criteria for abuse or dependence. From a public health perspective, the quantity of patients seen in these settings, along with the speed and ease of administering screening and intervention materials, has been critical to advancing the field. In primary care, brief interventions for alcohol misuse have ranged from a few simple, straightforward comments by the clinician to several short counseling sessions and telephone follow-up. Brief comments to a patient with at-risk or problem drinking might include stating concerns about the patient's drinking, informing the patient that his or her current consumption levels are above recommended limits, or recommending that the patient decrease or stop drinking (National Institute on Alcoholism and Alcohol Abuse, 2005b).

Most of the brief intervention trials have been conducted in primary care settings (Chick, Lloyd, & Crombie, 1985; Harris & Miller, 1990; Wallace et al., 1988). One of the largest clinical trials conducted in primary care practices, Project TrEAT (Trial for Early Alcohol Treatment), involved two brief in-person sessions conducted 1 month apart. Each session was followed 2 weeks later by a phone call (Fleming, Barry, Manwell, Johnson, & London, 1997). Individuals in the intervention group significantly reduced their use and had fewer hospital days and ED visits compared to controls after 2 years follow-up.

A number of meta-analytic studies have summarized brief intervention trials (Ballesteros, Gonzalez-Pinto, Querejeta, & Arino, 2003; Whitlock et al., 2004). All of the interventions in these studies included either personalized feedback based on the individuals' responses to screening questions or untailored (generic) messages to cut down or stop drinking. Meta-analyses of randomized controlled studies have found that these techniques generally reduce drinking in the intervention versus control groups. On average, intervention patients reduced their number of drinks per week by 13 to 34% more than controls.

There is some evidence that brief interventions may also be useful with primary care patients who report symptoms of substance abuse or dependence. Motivational interviewing techniques may help patients accept the need for and become motivated to pursue more intensive treatment for substance abuse. The primary care clinician can help facilitate the referral process to specialized treatment (National Institute on Alcoholism and Alcohol Abuse, 2005a).

Emergency Care Settings

In addition to the primary care settings for research, trials have been conducted in EDs with an even larger volume of patients at times of crisis often called "teachable moments" (Blow et al., 2006; see also Havard, Shakeshaft, & Sanson-Fisher, 2008; Maio et al., 2005; and Monti et al., 1999). Thus, the ED may be an ideal place to do substance use screening and brief interventions. Much of the brief intervention research in the ED has focused on patients presenting with injuries because early research found that up to 36% of injured patients presenting to the ED had positive blood alcohol concentrations (BACs) (MacDonald, Wells, Giesbrecht, & Cherpitel, 1999; Soderstrom et al., 1997). Additionally, positive BACs have been found in up to 47% of patients admitted to inpatient hospital care for trauma (Soderstrom, Dailey, & Kerns, 1994; Rivara et al., 1989). Alcohol use is present in nearly 50% of all motor vehicle crash deaths, suicides, and homicides. ED studies have found that among crash victims, 17–23% met criteria for alcohol abuse or dependence (Maio, Waller, Blow, Hill, & Singer, 1997; Soderstrom et al., 1997).

Brief interventions for adults in the ED take advantage of the teachable moment in which a patient needs urgent medical care for an injury or medical condition. An earlier study found that patients who received a brief intervention in the ED plus a booster session 7–10 days later had fewer alcohol-related injuries and problems after 1 year compared to patients receiving standard ED care (National Institute on Alcoholism and Alcohol Abuse, 1995). Some of the most innovative and efficient screening and brief interventions have been developed specifically for use in the ED (Substance Abuse and Mental Health Services Administration, 2007). Brief intervention approaches designed to encourage the participants to seek a substance abuse assessment and engage in treatment have been used with ED patients admitted to the hospital (Dyehouse & Sommers, 1995; Welte, Perry, Longabaugh, & Clifford, 1998), injured patients in the ED (Blow et al., 2006; Gentilello et al., 1999; Johnston, Rivera, Droesch, Dunn, & Copass, 2002; Longabaugh et al., 2001; Mello et al., 2005; Neuman et al., 2006), and with ED patients who met criteria for alcohol and drug abuse or dependence (Blow et al., 2011). One meta-analysis of ED studies found that ED-based interventions significantly reduce subsequent alcohol-related injury but found mixed results on whether or not patients decreased alcohol consumption (Havard et al., 2008).

Illicit Drug Use

A number of studies have discussed the need for brief interventions for illicit drug use, as well as alcohol abuse (Baker, Kochan, Dixon, Heather, & Wodak, 1994; Compton, Monahan, & Simmons-Cody, 1999; Greber, Allen, Soeken, & Solounias, 1997; Samet et al., 1995; Weaver, Jarvis, & Schnoll, 1999). However, there have been relatively few randomized, controlled brief intervention trials with illicit substance users. Promising results have been shown in studies investigating the effectiveness of brief interventions among cocaine, heroin, and amphetamine users from a variety of non-ED-based settings (Baker et al., 2005; Bernstein, Bernstein, & Levenson, 1997; Stotts, Schmitz, Rhoades, & Grabowski, 2001). For instance, Bernstein et al. (2005) reported on a brief intervention for heroin and/or cocaine users recruited from several walk-in clinics (an urgent care clinic, a women's clinic, and a homeless clinic) that included a motivational intervention session delivered by trained peer educators and a subsequent booster call 10 days later. Intervention patients had an increased likelihood of abstinence from these drugs at a 6-month follow-up visit. Similarly, Blow et al. (2010) conducted a brief intervention trial designed to help urban disadvantaged ED patients who met criteria for drug abuse or dependence to get a substance abuse assessment and move toward getting treatment. This trial compared a motivational interviewing group, a strengths-based case management group, and a control group. Preliminary results indicated that the most effective method to motivate ED patients with abuse and dependence for assessment was the structured-manual, strengths-based case management approach.

Stotts et al. (2001) found positive results with cocaine users in an outpatient detoxification treatment program. Baker and colleagues (2005) found an increased likelihood of abstinence from amphetamines among individuals receiving a cognitive-behavioral therapy-based intervention. Bashir, King, and Ashworth (1994) similarly found positive results from a brief drug intervention delivered by primary care providers in a small study (less than 100 patients). Positive results have been reported from brief motivational interventions among community cannabis-dependent adults. The Marijuana Treatment Project Research Group (Copeland, Swift, Roffman, & Stephens, 2001; Marijuana Treatment Project Research Group, 2004; Stephens & Roffman, 2000) studies also showed successful outcomes with community-based marijuana-dependent individuals, with positive outcomes reported at up to 15 months (Marijuana Treatment Project Research Group, 2004). Bernstein et al. (1997) found that an ED-based brief "negotiated" interview and an active referral process resulted in a 45% reduction in severity of drug problems, but only among patients who kept their follow-up treatment appointments. In sum, the evidence consistently supports the effectiveness of brief interventions to reduce illegal drug use, though there are admittedly fewer trials than for risky alcohol use. There is, unfortunately, much less research on changing psychoactive prescription drug use among those who misuse these substances.

Special Populations and Issues

Alcohol

Prenatal Care

For pregnant women who may be consuming alcohol or have mild to moderate alcohol problems, brief interventions are recommended as an initial step to change drinking behavior. First-trimester interventions to reduce or stop alcohol consumption can be well received among the other recommendations for healthy behaviors during pregnancy. Prenatal brief interventions have been shown to reduce drinking levels among pregnant women most effectively when a partner (generally the father of the unborn child) also participated in the intervention (National Institute on Alcoholism and Alcohol Abuse, 2005b). For women who report drinking during their last pregnancy, brief interventions have successfully reduced drinking during subsequent pregnancies compared to a control group.

Older Adults

Project GOAL (Guiding Older Adult Lifestyles) and the Health Profile Project are two brief alcohol intervention trials with adults ages 65 years and older that have tested advice protocols in primary care settings. These studies showed that the protocols were acceptable in this population and there was a substantial reduction in drinking among the at-risk drinkers receiving the interventions compared to control groups. Project GOAL (Fleming, Manwell, Barry, Adams, & Stauffacher, 1999) showed that an intervention group receiving physician-delivered advice and education drank significantly less than the control group at a 12-month follow-up. The Health Profile Project (Blow & Barry, 2000) contained both brief advice and discussion by either a psychologist or a social worker, delivered via motivational interviewing techniques and personalized feedback. The results were similar to those of Fleming et al. (1999) in terms of alcohol use and binge drinking at a 12-month follow-up, which demonstrates the potential of brief interventions for older adults.

A new study funded by the National Institute on Alcoholism and Alcohol Abuse has been completed identifying at-risk drinkers using the Comorbidity Alcohol Risk Evaluation Tool (CARET) screening instrument to screen for alcohol abuse, medication misuse, and comorbidities. The investigators, led by Moore (Lin, Karno, Barry, et al., 2010; Lin, Karno, Tang, et al., 2010; Moore et al., 2011) conducted a randomized, controlled trial with older adults attending nonacademic primary care clinics. The intervention consisted of very brief advice about at-risk drinking, comorbidities, and medication use by a primary care physician, as well as a telephone follow-up session with a health educator to address the particular reasons an individual was identified as being at risk. The control treatment consisted of a booklet on healthy behaviors. Within 2 weeks of receiving the intervention, 39% of the intervention participants had reduced their drinking. At 3 months, relative to controls, fewer intervention group participants were at-risk drinkers (odds ratio [OR] = 0.41; 95% confidence interval [CI] = 0.22–0.75). Moreover, at the 3-month follow-up, intervention participants reported drinking fewer drinks in the past 7 days (risk ratio [RR] = 0.79; 95% CI = 0.70–0.90), less heavy drinking occasions (OR = 0.46; 95% CI = 0.22–0.99), and had lower risk scores (RR = 0.77; 95% CI = 0.63–0.94). At 12 months, however, only the difference in number of drinks remained statistically significant (RR = 0.87; 95% CI = 0.76–0.99). Bivariate analyses showed that those who reduced drinking were more likely to be Hispanic or nonwhite, had lower levels of education, had worse self-rated health status, drank less alcohol, were identified for fewer categories of risk, and were less aware of alcohol-related risks. Multiple logistic regression showed increased odds of reduction in alcohol use at 2 weeks postintervention for individuals who were concerned about alcohol-related risks (OR = 2.03; 95% CI = 1.01–4.07), read through the educational booklet (OR = 2.97, 95% CI = 1.48–5.95), or perceived that their physicians discussed both risks of drinking and advised changing drinking behaviors (OR = 4.1; 95% CI = 2.02–8.32). Early reduction in drinking was common among older at-risk drinkers receiving intervention. This study was the first to assess a preventive intervention to reduce risks of alcohol use, alone or in conjunction with comorbidities and medication use among older adults in primary care.

Few studies address screening and brief interventions for older adults in settings other than primary care. The primary study in this area has been the Florida Brief Intervention and Treatment for Elders (BRITE) project, a 3-year pilot program of screening and brief intervention for older adult substance misusers. Agencies in four counties conducted screenings among 3,497 older adults for alcohol, medications, and illicit substance misuse problems and for depression and suicide risk. Screening occurred in elders' homes, senior centers, or other selected sites. Individuals who screened positive for substance misuse were offered a brief intervention using evidence-based practices derived from the Wisconsin GOAL Project (Fleming et al., 1999) and the Health Profiles Project (Blow & Barry, 2000), and rescreened at discharge, 6 months, and 12 months. Prescription medication misuse was the most prevalent substance use problem, followed by alcohol, over-the-counter medications, and illicit substances. Depression was prevalent among those with alcohol and prescription medication problems. Those who received the brief intervention generally improved on alcohol, medication misuse, and depression measures. The BRITE program effectively shaped state policy by responding to legislative mandates to address the needs of an increasing, but underserved, elder population. The pilot paved the way for a federally funded grant to expand BRITE to 21 sites in 15 counties in Florida (Schonfeld et al., 2010).

In addition, the federal Substance Abuse and Mental Health Services Administration recently funded a study to determine how to best implement SBIRT interventions for alcohol and/or psychoactive prescription medication misuse with adults ages 60 years and older. Because of the widespread use of alcohol and psychoactive medications in the baby boom cohort (the eldest of this cohort are 64 years of age), it will be important to find ways to implement and expand interventions to include prescription medications for pain, sleep, and anxiety.

Cost Effectiveness of Brief Interventions

Although brief interventions are effective in reducing use and improving some health outcomes, the issue of cost is particularly salient in an era of rapidly changing health care. Only been a few studies have measured the cost effectiveness of brief interventions. In the Fleming et al. (1997) primary care trial, a cost analysis found that the total cost per patient of the brief intervention was $205 (including both clinic and patient costs). The cost advantage between intervention and control groups was significant for subsequent medical and motor vehicle events. Overall, this suggested a $43,000 reduction in future health costs for every $10,000 invested in early intervention (Fleming et al., 2002).

Brief interventions in the ED have also been found to reduce costs in terms of injury and other alcohol-related health consequences, with savings of $3.81 for every $1 spent (Gentilello, Ebel, Wickizer, Salkever, & Rivara, 2005).

Components of Brief Interventions

Brief motivational interventions are designed to lessen the potential harm of continued at-risk use of alcohol and drugs. Specific goals will vary by individual patient characteristics and context. The FRAMES acronym summarizes strategies thought to be common to effective brief interventions. The following is adapted from Miller and Rollnick (2002):

- *Feedback* is given to the individual about risk.
- *Responsibility* for change is placed with the individual receiving the intervention,
- *Advice* for changing behavior is given by the clinician.
- *Menu* of alternative options for change is offered.
- *Empathic* listening style is used by the intervener.
- *Self-efficacy* or empowerment is promoted.

Brief intervention protocols often use a workbook containing the nine steps listed below. Workbooks provide opportunities for the patient and practitioner to discuss cues to use, reasons for the level of use, reasons to cut down or quit, a negotiated agreement for next steps, and daily diary cards for self-monitoring. Using the general clinical style of motivational interviewing (Miller & Rollnick, 2002), providers can be trained to administer the specific intervention protocol through role-playing and general skills-training techniques.

Manualized brief intervention protocols often include elements such as the following, adapted from Barry (2002):

1. *Identification of future goals for health, work, school, activities, hobbies, relationships, and financial stability.* This step provides information on what the patient is interested in achieving and can help to target goals for the intervention.

2. *Summary of health habits.* This element may provide customized feedback on screening questions relating to drinking and/or drug use patterns and other health habits (may also include questions about smoking, nutrition, tobacco use, seat belt use, safe sex, etc.). This health behaviors information can come from screening questionnaires or from the patient during the session.

3. *Discuss how the patient's use fits in with norms for alcohol/drug use in the population.* This step introduces drinking guidelines (women under 65: no more than one drink/day; men under 65: no more than two drinks/day; women and men 65 and over: no more than one drink/day or seven drinks/week) and the idea that the patient's misuse of alcohol, drugs, or psychoactive prescription medications can affect his or her physical and emotional health and put him or her at risk for additional health-related problems. It is very important to use an empathic manner to "roll with" any patient resistance to examining his or her use.

4. *Consequences of at-risk and problem drinking.* Relate this to any potential or ongoing health problem that is currently important in the person's care (e.g., hypertension, insomnia, gastrointestinal problems). The provider makes an explicit connection to present health concerns—for example, "I'm concerned about your [high blood pressure, sleep problem,

abdominal pain] and I think your alcohol use may have a negative effect on that."

5. *Reasons to quit or cut down on drinking*. This is a brief discussion of how changing one's substance use could have important benefits.

6. *Introduce the concept of standard drinks*. This discussion focuses on the equivalence of alcohol content across various beverage types. This concept provides the context for a discussion of sensible drinking limits, or the ways in which use of other drugs or medications can be affected by alcohol use.

7. *Negotiated drinking agreement*. Drinking limits in the form of an agreement can be negotiated and signed by the patient and the intervener. Patients take the workbook, including the agreement, with them when they leave the office. A follow-up visit or phone call can help the patient stay on track with any changes he or she is making. Key points include the following:

- *Giving guidance on abstinence versus cutting down*. Patients who have a serious health problem or take medications that interact with alcohol should be advised to abstain. Others may be appropriate candidates to cut down on drinking to below recommended limits. Individuals who use psychoactive prescription drugs or illegal drugs may need additional evaluation by primary providers to determine next steps. Pain clinics can be useful referrals for individuals experiencing serious pain or taking medications for pain. Based on clinical judgment regarding the seriousness of the problem, the clinician will decide if the patient should cut down on use or be abstinent. For instance, the provider might say, "I want you to stop drinking any alcohol for the next month so we can see if your stomach pain decreases. Then we can reevaluate the next steps when you come back," *or* "I want you to cut back your drinking to no more than one drink every other day. How do you feel about that?" This last statement provides the opportunity to negotiate and empowers the patient to be a part of the decision-making process. These approaches can also help to determine the seriousness of the patient's alcohol/drug/medication problem. If the patient cannot abstain or cut down, this may suggest a more serious problem that requires referral and follow-up.

- Throughout the process, it is important to be sensitive to patients' reactions including concern, embarrassment, defensiveness, or minimization of drinking problems.

8. *Coping with risky situations*. Social isolation, boredom, and negative family interactions can present special problems for individuals trying to change behavior. It helps if the individual can identify situations and moods that can be "risky" and to identify some individualized cognitive and behavioral coping alternatives.

9. *Summary of the session.* The summary should include a review of the agreed-upon goals and encouragement for change or for considering change.

Through all these processes, the practitioner communicates interest in and acceptance for what the patient is communicating. It is important to avoid behaviors that are not part of active, supportive listening and reflection. These include lecturing, criticizing, labeling, moralizing, or distracting. To help providers intervene effectively in time-sensitive settings, the National Institute on Alcoholism and Alcohol Abuse (2005b) has developed a booklet and guidelines for intervening.

Brief Therapies

Brief therapies are often used with either patients who are experiencing more consequences from their use, have difficulty changing their substance use behavior, or to promote relapse prevention. See Barry (1999) for further discussion of brief therapies for substance use/abuse. The most common brief therapies used in these situations are cognitive-behavioral therapies. There are a number of brief therapies that are used for individuals having more serious problems related to use. A provider's referral for additional assessments and brief therapy may be the step that helps someone change his or her behavior or may be an interim step to determine if more specialized substance abuse treatment is needed.

Conclusion

Primary clinical settings are ideal venues for screening and helping individuals with at-risk patterns of alcohol, drug, and medication use. Patients are receptive to dealing with health-related issues in these settings. The SBIRT model works well in primary clinical care because it focuses on quickly identifying risk, empowering individuals to work on changing their risk pattern and potential, and respecting and treating the "whole person." Research on screening and brief interventions for alcohol abuse (and more recently, illicit drug use and psychoactive prescription medications) indicates that brief interventions can reduce use and/or consequences over at least a 1-year period. The nonconfrontational, respectful approach used in motivational brief interventions is generally effective with both younger and older adults. Brief interventions are part of a *spectrum* of approaches to address alcohol and drug use/misuse/abuse. "Real-world" implementation strategies to address time and logistical barriers will be the key to their adaptation. The use of screening, brief interventions, brief therapies, and referral to substance abuse treatment, where appropriate, provides an evidence-based approach to improving outcomes and managing costs in a vulnerable population.

References

Adams, L. L., Gatchel, R. J., Robinson, R. C., Polatin, P., Gairai, N., Deschner, M., et al. (2004). Development of a self-report screening instrument for assessing potential opioid medication misuse in chronic pain patients. *Journal of Pain Symptom Management, 27*(5), 440–459.

Adrian, M., & Barry, S. J. (2003). Physical and mental health problems associated with the use of alcohol and drugs. *Substance Use and Misuse, 38,* 1575–1614.

Babor, T. F., Kranzler, H. R., & Lauerman, R. J. (1989). Early detection of harmful alcohol consumption: Comparison of clinical, laboratory, and self-report screening procedures. *Addictive Behaviors, 14*(2), 139–157.

Baker, A., Kochan, N., Dixon, J., Heather, N., & Wodak, A. (1994). Controlled evaluation of a brief intervention for HIV prevention among injecting drug users not in treatment. *AIDS Care, 6,* 559–570.

Baker, A., Lee, N. K., Claire, M., Lewin, T.J., Grant, T., Pohlman, S., et al. (2005). Brief cognitive-behavioral interventions for regular amphetamine users: A step in the right direction. *Addiction, 100,* 367–378.

Ballesteros, J., Gonzalez-Pinto, A., Querejeta, I., & Arino, J. (2003). Brief interventions for hazardous drinkers delivered in primary care are equally effective in men and women. *Health Psychology, 22*(2), 156–165.

Barry, K. L. (1999). *Brief interventions and brief therapies for substance abuse* (Treatment Improvement Protocol [TIP] Series No. 34). Rockville, MD: U.S. Department of Health and Human Services, Substance Abuse and Mental Health Services Administration, Center for Substance Abuse Treatment.

Barry. K. L. (2002). Alcohol and drug abuse. In M. Mengel & W. Holleman (Eds.), *Fundamentals of clinical practice* (2nd ed., pp. 689–716). New York: Plenum Medical Book Company.

Barry, K. L., & Fleming, M. F. (1993). The Alcohol Use Disorders Identification Test (AUDIT) and the SMAST-13: Predictive validity in a rural primary care sample. *Alcohol and Alcoholism, 2*(1), 33–42.

Barry, K. L., Milner, K., Blow, F. C., Impens, A., Welsh, D., & Amash, J. (2006). Screening for psychiatric emergency department patients with major mental illnesses for at-risk drinking. *Psychiatric Services, 57,* 1039–1042.

Bashir, K., King, M., & Ashworth, M. (1994). Controlled evaluation of brief intervention by general practitioners to reduce chronic use of benzodiazepines. *British Journal of General Practice, 44,* 408–412.

Bernstein, E., Bernstein, J., & Levenson, S. (1997). Project ASSERT: an ED-based intervention to increase access to primary care, preventive services, and the substance abuse treatment system. *Annals of Emergency Medicine, 30,* 181–189.

Bernstein, J., Bernstein, E., Tassiopoulos, K., Heeren, T., Levenson, S., & Hingson,

R. (2005). Brief motivational intervention at a clinic visit reduces cocaine and heroin use. *Drug and Alcohol Dependence, 77*, 49–59.

Blow, F. (1998). *Substance abuse among older adults* (Treatment Improvement Protocol [TIP] Series No. 26). Rockville, MD: U.S. Department of Health and Human Services, Substance Abuse and Mental Health Services Administration, Center for Substance Abuse Treatment.

Blow, F. C., & Barry, K. L. (2000). Older Patients with at-risk and problem drinking patterns: New developments in brief interventions. *Journal of Geriatric Psychiatry and Neurology, 13*(3), 115–123.

Blow, F. C., Barry, K. L., Walton, M. A., Maio, R. F., Chermack, S. T., Bingham, C. R., et al. (2006). The efficacy of two brief intervention strategies among injured, at-risk drinkers in the emergency department: Impact of tailored messaging and brief advice. *Journal of Studies on Alcohol, 67*, 568–578.

Blow, F. C., Walton, M. A., Barry, K. L., Murray, R. L., Cunningham, R. M., Massey, L. S., et al. (2011). Alcohol and drug use among patients presenting to an inner city emergency department: A latent class analyses. *Addictive Behaviors, 36*(8), 793–800.

Blow, F. C., Walton, M. A., Murray, R., Cunningham, R. M., Chermack, S. T., Barry, K. L., et al. (2010). Intervention attendance among ED patients with alcohol and drug use disorders. *Journal of Studies on Alcohol and Drugs, 71*(5), 713–719.

Booth, B. M., Kwiatkowski, C. F., & Chitwood, D. D. (2000). Sex-related HIV risk behaviors: Differential risks among injection drug users, crack smokers, and injection drug users who smoke crack. *Drug and Alcohol Dependence, 58*, 219–226.

Chen, K., Scheier, L., & Kandel, D. B. (1995). Effects of chronic cocaine use on physical health: A prospective study in a general population sample. *Drug and Alcohol Dependence, 43*, 23–37.

Chick, J., Lloyd, G., & Crombie, E. (1985). Counseling problem drinkers in medical wards: A controlled study. *British Medical Journal, 290*, 965–967.

Compton, P., Monahan, G., & Simmons-Cody, H. (1999). Motivational interviewing: An effective brief intervention for alcohol and drug abuse patients. *Nurse Practitioner, 24*, 27–28.

Copeland, J., Swift, W., Roffman, R., & Stephens, R. (2001). A randomized controlled trial of brief cognitive–behavioral interventions for cannabis use disorder. *Journal of Substance Abuse Treatment, 21*, 55–64.

Department of Health and Human Services & Department of Agriculture. (2005). *Dietary guidelines for Americans* (6th ed.). Washington, DC: U.S. Government Printing Office.

Dyehouse, J. M., & Sommers, M. S. (1995). Brief intervention as an advanced practice strategy for seriously injured victims of multiple trauma. *AACN Clinical Issues, 6*, 53–62.

Fiellin, D. A., Reid, M. C., & O'Connor, P. G. (2000). Screening for alcohol problems in primary care: A systematic review. *Archives of Internal Medicine, 160*(13), 1777–1989.

Fleming, M. F., Barry, K. L., & MacDonald, R. (1991). The Alcohol Use Disorders

Identification Test (AUDIT) in a college sample. *International Journal of Addictions, 26*, 1173–1185.

Fleming, M. F., Barry, K. L., Manwell, L. B., Johnson, K., & London, R. (1997). Brief physician advice for problem alcohol drinkers: A randomized controlled trial in community-based primary care practices. *Journal of the American Medical Association, 277*(13), 1039–1045.

Fleming, M. F., Manwell, L.B., Barry, K. L., Adams, W., & Stauffacher, E. A. (1999). Brief physician advice for alcohol problems in older adults: A randomized community-based trial. *Journal of Family Practice, 48*(5), 378–384.

Fleming, M. F., Mundt, M. P., French, M. T., Manwell, L. B., Stauffacher, E. A., & Barry, K. L. (2002). Brief physician advice for problem drinkers: Long-term efficacy and benefit–cost ratio. *Alcoholism: Clinical and Experimental Research, 26*(1), 36–43.

Garrity, T. F., Leukefeld, C. G., Carlson, R. G., Falck, R. S., Wang, J., & Booth, B. M. (2007). Physical health, illicit drug use, and demographic characteristics in rural stimulant users. *Journal of Rural Health, 23*, 99–107.

Gentilello, L. M., Ebel, B. E., Wickizer, T. M., Salkever, D. S., & Rivara, F. P. (2005). Alcohol interventions for trauma patients treated in emergency departments and hospitals: A cost–benefit analysis. *Annals of Surgery, 241*, 541–550.

Gentilello, L. M., Rivara, F. P., Donovan, D. M., Jurkocich, G. J., Daranciang, E., Dunn, C. W., et al. (1999). Alcohol interventions in a trauma center as a means of reducing the risk of injury recurrence. *Annals of Surgery, 230*, 473–480.

Grant, B. F. (1995). Comorbidity between DSM-IV drug use disorders and major depression: Results of a national survey of adults. *Journal of Substance Abuse, 7*, 481–497.

Greber, R. A., Allen, K. M., Soeken, K. L., & Solounias, B. L. (1997). Outcome of trauma patients after brief intervention by a substance abuse consultation service. *American Journal of Addictions, 6*, 38–47.

Harris, K. B., & Miller, W. R. (1990). Behavioural self-control training for problem drinkers: Components of efficacy. *Psychology of Addictive Behaviour, 4*(2), 90–92.

Havard, A., Shakeshaft, A., & Sanson-Fisher, R. (2008). Systematic review and meta-analyses of strategies targeting alcohol problems in emergency departments: Interventions reduce alcohol-related injuries. *Addiction, 103*, 368–376.

Holmes, C. P., Gatchel, R. J., Adams, L. L., Stowell, A. W., Hatten, A., Noe, C., et al. (2006). An opioid screening instrument: Long-term evaluation of the utility of the Pain Medication Questionnaire. *Pain Practice, 66*(2), 74–88.

Johnson, M., Brems, C., & Burke, S. (2002). Recognizing comorbidity among drug users in treatment. *American Journal of Drug and Alcohol Abuse, 28*, 243–261.

Johnston, B. D., Rivera, F. P., Droesch, R. M., Dunn, C., & Copass, M. K. (2002). Behavior change counseling in the emergency department to reduce injury risk: A randomized, controlled trial. *Pediatrics, 110*, 267–74.

Kandel, D. B., Huang, F.Y., & Davies, M. (2001). Comorbidity between patterns of substance use dependence and psychiatric syndromes. *Drug and Alcohol Dependence, 64*, 233–241.

Kristenson, H., Ohlin, H., Hulten-Nosslin, M., Trell, E., & Hood, B. (1983). Identification and intervention of heavy drinking in middle-aged men: Results and follow-up of 24–60 months of long-term study with randomized controls. *Alcoholism: Clinical and Experimental Research, 7*(2), 203–209.

Lin, J. C., Karno, M. P., Barry, K. L., Blow, F. C., Davis, J. W., Tang, L., et al. (2010). Determinants of early reductions in drinking in older at-risk drinkers participating in the intervention arm of a trial to reduce at-risk drinking in primary care. *Journal of the American Geriatric Society, 58*(2), 227–233.

Lin J. C., Karno M. P., Tang L., Barry K. L., Blow F. C., Davis J. W., et al. (2010). Do health educator telephone calls reduce at-risk drinking among older adults in primary care? *Journal of General Internal Medicine, 25*(4), 334–349.

Longabaugh, R., Woolard, R. E., Nirenberg, T. D., Minugh, A. P., Becker, B., Clifford, P. R., et al. (2001). Evaluating the effects of a brief motivational intervention for injured drinkers in the emergency department. *Journal of Studies on Alcohol, 62*, 806–816.

Macdonald, S., Wells, S., Giesbrecht, N., & Cherpitel, C. J. (1999). Demographic and substance use factors related to violent and accidental injuries: Results from an emergency room study. *Drug and Alcohol Dependence, 55*, 53–61.

Maio, R. F., Shope, J. T., Blow, F. C., Gregor, M. A., Zakrajsek, J. S., Weber, J. E., et al. (2005). A randomized controlled trial of an ED-based interactive computer program to prevent alcohol misuse among injured adolescents. *Annals of Emergency Medicine, 45*, 420–429.

Maio, R. F., Waller, P., Blow, F. C., Hill, E. M., & Singer, K. M. (1997). Alcohol abuse/dependence in motor vehicle crash victims presenting to the emergency department. *Academic Emergency Medicine, 4*, 256–262.

Marijuana Treatment Project Research Group. (2004). Brief treatments for cannabis dependence: Findings from a randomized multisite trial. *Journal of Consulting and Clinical Psychology, 72*, 455–466.

Mello, M. J., Nirenberg, T. D., Longabaugh, R., Woolard, R., Minugh, A., Becker, B., et al. (2005). Emergency department brief motivational interventions for alcohol with motor vehicle crash patients. *Annals of Emergency Medicine, 45*, 620–625.

Miller, W. R., & Rollnick, S. (2002). *Motivational interviewing: Preparing people to change addictive behavior* (2nd ed.). New York: Guilford Press.

Milner, K. K., Barry, K. L., Blow, F. C., & Welsh, D. (2010). Brief interventions for patients presenting to the psychiatric emergency service (PES) with major mental illnesses and at-risk drinking. *Community Mental Health Journal, 46*(2), 149–155.

Monti, P. M., Colby, S. M., Barnett, N. P., Spirito, A., Rohsenow, D. J., Myers, M., et al. (1999). Brief intervention for harm reduction with alcohol-positive older adolescents in a hospital emergency department. *Journal of Consulting and Clinical Psychology, 67*(6), 989–994.

Moore, A. A., Blow, F. C., Hoffing, M., Welgreen, S., Davis, J. W., Lin, J. C., et al. (2011). Primary care based intervention to reduce at-risk drinking in older adults: A randomized controlled trial. *Addiction, 106*(1), 111–120.

National Institute on Alcohol Abuse and Alcoholism. (1995). *Diagnostic criteria for alcohol abuse and dependence: Alcohol alert no. 30.* Retrieved from *pubs. niaaa.nih.gov/publications/aa30.htm.*

National Institute on Alcohol Abuse and Alcoholism. (2005a). *Brief interventions. Alcohol alert no. 66.* Retrieved from *pubs.niaaa.nih.gov/publications/AA66/ AA66.htm.*

National Institute on Alcohol Abuse and Alcoholism. (2005b). *Helping patients who drink too much: A clinician's guide,updated edition.* Retrieved from *pubs.niaaa.nih.gov/publications/Practitioner/CliniciansGuide2005/clinicians_guide.htm.*

Neumann, T., Neuner, B., Weiss-Gerlach, E., Tonnesen, H., Gentilello, L. M., Wernecke, K. D., et al. (2006). The effect of computerized tailored brief advice on at-risk drinking in sub-critically injured trauma patients. *Journal of Trauma, 61,* 805–814.

Prochaska, J. O., & Di Clemente, C. C. (1984). *The transtheoretical approach: Crossing the traditional boundaries of therapy.* Homewood, IL: Dorsey/Dow Jones-Irwin.

Prochaska, J. O., & Di Clemente, C. C. (1992). Stages of change in the modification of problem behavior. In M. Hersen, R. Eisler, & P. M. Miller (Eds.), *Progress in behavior modification* (Vol. 28). Sycamore, IL: Sycamore.

Rivara, F. P., Mueller, B. A., Fligner, C. L, Luna, G, Raisys, V. A., Copass, M., et al. (1989). Drug use in trauma victims. *Journal of Trauma, 29,* 462–470.

Substance Abuse and Mental Health Services Administration. (2008). Website at *sbirt.samhsa.gov/corecomp/index.htm, 2008.*

Substance Abuse and Mental Health Services Administration, Committee on Trauma Quick Guide. (2007). *Alcohol screening and brief interventions (SBI) for trauma patients* (DHHS Publications No. 07-4266). Washington, DC: U.S. Government Printing Office.

Samet, J. H., Libman, H., LaBelle, C., Steger, K., Lewis, R., Craven, D. E., et al. (1995). A model clinic for the initial evaluation and establishment of primary care for persons infected with human immunodeficiency virus. *Archives of Internal Medicine, 155,* 1629–1633.

Saunders, J. B., Aasland, O. G., Babor, T. F., DeLa Fuente, J. R., & Grant, M. (1993). Development of the Alcohol Use Disorders identification Test (AUDIT): WHO collaborative project on early detection of persons with harmful alcohol consumption—II. *Addiction, 88,* 791–804.

Schmidt, A., Barry, K. L., & Fleming, M. F. (1995). Detection of problem drinkers: The Alcohol Use Disorders Identification Test (AUDIT). *Southern Medical Journal, 88*(1), 52–59.

Schonfeld, L., King-Kallimanis, B., Duchene, D., Etheridge, R., Herrera, J., Barry, K. L., et al. (2010). The Florida BRITE Project: Screening and brief intervention for substance misuse in older adults. *American Journal of Public Health,100*(1), 108–114.

Soderstrom, C, A., Dailey, J. T., & Kerns, T. J. (1994). Alcohol and other drugs: An assessment of testing and clinical practices in U.S. trauma centers. *Journal of Trauma, 36,* 68–73.

Soderstrom, C. A., Smith, G. S., Dischinger, P. C., McDuff, D. R., Hebel, J. R.,

Gorelick, D. A., et al. (1997). Psychoactive substance use disorders among seriously injured trauma center patients. *Journal of the American Medical Association, 277,* 1769–1774.

Stephens, R. S., & Roffman, R. A. (2000). Comparison of extended versus brief treatments for marijuana use. *Journal of Consulting and Clinical Psychology, 68,* 898–908.

Stotts, A., Schmitz, J. M., Rhoades, H. M., & Grabowski, J. (2001). Motivational interviewing with cocaine-dependent patients: A pilot study. *Journal of Consulting and Clinical Psychology, 69,* 858–862.

U.S. Department of Health and Human Services. (1990). *Healthy people 2000* (PHS No. 91-50212). Washington, DC: Author.

Vincent, N., Shoobridge, J., Ask, A., Allsop, S., & Ali, R. (1998). Physical and mental health problems in amphetamine users from metropolitan Adelaide, Australia. *Drug and Alcohol Review, 17,* 187–195.

Wallace, P., Cutler, S., & Haines, A. (1988). Randomized control trial of general intervention in patients with excessive alcohol consumption. *British Medical Journal, 297,* 663–668.

Weaver, M. F., Jarvis, M. A., & Schnoll, S. H. (1999). Role of the primary care physician in problems of substance abuse. *Archives of Internal Medicine, 159,* 913–924.

Welte, J. W., Perry, P., Longabaugh, R., & Clifford, P. R. (1998). An outcome evaluation of a hospital-based early intervention program. *Addiction, 93,* 573–581.

Whitlock, E. P., Polen, M. R., Green, C. A., Orleans, T., & Klein, J. (2004). Behavioral counseling interventions in primary care to reduce risky/harmful alcohol use by adults: A summary of the evidence for the U.S. Preventive Services Task Force. *Annals of Internal Medicine, 140*(7), 557–568.

Chapter 14

Integrating Theory, Research, and Practice
A Clinician's Perspective

Edward M. Rubin

Recently, as I was walking from my office in the primary care clinic back to the printer, I encountered two of my colleagues in the midst of a determined, serious discussion. As I wandered past, the attending physician who had been talking with one of the internal medicine residents grabbed my arm and said, "Oh, thank God! I'm glad you're here!" Puzzled, of course, I stopped. This conversation was taking place in the Internal Medicine Clinic at Aurora Sinai Medical Center, a teaching clinic for internal medicine residents through Aurora Health Care and the University of Wisconsin School of Medicine and Public Health, where my office is located. The attending physician said that she had just been called into an exam room by the resident to supervise him with his next patient. As it turns out, the patient had said that he was suicidal and had been trying to kill himself by drinking (alcohol) and smoking cocaine. Immediately engrossed and concerned, I asked for the details of this gentleman's care to try to determine the best course of treatment.

This sort of "curbside consult" occurs often for me, and I must say, I love this type of practice. This style of practice is a sea change in my experience. For over 30 years, I had been practicing in traditional outpatient behavioral health clinics, both for Aurora Health Care and privately. For the past several years, however, my practice has been located and integrated, as much as possible, into the general medical practice of this primary care clinic located in the central city of Milwaukee, Wisconsin.

As this change has occurred for me personally, the state of the art and knowledge of addiction treatment has continued to grow exponentially. Recently, it seems that the addiction treatment field is much more willing to take suggestions for treatment approaches from the scientific literature and accept the reality that "science-based treatments are effective" (Volkow, 2009, p. 2). In addition, the character of my own practice has changed dramatically over the past several years. I now practice primarily from within a primary care clinic that is a clinical training site for internal medicine residents through the University of Wisconsin School of Medicine and Public Health. As the clinic moves toward establishing itself as a patient-centered medical home (McDaniel & Fogarty, 2009), my role as a psychological treatment facilitator has become more integrated into the process of serving these primary care patients and their providers, in a setting generally unused to having a psychologist or other behavioral health provider as part of the treatment team. In fact, behavioral health has often been a "last resort," or an afterthought, for many frustrated primary care providers who no longer have any idea what to do for a patient. My presence has been welcomed with varying degrees of acceptance by the diverse group of attending physicians who practice and supervise in the clinic. Even now, after practicing at the clinic for a number of years, I know who understands the value of behavioral health with their patients . . . and who does not.

This chapter illustrates how current research and a variety of treatment approaches can be integrated into a coherent approach to clinical practice. The challenge addressed here is to bring the thinking, clinical understanding, and decision making of the psychologist directly into this interesting and diverse clinical situation. The chapter provides firsthand clinical experiences and my thinking about each one as I attempt to meet the needs of the patient as well as those of the medical provider and the clinical setting. That way, I hope to show how treatment research has influenced my thinking and approaches to my work.

Getting Started

I have for many years believed that the traditional substance abuse treatment approach of "confrontation" is a mistake. I had reached this conclusion, in part, because I was personally uncomfortable doing what had been demonstrated to me as part of my early training. I also thought that I would not like to be treated that way, by anyone whose basic assumption is illustrated by the old joke: "How can you tell if an alcoholic is lying? His lips are moving." Later, it became clear from the research that *therapist* effects can account for a moderate amount of the variance in outcome

(Lutz, Martinovich, Lyons, Leon, & Stiles, 2007). As a therapist, this is the part that I can control. You may also note that nowhere in this chapter do I refer to the "disease" of alcoholism or drug addiction. Frankly, it doesn't really matter to me *what* it is when I am treating patients. It is much more important how the client conceptualizes his or her problem. If someone understands his or her drinking or drug use as a disease (which in fact may be more likely in a physician's office), I can certainly use that concept in our work together. If he or she finds a different way to understand the problem, such as drinking or drug use as a bad habit, I can certainly work with that concept as well. Others have admitted to me that they might, in fact, have a problem with alcohol, but *certainly* are not an alcoholic. In this sense, I have been described as "nontraditional" in my approach (Washburne, 2001), although, despite this, or perhaps because of it, my behavioral health colleagues have said that "I know the ropes" (Washburne, 2001) and that "people just seem to do well when working with [me]" (Washburne, 1994) and have twice selected me as a "trusted [psychologist] the pros would chose [*sic*] to help friends and family cope with life's sometimes distressing problems" (Washburne, 2001, p. 42).

Treatment can begin in a couple of ways. Some referrals come to me from other providers or through insurance companies. As I generally make my own appointments, when I first speak with the person on the phone I have an opportunity to begin the engagement process:

> "I'm glad you called. It seems you've made a decision to begin to look at your drinking. I'm sure it took some courage to do this, and I appreciate your effort on your own behalf. I can also offer some reassurance that other people have found our work together helpful."

In the clinic, it is not uncommon for providers or residents to come looking for me in my clinic office. At that point, they may ask for a quick consult about a patient and wonder if it might be helpful for me to meet the patient. I always check to see if they have spoken first with the patient to see if she or he is willing to meet with me, either right there in the exam room, or, if they happen to be in the waiting room after their appointment, to come into my office briefly. As you may assume, it is important how medical providers addresses their concerns with the patient, how they tell the patient why and to whom they want to make a referral, and how they discuss my role. If I am introduced as an "integral member of the team" (McDaniel & Fogarty, 2009, p. 483), it is often much easier to make a successful referral. Also, as my office is located in the same clinic where the patient just saw his or her medical provider, the stigma that sometimes accompanies going to a "mental health clinic" is reduced. Whether I see the patient in the examination room or in my office right after (or before) his or her medical visit, this process is the same as on the phone. In the clinic, I have the advantage of seeing the person, shaking his or her hand (if appropriate), and having the support of his or her medical provider for my intervention.

An introduction to my therapy style often begins with an inquiry about why the client called or why the client thinks he or she was referred to me, and by whom. My referrals come from a multitude of places including the primary care clinic where my office is located, colleagues, other professionals in the field, insurance or managed care organizations, and self-referrals of clients having found me on the Internet through various websites where my skills and interests are listed (*www.behaviortherapy.com/moderate. htm#therapists*). Before I see a patient from the Internal Medicine Clinic in the exam room or in my office in the clinic, I have usually had a chance to speak, at least briefly, with the referring physician. Also, as part of my role in the clinic, I find it invaluable to attend any "preclinic conference" being held for all of the residents providing service. Seeing my face reminds the residents as well as the attending physicians of the importance of psychological factors in many of the issues they address. And I often get to "eavesdrop" on the clinical case presentations between residents and attending physicians and remind them about the potential role of psychological factors. I often will inquire about alcohol or drug use if certain physical findings are being discussed such as hypertension, liver concerns, gout, or sleep difficulties. As the Center for Substance Abuse Treatment (2005a, p. 4) reported, "national surveys suggest COD [co-occurring disorders] are common in the adult population." The Center for Substance Abuse Treatment (2005a) goes on to report that more clients can be engaged and retained in substance abuse treatment if that treatment is integrated with medical care than if clients are referred to a separate substance abuse treatment program. Some brief interventions have been specifically designed for primary care clinics, and can be done by the primary care provider or a behavioral health provider in the clinic (National Institute on Alcohol Abuse and Alcoholism, 2007).

Asking the patient about his or her understanding of the reason for the referral or self-referral gives him or her a chance to reveal a bit of an understanding of his or her issues. In any case, it gives me an opportunity to begin to establish rapport. My motivational approach is to express empathy, respect, and acceptance of the individual and his or her concerns. I almost always also find something in the discussion to compliment him or her about as part of the engagement process. I communicate my conviction that change is always possible and that the ability to do that ultimately lies within him or her (Miller & Rollnick, 2002).

I have specialized in the treatment of addictions for many years. It is not uncommon for many of the referrals I see to be people who have had previous addiction treatment experiences and are struggling with their addictive behavior yet another time. I often convey to my clients that there is no one right approach to successful treatment of addictive disorders and our job is to find the right one *for them*. This is my attempt to convey a sense of optimism about the treatment experience and to give the patient a further taste of my approach and style. The client is often expecting a much more challenging, confrontational, and directive style from the therapist. After this brief exchange, I ask if the person wants to make an appointment with me. Logistics are then handled for phone contacts with directions to my office provided, parking, insurance issues, and the like. I reiterate contact information to the client at that time to make sure he or she can get in touch with me, should the need arise. In addition to the convenience of my office location for primary care referrals, I have generally found that this process significantly reduces my "no show" rate for initial appointments.

Potential Brief Intervention

I am fortunate to be able to meet patients who are being referred to me right in the clinic examination room with the attending physician and/or medical resident present. At that point, I can engage the patient and provide a brief, motivational intervention. It may be about drinking, or it may be about coming to meet with me at a later time in my office. In fact, a number of studies show that brief interventions can be effective for a range of problems (Center for Substance Abuse Treatment, 1999a). In either case, I provide some feedback along with the medical provider about his or her findings and concerns from the examination. I also may offer advice about safe, lower drinking (or safer drug-using) consumption limits and suggest some things that they may want to consider to help them change their behavior, if they have accepted change as a goal. At this point, I also assess their level of motivation or readiness to change this behavior. We can then negotiate some intermediate goals and change strategies they might employ or inquire about their interest in a subsequent follow-up appointment. All of this takes place with the patient's permission, meaning that I have asked for and they have agreed to our conversation, advice, and suggestions (Center for Substance Abuse Treatment, 2005b). There are also times when I will "piggyback" an appointment with me in conjunction with a follow-up appointment with the person's medical provider, again reducing appointment failures. I also have adjusted my appointment times for medical clinic patients, seeing them initially for 20–30 minutes, mimicking their primary care experience.

Initial Assessment

The content of the initial information gathered from new clients is partly determined by licensing and governing bodies as well as by various codes of ethics (American Psychological Association, 2010). These guidelines mandate that enough clinical information be gathered about the person seeking services so that clinical decisions can be made with confidence and so that the practitioner can know that he or she is practicing within the scope of his or her expertise and training.

Data gathering most often takes the form of a clinical interview, but may also include information from collateral sources. Aside from talking with others in the client's life, I have the opportunity to speak directly with the referring physician and to consult the patient's medical record, both of which have become increasingly important sources of collateral information for me. I then have multiple options: I can get insight into the patient's perception of the reason for referral, review physician's notes about it, access any referrals to other specialists, see the entire list of prescribed medications, and communicate through the electronic medical record with the referring physician. Providers are often immensely grateful for this communication about their referral. One provider told me that in 80–90% of the referrals she makes, she never knows what happens to the patient once the referral is made. Often with patients, my asking for permission to view and then access their medical record with them present reassures them that I will be talking with their physician about their care. Of course, there is the occasional patient who refuses, causing a clinical issue regarding his or her reason for not allowing this communication and coordination.

I also make liberal use of some psychological screening and assessment instruments (Allen & Wilson, 2003; Rubin, 2010; Center for Substance Abuse Treatment, 1999b). The decision about the use of assessment instruments depends upon the reason for the referral, one's usual practice patterns, and reimbursement considerations. There are a number of instruments that I have found helpful in this regard. They include the Drinkers Inventory of Consequences/Inventory of Drug Use Consequences (DrInC/InDuc); the Alcohol Use Disorders Identification Test (AUDIT); the CAGE Questions; and the RTC (Readiness To Change Questionnaire) (Rubin, 2010). These all provide additional opportunities for more individualized feedback to the client about his or her drug or alcohol use and its effect in his or her life. I also sometimes use assessment instruments later in the process to aid in increasing motivation to change (Hester & Miller, 2003).

In making assessment choices, I gather information that I may want to use later as part of engagement and motivational strategies (Miller, Zweben, DiClemente, & Rychtarik, 1994). For example, it is often important to inquire about previous periods of abstinence, sobriety, or moderation. This can lead the client to recognize that he or she has been able to stop or moderate his or her drinking (or other addictive behavior) in the past. I am then able to take the position of supporting past success(es) to express optimism and hope and strengthen his or her self-efficacy. The testing and assessment in which I engage can also provide useful individualized feedback and information to the patient. If the patient is a referral from one of the medical clinics in which I work, there is also the additional laboratory information the patient has already received from his or her physician.

Challenge, confrontation, or "breaking through denial" are not part of my therapeutic approach. I utilize a motivational enhancement approach (Center for Substance Abuse Treatment, 1999b) and conceptualize therapeutic movement through the transtheoretical-stages-of-change model (Connors, Donovan, & DiClemente, 2004). From this position, I do not find it helpful or therapeutic to "argue" with the client about whether he or she has an alcohol or drug problem. In addition, I have found little value in having someone accept a label such as "alcoholic" or "addict."

> Similarly, in the substance use arena, there is a trend to avoid labeling persons with substance abuse disorders as "addicts" or "alcoholics." Clinicians who use a motivation style avoid branding client with names, especially those who may not agree with the diagnosis or do not see a particular behavior as problematic. (Center for Substance Abuse Treatment, 1999b, p.11)

If the client and I engage in a power struggle about accepting a label or a name, ultimately I will always lose. Alternatively, it enhances engagement and client empowerment to accept his or her own view, philosophy, or explanation of the problem and to use that as a starting point for our work together.

Shaping the Relationship

Interestingly, I have generally found that substance-abusing clients are already quite self-critical upon entering treatment. This is especially true if the person has had previous treatment experience(s) or has encountered criticism or confrontation from family members. Past treatment attempts are often interpreted as failures now that he or she is again seeking professional help for the same problem. In this circumstance, I find myself commonly using the metaphor of learning how to ride a bicycle. It is rare, I point out, that someone learning this new behavior gets it right the first, the second, or even the third time. Most often, learning entails stopping or falling off the bicycle until the individual finally masters the multitude of new behaviors needed to get this complex skill correct. To succeed, the client must continue to work until he or she gets it "right." This image will often soften thoughts of failure about previous unsuccessful efforts as the individual can see earlier treatments as part of a learning process not yet complete. The same metaphor may also prove useful later in treatment if we must address lapses or relapses.

One of my goals throughout treatment is to shape my relationship with the individual so that it is different from any other that he or she has encountered in life. I do not want our relationship to mirror that which he or she may have with a parent, sibling, boss, spouse or lover, child, neighbor, or anybody else; rather, I want this therapeutic relationship to be unique. I do not deny the possibility of transference (or countertransference), but I recognize that there are likely already many people in this person's life who have coaxed, criticized, cajoled, confronted, or otherwise told him or her what, when, where, and how to do things better. Our relationship needs to be different: it needs to be uncritical and empathic so that motivation to change can be increased. Further, as Hester and Miller (2003, p. 39) point out, "therapist empathy is one of the better-specified determinants of effective treatment."

As part of the assessment process, I gather both quantity and frequency data about drinking or drug use. This can then be annualized to provide a dollar estimate of the cost per year of his or her drinking or drug use. When annualized, it is often quite amazing to the patient how much this behavior is actually costing. After receiving permission to share this information with the patient, the response is frequently that he or she "never thought about it like that before." After providing this revelation, I ask what else he or she might have done with that money. This begins to create some discrepancy between the client's reality of drug use or drinking and what he or she might have as future goals or plans. I often also provide a comparison of his or her drinking to general adult drinking norms in the United States (U.S. Department of Justice, 2002). The other information that is of interest to some is the caloric value of the alcohol they are consuming (Anonymous, n.d.). For a patient concerned about their weight, blood pressure, diabetic control, and so on, this is often an eye-opening statistic. I am able to translate the total annual calories consumed in alcohol converted to pounds potentially gained from drinking. Another very helpful piece of individualized data can be an estimate of blood alcohol concentration (BAC) on any one drinking occasion (Markham, Miller, & Arciniega, 1993).

Most often, people have little sense about how their own level of intoxication compares to the legal limit of alcohol consumption if they were driving, for example. In fact, it is not uncommon for the client to tell me *emphatically* that he or she was *not* drunk as I am estimating his or her BAC.

All this is designed to provide specific and individualized feedback, unique to the particular person, and can be highly motivating as he or she considers changing addictive behavior. As part of this process of providing feedback, I inquire about the client's reaction to the individual pieces of information that the medical staff or I have provided. This allows an opportunity to heighten any discrepancies between what the client believes about his or her substance use and what the data are suggesting about it, further enhancing change motivation.

Agreeing on a Plan of Action

After an initial assessment period of gathering data, it is useful to establish a treatment plan. Often, this is required by state certification and licensing authorities or by third-party payers, but beyond that, it is a very powerful tool for establishing rapport and engagement with the client as well as providing a clearer direction for the treatment. After providing feedback from the initial assessment procedure (Connors et al., 2004), I ask the client what he or she would like to work on. By asking what the *client* wants to focus on, I model a collaborative relationship and make it clear that the ultimate responsibility for any changes rests with the client (Hester & Miller, 2003). Of course, none of this precludes my sharing with the client my opinion about these matters—it is just that I find the timing of that interaction to be very important.

When my initial, brief meeting with the patient occurs in the presence of the medical provider(s), my treatment style models for the medical provider(s) a collaborative, consultative relationship with his or her (their) patient. This attitude and approach on behalf of the provider is sometimes lacking, but it is important to set an example in the context of the patient-centered medical home model (*www.ncqa.org/tabid/631/default.aspx*) now being encouraged and promoted in primary care settings throughout the United States, including the clinic in which I work.

I always hope that the patient will establish at least one goal regarding the use of alcohol or other drugs, but there are times when I am surprised by the goals that some want to set for themselves. It is not uncommon for a person to decide that his or her substance use is not a problem. Rather, people may identify a variety of other problems as the primary concern, despite what feedback they may have already received either from me or the medical provider about their health and other circumstances. Whatever starting point the patient identifies, that is where I endeavor to begin, addressing his or her primary concern.

More than two decades ago, Milwaukee County (1990) funded a study to examine the reason for dropout of publically funded clients referred to substance abuse treatment. The study concluded that two factors accounted for the majority of the treatment dropouts. The first had to do with access and ease of service delivery. The second factor influencing treatment dropout was the perception of clients that their therapist or counselor was not listening to what the client had to say. Many clinicians were seen as having their own agenda and therefore did not seem to value the issues the clients said were important to them. Conversely, Hester and Miller (2003, p. 140) point out that

> one of the strongest predictors of therapist success in motivating and treating alcoholic clients is *empathy*. An empathic therapist, in this definition, is one who maintains a more client-centered approach, listening to and reflecting the client's statements and feelings. Empathic counselors in this sense are characterized as warm, supportive, sympathetic, and attentive.

Accepting the client's agenda means that, at times, abstinence may not be the goal. A goal of moderation or controlled drinking or drug use may need to be seriously considered and, at least initially, become part of the treatment plan. In my experience, this is not uncommon. This goal may include a desire to stop using one drug (e.g., cocaine or narcotics), but not another (e.g., alcohol). If the treating clinician cannot incorporate this harm-reduction approach (Tatarsky & Marlatt, 2010) into his or her treatment philosophy, he or she should have a frank discussion with the client and then make a referral to a clinician who can pursue harm reduction as a legitimate goal of treatment.

That is not to say that the therapist has to blindly agree that controlled drinking or drug use is the only, best, or safest treatment goal. However, if the agenda of the therapist (e.g., only and always abstinence) is not a goal that the client is willing to acknowledge and accept, chances are that the client will terminate treatment prematurely because his or her issues are not being adequately addressed, or will continue to sit in the therapist's office, but be passively unengaged in treatment. In either case, therapy will likely be of little help to the client. At this early point in the treatment process, the therapist needs to make a decision about whether he or she is willing to work on a non-substance-abuse goal or to take a harm reduction or moderation approach (Rotgers, Kern, & Hoeltzel, 2002) with this client. This willingness to work with articulated client goals reflects a number of the six elements identified as integral to the brief motivational counseling approaches associated with positive change in behavior (Connors et al., 2004). The acronym FRAMES describes them:

- **F**eedback of information from assessment about risk or impairment.
- Emphasis on personal **R**esponsibility for change.
- **A**dvice to change.
- Providing a **M**enu of strategies for change.
- Therapist **E**mpathy.
- Facilitation of client **S**elf-efficacy or optimism.

Advice giving can sometimes be an integral part of the treatment approach. If the therapist finds that he or she disagrees with the client's goals, the therapist can certainly make that opinion known, but the therapist should not simply dismiss the client's goals out-of-hand because of this disagreement. It is also noteworthy that Miller, Wilbourne, and Hettema (2003) have found that many different treatment approaches can be effective in a variety of treatment settings and systems. When a client helps to select his or her own treatment goals and approach, this increases his or her motivation and commitment to the change behavior. My style and therapeutic interventions described here are designed to match a client earlier in the change process (Center for Substance Abuse Treatment, 1999b).

Various therapeutic tasks and interventions are appropriate for clients as they progress through the stages of change, as illustrated in Table 14.1.

In terms of the transtheoretical model (Prochaska, DiClemente, & Norcross, 1992), when a client has decided that there is indeed a problem that he or she wants to address, my therapeutic stance shifts a little. Although I continue to utilize some of the techniques listed above, I generally also include a more cognitive-behavioral approach (Kadden et al., 1992).

Of course, establishing goals for treatment begs the question about how the goals can be accomplished. This, too, is a question that should be posed to the client. This change model suggests that if someone moves *too quickly* into action, without adequate planning, there can be a higher risk for relapse or recurrence of the problem behavior. If desired by the client, the therapist might offer information about what to consider as well as suggestions and advice for change. However, the primary ideas should still come from the client. This style further reinforces the collaborative and respectful nature of the therapeutic relationship.

Once it has been decided that there is, in fact, a problem to be addressed and a decision has been made to address it (two distinct and different parts of the decision-making process), and after inquiring about what the client thinks will be helpful, I will generally present a menu of choices or treatment approaches. We may discuss options or treatment modalities about which the client has expressed some earlier interest, or perhaps something he or she has tried in the past with some success in changing other behaviors.

Treatment options selected by the client are more likely to be carried through than those initially suggested, recommended, or insisted upon by the therapist. Choices may include the obvious alternatives, such as individual or group therapy; couple or family treatment; and services with a variety of intensities, such as a partial hospitalization program, an intensive outpatient program, or a level of involvement that is at the lowest intensity of care, which might include weekly individual, group, couple, or family treatment. Inpatient or outpatient detoxification is also discussed at this juncture, if warranted, as well as the use of medications for the treatment of

TABLE 14.1. Motivational Strategies Based on Stage of Change

Client's stage of change	Appropriate motivational strategies for the clinician

Precontemplation
The client is not yet considering change or is unwilling or unable to change.
	• Establish rapport, ask permission, and build trust.
	• Raise doubts or concerns in the client about substance-using patterns by:
	  ○ Exploring the meaning of events that brought the client to treatment.
	  ○ Eliciting the client's perceptions of the problem.
	  ○ Offering factual information about the risks of substance use.
	  ○ Providing personalized feedback about assessment findings.
	  ○ Exploring the pros and cons of substance use.
	  ○ Helping a significant other intervene.
	• Express concern and keep the door open.

Contemplation
The client acknowledges concerns and is considering the possibility of change but is ambivalent and uncertain.
	• Normalize ambivalence.
	• Help the client "tip the decisional balance scales" toward change by:
	  ○ Eliciting and weighing pros and cons of substance use and change.
	  ○ Examining the client's personal values in relation to change.
	  ○ Emphasizing the client's free choice, responsibility, and self-efficacy for change.
	• Elicit self-motivational statements of intent and commitment from the client.
	• Elicit ideas regarding the client's perceived self-efficacy and expectations regarding treatment.
	• Summarize self-motivational statements.

Preparation The client is committed to and planning to make a change in the near future but is still considering what to do.	• Clarify the client's own goals and strategies for change. • Offer a menu of options for change or treatment. • Negotiate a change—or treatment—plan and behavior contract. • Consider and address barriers to change. • Help the client enlist social support. • Elicit from the client what has worked in the past either for him or others whom he knows. • Assist the client to negotiate finances, child care, work, transportation, or other potential barriers. • Have the client publicly announce plans to change.
Action The client is actively taking steps to change but has not yet reached a stable state.	• Engage the client in treatment and reinforce the importance of remaining in recovery. • Support a realistic view of change through small steps. • Acknowledge difficulties for the client in early stages of change. • Help the client identify high-risk situations through a functional analysis and develop appropriate coping strategies to overcome these. • Assist the client in finding new reinforcers of positive change. • Help the client assess whether he or she has strong family and social support.

(cont.)

TABLE 14.1. *(cont.)*

Client's stage of change	Appropriate motivational strategies for the clinician
Maintenance The client has achieved initial goals such as abstinence and is now working to maintain gains.	• Help the client identify and sample drug-free sources of pleasure (i.e., new reinforcers). • Affirm the client's resolve and self-efficacy. • Help the client practice and use new coping strategies to avoid a return to use. • Maintain supportive contact (e.g., explain to the client that you are available to talk between sessions). • Develop a "fire escape" plan if the client resumes substance use. • Review long-term goals with the client.
Recurrence The client has experienced a recurrence of symptoms and must now cope with consequences and decide what to do next.	• Help the client reenter the change cycle and commend any willingness to reconsider positive change. • Reframe the recurrence as a learning opportunity. • Assist the client in finding alternative coping strategies. • Maintain supportive contact.

Note. Adapted from Center for Substance Abuse Treatment (1999b).

addictions, for example, Antabuse, naltrexone, acamprosate and Vivitrol (Smith, 2007).

After discussion of the choices available to the client, I often ask if I may offer some advice or suggestions. With the client's permission, I may suggest a particular service or intensity of treatment based on my knowledge of the literature and experience in working with others with similar problems. I do not insist that the client accept the form of treatment that I recommend. I only offer my recommendations based on my observations and personal experience. However, no matter what the client's choices may be, it is always worth asking how the client thinks that he or she will follow through with those choices. If the client decides that part of his or her program will include attendance at a community-based self-help meeting, for example, I will invariably inquire about his or her ideas about frequency of attendance. In fact, I may also challenge the client a bit, asking if he or she thinks that that particular frequency is enough, too much, and so on. I ask about which particular meetings he or she thinks that he or she will attend as a way to help focus on issues of geography, time, and travel. I ask the client when he or she thinks he or she might actually begin attending, as well. Finally, I often ask what things he or she thinks might interfere with meeting attendance. All of this is designed to help the client think about logistics and how meeting attendance will impact the rest of his or her life. In this way, any "bumps in the road" are less likely to destroy positive plans for behavior change. This discussion is also a model for how I approach other involvements in which the client may be willing to participate as part of his or her treatment. We discuss therapy time, schedules, frequency, and anticipated interference in the same way that we discuss meeting attendance.

Beginning Treatment

Whether or not the client accepts *my* suggestions, we proceed by arranging to begin that treatment to which he or she does agree. This is when the client moves into the action stage of change. As part of this stage, I will accept the level of care in which the individual is willing to participate. Although I may disagree, accepting the client's own sense about the level of care that he or she needs is much more likely to encourage the client to continue to participate in treatment. I find that this approach also reinforces the idea that the client is always the final arbiter of his or her own fate, and so places in a very real way the ultimate responsibility for change upon the client. In addition, it acknowledges that the client knows him- or herself better than I ever can. Too often I have seen an individual dropping out of treatment prematurely as a result of a mismatch between what the therapist wanted and what the client was willing to accept. If a client does leave treatment prematurely, I have no hope of being able to help him or her with change. However, if he or she is willing to engage in *some* form of treatment experience (e.g., harm reduction), I can engage, motivate, and encourage change at the level the client is willing to accept. As a result, I hope the client will eventually accept a different level of treatment if the original choice is inadequate.

If I can begin with issues that are important to the client (after all, that is what brought him or her in to see me or his or her physician in the first place), I can often later bring up the relationship between these problems and any addictive behaviors. I can also comment on whether or not it appears that we are making progress in treatment. This can be done as part of the ongoing dialogue between client and therapist or as part of the regular review of the treatment plan. If we seem to be foundering, I am not unwilling to point this out to the client. Hopefully, this will encourage a further discussion of treatment goals and what we each see may be interfering with treatment progress. This will allow me to discuss the role that substance use may be playing. Ultimately, I am free to continue or not continue therapy with someone. If we do not seem to be making progress, my decision can be to end treatment and make an appropriate referral.

When creating a menu of options for treatment services, a variety of treatment modalities are available. These range from services that are most intensive (e.g., inpatient detoxification) through decreasing levels of care and intensity. The system for which I work provides the entire range of services and offers treatment in individual, group, family, or couple modalities.

Support Groups and Treatment

An array of community-based self-help groups are available. Although there are primarily 12-step programs (Alcoholic Anonymous, 1976) in Milwaukee, there are also a few Women for Sobriety (1993) and Secular Organization for Sobriety (Christopher, 1992) groups available. More recently, a growing number of S.M.A.R.T. Recovery (1996) groups have also become available.

A discussion of the value of community-based self-help groups is always part of my practice with clients suffering from addiction problems. Over time, my enthusiasm for these programs has waxed and waned. When I was first employed at a center for the treatment of substance use disorders, I worked at a traditional, 12-step-based treatment facility. My impression is that this was and continues to be the treatment approach of the majority of treatment centers available in the United States. At that time, virtually every clinician had, at the core of his or her clinical repertoire, a 12-step-based philosophy as part of his or her treatment approach. Also at that time, virtually every clinician had *his or her own* 12-step experience as part of *his or her* own recovery on which to draw and share with clients. At that time, it was clear to me how the 12 steps were integrated into the universal, standard treatment program for alcohol and other drug abuse. Every patient at this facility was expected to attend 12-step meetings while in treatment and everyone was expected to complete a certain number of the 12 steps prior to successful discharge. This included "doing" a fourth and fifth step (Alcoholics Anonymous, 1976). If patients failed to do what was expected, they could be "unsatisfactorily" discharged from the program. As I gained experience, however, and read more of the research, I began to see how this approach did not fit everyone. In the context of this first treatment setting in which I was working, however, this was a thorny issue.

I think now that I have a more balanced view of the role of self-help groups. Both anecdotally and in reviewing the findings of the Project MATCH Research Group (1997), I see that there are certain people for whom 12-step groups can be of great use. There are also some for whom 12-step support is not a good fit.

Some have difficulty with the spiritual/religious nature of the program; others have difficulty with the apparent rigid structure and mandate of following the 12 steps; still others struggle with the group format. However, I also understand the value of community or social support to mitigate the risk of relapse to addiction. As a result, 12-step groups have become part of a larger discussion I have with clients about community connections and support. This might also include mention of other types of community support groups available. For example, involvement in religious, social, or educational activities can also be very helpful. The importance of these options varies depending upon each individual client, and what he or she brings into the treatment and the choices he or she makes about his or her own life and community.

Choosing Specific Modalities

At the site where I practice, there is no standard substance abuse treatment program that everyone gets if they have the *proper* diagnosis. I present the array of services to the client, and then a negotiation takes place as to what seems to be indicated by the clinical aspects of the case and what the client is willing to do. Part of the initial assessment protocol for substance abuse problems that I helped develop for Aurora Behavioral Health Services specifically asks, "What does the *client* think will be helpful?' Often, in accepting the client's choice about treatment options, I will suggest that if what he or she has decided upon does not achieve the desired results, I will want to revisit this initial treatment decision in the future, when I may suggest other treatment options. In addition, I point out that not achieving treatment goals at one particular level of care does not automatically result in a referral to a higher, more intensive level of care. In fact, sometimes it is just the opposite. One of the assumptions that I make—and that I have helped integrate into the thinking and philosophy of other substance abuse treatment providers within Aurora Health Care—is that if one does not achieve his or her stated treatment goals at one treatment level, it may be because there has been a mismatch between what the client wants or is willing to do and the treatment provided. Therefore, at times this can result in a referral to a *less* intensive level of care (corresponding to an earlier stage of change).

With this in mind, one of the treatment experiences in which clients have sometimes been willing to enter when they are unwilling to do something else is called a "decision group." This group experience does not require abstinence prior to or even during participation, participants do not have to label themselves with any particular diagnosis, and no random urine drug screens are performed. The only requirements, as explained to the participants, are that they agree to attend regularly, not to be intoxicated in group, and be willing to discuss the role of addiction in their lives. I have found the book *Group Treatment for Substance Abuse* by Velasquez, Maurer, Crouch, and DiClemente (2001) very helpful in this regard. It supports the notion that treatment should not be uniform throughout the change process or consist of simply doing more of the same at later stages, but rather should consist of doing the right thing at the right time in the process of change. This group model has been adopted within the behavioral health system in which I work, and is a "least restrictive" treatment option available to clients who do not seem to be ready for more intensive or demanding services. It provides an additional referral so that people do not have to be discharged from services as "unmotivated" or "in denial." As Miller et al. (2003, p. 131) states "over the past three decades, however, there has been a gradual yet dramatic change in thinking about motivation for change." Clients who have had previous treatment experiences elsewhere are often dumbfounded by this particular group and treatment approach. It is nonconfrontational, encouraging, and positive about client participation. There are no overriding group goals or agendas except to enhance motivation for change. Rather, individual participants are able to set their *own* goals with regard to their addictive behavior. Therefore, it is not unusual to have some group members exploring the possibility of abstinence from some drug, others working on moderating their use, and yet others working on abstaining from one drug while moderating another. Most interesting to me is that the group members seem to have little problem dealing with different and varying treatment goals. It seems that as much as I am able to model acceptance of a variety of goals as reasonable, the group members are also able to do the same.

The initial reactions of the substance abuse treatment staff to the decision group were different. The staff and former medical director accused me of being an "enabler." I was told that what I was proposing was unethical since I would be encouraging and permitting people to use drugs or drink. Also, by not taking a strong, confrontive stance, I would be exposing the medical center and myself to liability if something untoward were to occur. Over time, staff and administrative attitudes have changed significantly. Through training, consultation, ongoing seminars, and exposure to current literature (as well as some staff turnover), this treatment group model, and the attitude and philosophy behind it, has become an accepted treatment modality, and is now seen as an evidence-based practice (American Psychological Association, 2005) throughout Aurora Behavioral Health substance abuse treatment services.

As mentioned previously, discussion takes place with the client about possible future renegotiations of treatment goals and approaches, depending upon the outcome of the current plan at the current level of intensity. That is, if an agreement is reached that the current goal of treatment is moderation of drinking, we also agree on a period during which we will work together on this goal. I then work *actively* with the client to teach behavioral ways to moderate his or her drinking or other drug use. At the end of that time, as part of the review of the treatment plan, a new goal may be established. Often what occurs is that if the moderation goal is not achieved after the agreed-upon time, the goal of abstinence might then be reconsidered as more reasonable. Even if moderation is ultimately achieved, it is not unusual for the individual to decide that abstinence is really the outcome he or she seeks. Frequently, the client realizes while working on moderation that this particular goal requires significant energy and concentration. It necessitates, for example, that the individual decide if he or she wishes to drink on any particular day. If so, on that day he or she may have to count his or her drinks, watch the passage of time, alternate alcoholic with nonalcoholic drinks, and so on. Individuals sometimes conclude that it is easier to quit entirely than to go through a rather elaborate formula each time they decide to drink. Nonetheless, from the perspective of engagement and motivation, it is much more powerful and respectful to work on the client's stated goal rather than to impose my own on the client. In addition, I know that it is possible for some people to moderate successfully. Because of my willingness to acknowledge and respect the client's goals, and engage with each client in working on those goals, I find that my clients are more likely to continue to work with me even if their goals are not accomplished, and so dropout is reduced. Also, they are more likely to consider abstinence at a later point in the treatment process, even though they may have been reluctant to do so earlier.

Involving Others

Another service I frequently offer clients is meeting with a significant other. This is not "marriage" or "couple counseling," although that may also be needed. The addiction treatment field recognizes that there is tremendous power in a collateral person to either positively or negatively influence behavior change, and "there is . . . clinical and research evidence of reciprocal relationships between marital/family interaction and abusive drinking," (O'Farrell & Fals-Stewart, 2003, p. 188). Thus, the value of meeting with a significant other in an attempt to engage her or him in supporting and contributing to the behavior change can be quite potent in enhancing motivation and commitment to change (Fals-Stewart, O'Farrell, Birchler, Córdova, & Kelley, 2005). Such a meeting affords the spouse or partner a chance to relate directly to the substance abuser in a controlled environment how his or her drinking or drug use has affected the couple and their relationship. It also provides an opportunity for the spouse or significant other to gain a clearer understanding of the problem, and to have input into the development of treatment goals.

One of my goals in involving others is to help change "poor communication and problem solving, arguing, financial stressors, and nagging" which "are common antecedents to substance use" (Fals-Stewart et al., 2005, p. 230). Positive interactions that can enhance and support the behavior change of the client can be identified and reinforced. Identification of interactions that interfere with or impede the treatment goals can also occur, and then be modified. "Communication problems are routinely found in relationship involving individuals who abuse substances" (Smith & Meyers, 2004, p. 108). Fletcher (2001) includes a chapter in her book on the role family members can play in supporting or hindering the recovery of a loved one, written from the perspective of the addicts themselves. All this can serve to increase marital or relationship satisfaction, which further enhances motivation to change and reduces the risk of relapse.

The Process of Change

It is rewarding to see someone proceed through the stages of change from precontemplation to action and beyond. Although this process can take some time, it can also proceed relatively quickly. I have seen patients pass through two or three stages within one or two therapy sessions.

Some years ago, I met with a man who had been arrested for his first OWI (operating while intoxicated). He had gone through a standard, state-mandated assessment, as all who are arrested in Wisconsin for drunken driving must do. As a result, he had been mandated to attend outpatient treatment for several months, something he did not believe he needed. Failure to do so would have resulted in loss of his license until the mandate was fulfilled, however, so he began to attend an outpatient treatment group that was the "standard treatment" in this particular agency. He came to me several months after having dropped out of that program, having previously decided that he would live without a driver's license for failure to fulfill the state treatment requirement. He came because he finally decided that he wanted his operator's license back. I agreed to see him. For the entire first session I was unable to even begin the assessment process because he could only rant and rave about his "horrible" past treatment experience. He felt he had been mistreated and misunderstood by the therapist who had challenged virtually every explanation he had made about his drinking, telling him he was a "drunk" and to "take the cotton out of your ears and put it in your mouth!" He was incredulous that this counselor made so many assumptions about him without having taken the time to really understand and get to know him. He was clear to me that he was *not* going to let that happen again with me. So, for the first session I listened and empathized with how difficult this must have been for him to sit through, feeling so misunderstood. He explained that he was not at all sure he actually had an alcohol problem and certainly did not think he needed to stop drinking. I told him I could certainly understand how he could feel that way, and how he must have felt quite different from the others in the group. In the second session, he was much less angry and more willing to explore various aspects of his drinking, including the fact that this was the first time he had been *caught* drinking and driving, but not the first time he had done it.

Over the course of the next several sessions, this young man went from the position of not thinking he had any problem with alcohol and being irate at the entire process, to ultimately deciding that he should stop drinking, at least for a while, as his drinking had created some additional problems in his life aside from this legal one. All of this occurred without my ever telling him to consider that option, and without ever labeling him. I only saw him for a few sessions, but in those few meetings, he proceeded from precontemplation through contemplation, to preparation to action. Ultimately, he did reobtain his driver's license.

Early in treatment, I may not meet weekly with an individual. He or she may not be ready for even that level of intensity of service, as with the young man noted above. Of course, levels of treatment intensity can be modified as the client moves through the stages. It is rare, however, for me to see someone through to the maintenance stage. Obviously, this takes place much later in his or her process of recovery. It may be as many as 6–9 months after recovery begins that someone reaches and settles into the maintenance stage. Because of the time frame, my practice location inside an internal medicine primary care clinic, and the vicissitudes of behavioral health reimbursement, clients who do that well at sustaining change seldom remain in treatment this long unless there are other, co-occurring disorders (Center for Substance Abuse Treatment, 2005a). My hope, assumption, and experience are, however, that if they run into trouble, they will feel that they can recontact me for additional help.

Things seldom go perfectly. Changing problematic substance use is difficult and there is no reason to expect that the client will "get it right" the first, the second, or even the third time. Because of this reality, I want to be encouraging and support repeated attempts. I may see the client when change efforts have broken down, he or she has returned to drinking or drug use, and is feeling ashamed, guilty, and demoralized. It is important for the client to understand that I see this lapse as a natural part of the change process for most people. My usual manner of addressing setbacks is to be supportive and encouraging. My language can help to convey my attitude. As do others in the field, I often speak about "slips" or "lapses" rather than use the word "relapse." The latter, I teach, has the connotation of a full return not only to drinking or drug use, but to the entire lifestyle engendered by that behavior. The other words (e.g., "slip," "lapse") I define as being of much shorter duration with many fewer consequences. I am also very encouraging and supportive about the client's willingness to return to address this concern with me rather than simply disappearing from treatment.

I take a positive, nonjudgmental attitude about the experience of slips or lapses (e.g., the client stopped drinking or using drugs after a very short time; the client came in right away to discuss it), finding ways to reframe the behavior to provide a sense of optimism and hope rather than shame and embarrassment. I focus instead on helping the patient to see that somehow he or she managed *this* use differently than previously in his or her addiction experience. I also remind the person that setbacks are a natural part of changing almost *any* behavior or habit, and then refocus the client's attention on how the slip happened. I try to reframe the client's perspective on the return to drinking or drug use as a learning experience. I wonder with the client about what he or she learned from this slip that he or she did not know before it happened or had forgotten. I wonder with the client what he or she might do differently in the future if encountering similar circumstances. Often, there are similarities between this discussion and others that have taken place during the preparation stage of change. Under the rubric of "relapse prevention," treatment often must include some training in behavioral self-control. "It consists of behavioral techniques of goal setting, self-monitoring, managing consumption, rewarding goal attainment, functionally analyzing drinking situations, and learning alternate coping skills" (Hester, 2003, p. 152). All this I hope to do without the client becoming so demoralized that he or she returns to and becomes stuck in earlier stages of change. Rather, I hope to encourage the client to keep moving on from the stage he or she currently is at back to action again.

The Role of Medication in Treatment

It is important to discuss the role of medication in the treatment process. My perspective is that the hard work of recovery rests with my client. Ultimately, he or she is the one who must make the cognitive and behavioral changes that will result in abstinence or moderation of his or her drinking or drug use. Nonetheless, I think that medication can play an important role in this process. I am not speaking to the role of medication in the treatment of withdrawal symptoms or the role that medication can play in the treatment of co-occurring psychological disorders, although the majority of my work has been with people suffering from both addictions and multiple psychological problems. The complexity of this latter, multifaceted problem is well addressed by the Center for Substance Abuse Treatment (2005a). Rather, I particularly address the role that I see medication can play in helping an individual maintain abstinence from alcohol (e.g., Antabuse), the reduction in urges and cravings for cocaine (e.g., Seroquel), the medication treatment options for narcotics addiction (e.g., methadone, Suboxone, Subutex), or in the reduction of urges or cravings, as well as in the ultimate effect of alcohol (e.g., ReVia, acamprosate, Depade, Vivitrol, topamax). These medications become part of the menu of options that I discuss with my client during various phases of treatment.

Often, I have found that patients are not initially interested in medication. They see its use as a "crutch," suggesting that they are not strong enough to do this on their own. Although not necessarily accepting their characterization of the use of medication, I will go with their particular and unique treatment preferences, reminding them that if things don't go as planned, they always have these additional options available at another time to reconsider. In the course of my practice, I have found that there is little awareness of naltrexone or acamprosate and the apparent value of these medications in reducing the urges, craving, and effect of alcohol in some people. Once explained, however, I have found that there is more interest in those medications than in Antabuse. The work by Volpicelli, Alterman, Hayashida, and O'Brien (1992) has convinced me that medication should be an integral part of the menu of options offered for alcohol treatment. In any case, medication is most often seen by my clients as a secondary option in their recovery. That has changed a bit lately, however. As I see many of my clients in the Internal Medicine Clinic, they seem to be more willing to consider these addiction medications earlier in the treatment process. The more options available to someone who is trying to recover, the more likely he or she will be able to find an approach, or combination of approaches, that will be successful.

I should also mention that I am not at all opposed to working with people who may be taking methadone as part of a treatment program for opiate addiction or chronic pain. I have found a certain prejudice among some substance abuse treatment professionals and programs against those who may be using methadone as part of their recovery. Research (National Institute on Drug Abuse, 2000) leads me to conclude that methadone maintenance is one of the most successful treatment approaches for opiate addiction. I examined this prejudice against people taking methadone, where the primary treatment goal for many is abstinence from some other drug. I have been told by some counselors that the person using methadone is "stoned," "high," or intoxicated, and therefore unable to fully utilize therapy. In addition, others have said that they are "still using drugs," having only substituted one opiate for another. In my view, this latter perspective is a gross oversimplification, and I have not found the former view to be true, once the appropriate dosage has been found and stabilized. I will work toward *sobriety, recovery and abstinence* with them, as well as on whatever other recovery issues may arise.

If the client is taking medication as prescribed, and is not using any other illicit drugs, I have no difficulty describing this as abstinence, seeing methadone as the harm-reduction technique that it is. There have also been times in my clinical experience where I have, paradoxically, challenged a client's motivation by suggesting that he or she may not yet be ready for abstinence, or that it might be too difficult of a goal at this time. Further, I might suggest that he or she may want to wait a while before tackling abstinence. This tends to elicit a great deal of change talk. As part of the discussion about "waiting," I have sometimes suggested methadone maintenance or Suboxone treatment as viable alternatives. Although generally not accepted by the client, it has allowed for a good discussion of the role of methadone (or other medications) in treatment as well as an examination of the client's current motivation and goals. There have also been times when the client thought about my suggestion, and returned later wanting to pursue it. At those times, I have been more than willing to provide a referral to a local methadone maintenance program and also to continue working with the patient. Continuing to maintain my therapeutic relationship with that client becomes more difficult in this circumstance, however. This is because it may not be permissible in the context of the methadone program for the client to continue treatment elsewhere while also getting services from them. If the client is getting methadone from a private, trained physician not affiliated with a program, continuing my treatment with him or her is not a problem, and is often endorsed by the prescriber, permitting close collaboration between treaters and the patient.

Conclusion

This chapter provides a sense of my style, thinking, and approach to the treatment of addictions. There may also be a sense of how I have grown and evolved into my current approach over the past 30 years of practice. When I first entered the field of addiction treatment, it seemed much more simple; virtually everyone got the same thing: 30 days of inpatient treatment in a hospital setting. The longer I have been in the field, the more complex it has become. Beginning with counselors who had their own personal recovery experience, principally with AA as their only resource, to the current level of sophistication in therapists, primarily with graduate degrees and with a much more complex understanding of addictive behavior and behavior change, what we have today has represented a quantum shift in addiction treatment, philosophy, and approach. What has been a personal and professional evolution for me has been a revolution in the substance abuse treatment field. The dedicated professionals entering the addiction treatment field have changed over time and the clinicians' hunger for research and advances in the field has increased. We have rightly become much more interested in the integration of research and technology into practice and now look to evidence-based practices to enhance our treatment and outcomes. Clearly, now we see more of the individual differences among those with addiction problems rather than seeing all addictions, and addicts, as the same. The treatment models I have discussed in this chapter not only respect the individual differences and uniqueness of the individual being treated, but are gender- and culturally sensitive as well.

The latest revolution for me is a personal one: my corelocation into a primary care clinic in the central city of Milwaukee, Wisconsin, and my integration into a primary care treatment team. This represents not only a change in the delivery of addiction treatment services, but in provision of behavioral health services generally. This has served to enhance my practice, allowing me to meet with, and intervene, much earlier in the process than previously, and to see many patients who would otherwise *never* accept a referral to an addiction specialist or psychologist. It has allowed and encouraged a much closer collaboration between the primary care providers and myself, which also enhances treatment outcomes. As much as I have enjoyed my career to date, and as long as I have been practicing, this latest change has me even more engaged. It is the most fun I have had so far in my practice of treating addiction!

References

Alcoholics Anonymous. (1976). *Alcoholics Anonymous: The story of how many thousands of men and women have recovered from alcoholism* (4th ed.). New York: Alcoholics Anonymous World Services. Available online at *www.aa.org/bigbookonline*.

Allen, J. P., & Wilson, V. B. (Eds.). (2003). *Assessing alcohol problems: A guide for clinicians and researchers* (2nd ed., National Institute on Alcohol Abuse and Alcoholism Treatment Handbook Series 4). Bethesda, MD: U.S. Government Printing Office.

American Psychological Association. (2005). American Psychological Association policy statement on evidence-based practice in psychology. Retrieved December 12, 2010, from *www.apapracticecental.org/ce/courses/ebpstatement.pdf*.

American Psychological Association. (2010). *Ethical Principles of Psychologists and Code of Conduct.* Retrieved December 19, 2010, from *www.apa.org/ethics/code/index.aspx*.

Anonymous. (n.d.). *Alcohol calories.* Retrieved December 19, 2010, from *www.personal-nutrition-guide.com/alcohol-calories.html*.

Center for Substance Abuse Treatment (CSAT). (1999a). *Brief interventions and brief therapies for substance abuse* (Treatment Improvement Protocol [TIP] Series 34). Rockville, MD: Substance Abuse and Mental Health Services Administration.

Center for Substance Abuse Treatment. (1999b). *Enhancing motivation for change in substance abuse treatment* (Treatment Improvement Protocol [TIP] Series 35). Rockville, MD: Substance Abuse and Mental Health Services Administration.

Center for Substance Abuse Treatment. (2005a). *Substance abuse treatment for persons with co-occurring disorders* (Treatment Improvement Protocol [TIP] Series 42). Rockville, MD: Substance Abuse and Mental Health Services Administration, 2005.

Center for Substance Abuse Treatment. (2005b). *A guide to substance abuse services for primary care clinicians* (Treatment Improvement Protocol [TIP] Series 24). Rockville, MD: Substance Abuse and Mental Health Services Administration.

Christopher, J. (1992). *SOS sobriety: The proven alternative to 12–step programs.* Buffalo, NY: Prometheus Books.

Connors, G. J., Donovan, D. M., & DiClemente, C. (2004). *Substance abuse treatment and the stages of change: Selecting and planning interventions.* New York: Guilford Press.

Fals-Stewart, W., O'Farrell, T. J., Birchler, G. R., Córdova, J., & Kelley, M. L. (2005). Behavioral couples therapy for alcoholism and drug abuse: Where we've been, where we are, and where we're going. *Journal of Cognitive Psychotherapy: An International Quarterly, 19*, 229–246.

Fletcher, A. M. (2001). *Sober for good: New solutions for drinking problems— Advice from those who have succeeded.* Boston: Houghton Mifflin.

Hester, R. (2003). Behavioral self-control training. In R. K. Hester & W. R. Miller (Eds.), *Handbook of alcoholism treatment approaches: Effective alternatives* (3rd ed., pp.152–164). Boston: Allyn & Bacon.

Hester, R. K., & Miller, W. R. (Eds). (2003). *Handbook of alcoholism treatment approaches: Effective alternatives* (3rd ed.). Boston: Allyn & Bacon.

Kadden, R. M., Carroll, K., Donovan, D., Cooney, N., Monti, P., Abrams, D., et al. (Eds.). (1992). *Cognitive-behavioral coping skills therapy manual: A clinical research guide for therapists treating individuals with alcohol abuse and dependence* (Project MATCH Monograph Series, Vol. 4). Rockville, MD: National Institute on Alcohol Abuse and Alcoholism.

Lutz, W., Martinovich, Z., Lyons, J. S., Leon, S. C., & Stiles, W. B. (2007). Therapist effects in outpatient psychotherapy: A three-level growth curve approach. *Journal of Counseling Psychology, 54*(1), 32–39.

Markham, M. R., Miller, W. R., & Arciniega, L. (1993). BACCuS 2.01: Computer software for quantifying alcohol consumption. *Behavioral Research Methods, Instruments, Computers, 25*, 420–421.

McDaniel, S. H., & Fogarty, C. T. (2009). What primary care psychology has to offer the patient-centered medical home. *Professional Psychology: Research and Practice, 40*(5), 483–492.

Miller, W. R., & Rollnick, S. (2002). *Motivational interviewing: Preparing people for change.* New York: Guilford Press.

Miller, W. R., Wilbourne, P. L, & Hettema, J. E. (2003). What works?: A summary of alcohol treatment outcome research. In R. K. Hester & W. R. Miller (Eds.), *Handbook of alcoholism treatment approaches: Effective alternatives* (3rd ed., pp. 13–63). Boston: Allyn & Bacon.

Miller, W. R., Zweben, A., DiClemente, C. C., & Rychtarik, R. G. (1994). *Motivational enhancement therapy manual: A clinical research guide for therapists treating individuals with alcohol abuse and dependence* (Project MATCH Monograph Series, Vol. 2). Rockville MD: National Institute on Alcohol Abuse and Alcoholism.

Milwaukee County. (1990). *Treatment of publically funded substance abuse clients in Milwaukee County.* Unpublished raw data.

National Institute on Alcohol Abuse and Alcoholism. (2007). *Helping patients who drink too much: A clinician's guide.* Retrieved from *pubs.niaaa.nih.gov/ publications/practitioner/cliniciansguide2005/guide.pdf.*

National Institute on Drug Abuse. (2000). *High success rates for a variety of heroin addiction treatment medications.* Retrieved December 12, 2010, from *archives.drugabuse.gov/newsroom/00/NR11–1.html.*

O'Farrell, T. J., & Fals-Stewart, W. (2003). Marital and family therapy. In R. K. Hester & W. R. Miller (Eds.), *Handbook of alcoholism treatment approaches: Effective alternatives* (3rd ed., pp. 188–212). Boston: Allyn & Bacon.

Prochaska, J. O., DiClemente, C. C., & Norcross, J. C. (1992). In search of how people change: Applications to addictive behaviors. *American Psychologist, 47*(9), 1102–1114.

Project MATCH Research Group. (1997). Matching alcoholism treatment to client heterogeneity: Project MATCH posttreatment drinking outcomes. *Journal of Studies on Alcohol, 58,* 7–29.

Rotgers, F., Kern, M. F., & Hoeltzel, R. (Eds.). (2002). *Responsible drinking: A moderation management approach for problem drinkers.* Oakland, CA: New Harbinger.

Rubin, E. M. (2010). Essentials of substance abuse assessment. In M. J. Ackerman (Ed.), *Essentials of forensic psychological assessment* (2nd ed.). New York: Wiley.

S.M.A.R.T. Recovery. (1996). *S.M.A.R.T. recovery: Self-management and recovery training* [Member's manual]. Beachwood, OH: S.M.A.R.T. Recovery Self-Help Network. Available online at *www.smartrecovery.org.*

Smith, J. E., & Meyers, R. J. (2004). *Motivating substance abusers to enter treatment: Working with family members.* New York: Guilford Press.

Smith, J. K. (2007). *Drugs for drugs: Medications to treat addictions.* Retrieved December 9, 2010, from *www.fortherecordmag.com/archives/ftr_11262007p21.shtml.*

Tatarsky, A., & Marlatt, G. A. (2010). State of the art in harm reduction psychotherapy: An emerging treatment for substance misuse. *Journal of Clinical Psychology, 66,* 117–122.

U.S. Department of Justice. (2002). *Drinking in America: Myths, realities, and prevention policy.* Retrieved December 19, 2010, from *www.udetc.org/documents/Drinking_in_America.pdf*

Volkow, N. D. (2009). Suiting treatment to the nature of the disease. *NIDA Notes, 22*(4), 2. Retrieved December 19, 2010, from *www.nida.nih.gov/NIDA_notes/NNvol22N4/DirRepVol22N4.html.*

Velasquez, M. M., Maurer, G. G., Crouch, C., & DiClemente, C. C. (2001). *Group treatment for substance abuse: A stages-of-change therapy manual.* New York: Wiley.

Volpicelli, J. R., Alterman, A. I., Hayashida, M., & O'Brien, C. P. (1992). Naltrexone in the treatment of alcohol dependence. *Archives of General Psychiatry, 49,* 876–880.

Washburne, C. K. (1994, December). Mind healers: The city's top therapists. *Milwaukee Magazine,* pp. 30–45.

Washburne, C. K. (2001, February). Mind healers. *Milwaukee Magazine,* pp. 42–53.

Women for Sobriety. (1993). *Welcome to WFS and the new life program.* Quakertown, PA: Author.

Chapter 15

Case Management in Substance Abuse Treatment

Allen Zweben

Case management is an approach that is used across health care, mental health, and social service settings to help clients gain access to services. In the addictions field, case management is especially important for those deemed to be at risk for early relapse. This chapter provides the rationale and support for case management in the treatment of addiction problems. In addition to discussing practical case management strategies, it provides case examples to show how these strategies can be applied to resolve issues that often arise in substance use treatment. The chapter shows how case management can be incorporated into an integrated system of care to serve a liaison function between services that address different aspects of substance use problems. Finally, the chapter ends with a presentation of issues that need to be investigated for the improvement of case management services.

Models of Case Management

Several models of case management have been used with different client populations in various settings, ranging from a broker/generalist model to a strengths-based, assertive community treatment (ACT) approach (Rapp, 2002; Rothman, 2003; Substance Abuse and Mental Health Services

Administration, 1998; Test, 2003; Walsh, 2003). The differences between these models pertain mainly to the intensity of services offered. For example, the broker/generalist model focuses primarily on assessment, information sharing, and an active referral to a community agency. The strengths-based ACT approach is more comprehensive than the broker/generalist model. It is focused on forging strong therapeutic ties with clients and advocating for clients by working to establish new resources that are necessary to fulfill case management goals. Unlike the broker/generalist approach, ACT typically employs professionals with more advanced degrees (e.g., master of social work) and is more likely to be utilized with clients who have a high severity of addiction problems, such as addicted individuals who also have other serious mental health conditions.

Research on Case Management

There is strong evidence that addressing medical and social service issues while dealing with addictive behaviors is more likely to produce better posttreatment outcomes than treating addictive behaviors alone (Conrad et al., 1998; Cox et al., 1998; Kirby et al., 1999; Najavits, Weiss, Shaw, & Muenz, 1998; Siegel, Li, & Rapp, 2002; Siegel et al., 1995; Siegel, Rapp, Li, Saha, & Kirk, 1997; Sullivan, 2003). Such interventions have often combined pharmacological and behavioral approaches along with case management services. Case management is an effective way to help clients gain access to and engage in services (McLellan et al., 1999), while focusing on a range of factors such as reducing cravings, improving individual coping resources, and providing concrete supports to lessen the everyday hardships associated with serious alcohol and drug use problems.

In a recent study, Morgenstern compared case management with usual care (UC) for welfare recipients with substance use problems (Morgenstern et al., 2008). In case management, more effort was made to link clients with employment, mental health, and medical services during the first 3 months relative to UC. Case management also included linking clients to concrete services at the point of crisis. At the 15-month follow-up, case management clients had significantly higher rates of treatment entry, engagement, and retention compared to UC clients. More significantly, case management clients had double the abstinent rates of UC clients.

The above findings were supported by a meta-analysis of case management with substance use clients (Vanderplasschen, Wolf, Rapp, & Brockaert, 2007). This review suggested that case management tends to extend treatment duration, forestall readmission to detoxification, and improve outcomes in a number of areas such as substance use, employment, physical health, and legal problems.

McLellan et al.'s (1999) study on case management underscores the utility of the approach. They evaluated the impact of case management in eight methadone maintenance settings. Due to the large numbers of clients in these agencies, not all could receive case management. This allowed for a natural experiment since clients' receipt of case management was essentially determined by "chance." At follow-up, case management clients tended to do better on measures of drinking, drug use, psychiatric symptoms, and legal and employment outcomes. McLellan et al. (1999), attributed such differences to the fact that case management clients had made greater use of community services—that is, housing, training, and employment opportunities—than non-case management clients did.

Employing Case Management in Addiction Services

Providers have increasingly recognized that dealing solely with drinking or drug use may not necessarily result in the resolution of accompanying problems. Failure to deal with these concomitant difficulties increases the likelihood that such matters will eventually lead to a resumption of substance abuse (Alexander, Pollack, Nahra, Wells, & Lemak, 2007). To produce lasting change, providers need to attend to both the substance use and concomitant difficulties. To illustrate:

> Ted has been drinking problematically for the past 10 years. As a consequence, he has been confronted with a variety of problems such as unemployment and family difficulties. He recently entered a 12-step treatment program and consequently has been able to remain abstinent for the past 6 months. Despite this improvement, Ted has been unable to find a job and continues to rely on this wife, Helen, for financial support.
>
> Although Helen is pleased with Ted's improvement, she is unhappy about having to be the breadwinner in the household. She continues to pressure Ted to find a job and remains suspicious about his sobriety. Helen wonders whether Ted is actively looking for work or just hanging out with "friends" in the local bar as he has done in the past.
>
> Ted has become very frustrated about not finding a job. He has also become demoralized about Helen's pressure to find a job. He tells the case worker, "It is not enough that I stopped drinking. I cannot take Helen's suspiciousness and nagging anymore."
>
> One night after a heated episode with Helen, Ted joined his "drinking buddies" at the local tavern. He came home intoxicated and Helen asked him to leave. Ted did not talk with the case worker about the incident because he was ashamed about his behavior. He felt that the case worker would be very disappointed with him which would further exacerbate his negative feelings about the drinking episode.

Rather than continuing to hide information from the worker, he stopped coming to the sessions.

In this vignette, making changes in drinking patterns did not affect the accompanying problems. Ted's inability to find a job had a negative impact on Helen who, in turn, questioned his sobriety and his motivation to change. Ted's frustration with not finding employment along with his inability to maintain Helen's trust contributed to the recent setback. He did not have sufficient trust in the clinician to talk about these difficulties, thereby causing him to eventually drop out of the program.

In the addiction field, entry to treatment usually starts in detoxification. However, detoxification is usually not a stand-alone treatment. To facilitate recovery, individuals need to be connected with additional services. case management is an essential ingredient in linking clients with services that might help address factors such as housing, employment, and financial problems that can interfere with cessation of drinking or drug use. Case management is not an alternative to individual or group therapy but a complement to it (Miller, Forcehimes, & Zweben, 2011). Case management also enables clients to connect with adjunctive services ranging from pharmacotherapy to behavioral marital therapy. Such issues often occur once abstinence has been achieved (Rapp et al., 2008).

The case manager helps to identify "early warning signs" such as interpersonal stress that may precipitate alcohol or drug use (Zweben, Rose, Stout, & Zywiak, 2003). He or she makes a referral to the appropriate service to address these early warning signs or may enlist family, friends, employers, or pastors as resources to help prevent a recurrence of drinking or drug use.

Delivery of Case Management Services with Substance Use Clients

There are a number of issues to consider in delivering case management effectively with substance use clients. First, case management works better if a strong working relationship has developed between case managers and clients (Morgenstern et al., 2008). Second, it is often useful to use a structured (or manualized) approach (Morgenstern et al., 2008; Vanderplasschen, Rapp, Broekaert, & Fridell, 2009). Third, the amount of time spent in case management core functions such as goal setting, case monitoring, client advocacy, and service coordination seems to be related to improved treatment outcomes (Alexander et al., 2007; Morgenstern et al., 2008; Noel, 2006; Vanderplasschen, Rapp, Broekaert, & Fridell, 2004). Finally, readiness for change predicts whether or not clients will connect with essential services, and thus it is an important target for case managers (Zweben & Zuckoff, 2002).

Several issues should be considered in evaluating client readiness:

- In terms of importance, how does the individual feel about the needed service? Does he or she view the service as essential for recovery? Does the person make the connection between the service and addiction problems? For example, does the person realize that the referral for job counseling may help alleviate marital conflict, which in turn might enhance commitment to abstinence?
- How confident does the individual feel about using the service? For example, is he or she ready to participate in a job-training program 5 days a week?
- What are the obstacles that need to be addressed in order for the person to enter and participate in a needed service—child care arrangements, health care, psychiatric symptoms, and so on?

In sum, clients are more likely to enter, participate, and remain in a service if they perceive the service as relevant and important and, at the same time, are confident about utilizing the service (Zweben & Zuckoff, 2002).

Practical Case Management Strategies

For clients who view services as important to their treatment goals and feel confident about utilizing the needed service, a strengths-based, broker-generalist model may be sufficient to link them with essential services (Zweben & Zuckoff, 2002). Sharing relevant data on their case management needs and providing referral information may be all that is necessary to achieve case management goals.

However, for clients who are uncertain or ambivalent about their alcohol or drug use, it may not be sufficient to simply provide information, contact referral sources, and/or escort clients to services (Substance Abuse and Mental Health Services Administration, 1998). This group of clients represents a sizable proportion of individuals seen in addiction treatment.

The strategies discussed below are primarily aimed at individuals who are at risk for referral failure (Conrad et al., 1998). Such strategies, mainly derived from the motivational interviewing (MI) literature, have been consistently found to be effective in addressing adherence issues with substance use clients (Miller et al., 2011; Zweben et al., 2008; Zweben & Zuckoff, 2002). Consequently, these strategies have been adapted and incorporated into the referral compliance strategies that are often used in case management settings.

There are several considerations when dealing with this at-risk group:

1. How do you increase the individual's awareness and acceptance of the need for a particular service?
2. How do you raise the individual's confidence that he or she will be able to attend and complete the service?
3. What strategies are most effective in resolving these matters?

Table 15.1 provides a list of major case management strategies that are used to address these issues.

Assessing Case Management Needs

The first step in identifying and addressing clients' ancillary needs is to conduct an assessment of the areas needing additional help. Consider using a service request form to identify resources needs. A service request form was developed for this purpose and was employed in the COMBINE study for individuals with alcohol problems (Miller, 2004; Miller et al., 2011). A modified version is included in Figure 15.1. The service request form covers a wide range of items that are often seen with clients, such as finances, child care, residential needs, employment interests, and medical and psychosocial concerns.

People in case management settings vary considerably. Individuals coming from mainly lower socioeconomic backgrounds tend to have different needs than those coming from middle-class backgrounds. Individuals with co-occurring disorders (e.g., mental health and substance use problems) have different needs than those having substance use problems without other mental health conditions. With dually diagnosed clients, greater emphasis might be placed on medication-assisted treatment to stabilize their mental conditions. For individuals just released from prison (parolees), greater efforts may be devoted to locating and building a prosocial support network. In completing the form, clients are asked to check all the items that they think are relevant to their service needs, rank the importance of

TABLE 15.1. Case Management Strategies

- Assess case management needs.
- Provide feedback.
- Formulate goals.
- Negotiate tasks.
- Address barriers.
- Conduct follow-up.

Would you like assistance in any of these areas? If YES, mark with an X and indicate how important it is for you on a scale from 1 (least important) to 10 (most important).	If YES, mark X	How important (1–10)	Formulate goal	Task to be completed
1. Housing (location, landlord, etc.)				
2. Employment (finding a job, better job, etc.)				
3. Legal problems or advice				
4. Health care or medical problems				
5. Medications or managing medications				
6. Self-help or support groups				
7. Child care (or other dependent care)				
8. Parenting and family issues				
9. Obtaining or keeping benefits or insurance (disability, Medicaid, SSI, VA, etc.)				
10. Financial assistance (debt, budgeting, food stamps, welfare, etc.)				
11. Work or employment training				
12. School, education, GED, etc.				
13. Personal or family safety				
14. Mental health or psychological problems				
15. How I spend my free time				
16. Advocacy with another system				
17. Utilities (telephone, heat, water, etc.)				
18. Food				
19. Clothing and household needs				
20. Transportation				
Are there other areas (not listed) in which you need assistance? Please write these below.				
21.				
22.				
23.				

FIGURE 15.1. Services request form. Adapted from Miller, Forcehimes, and Zweben, (2011). Copyright 2011 by The Guilford Press. Adapted by permission.

items, formulate goals related to each of the items, and develop tasks that need to be accomplished to achieve those goals.

Giving Feedback

Reviewing the findings on the service request form will help raise the client's awareness and motivation to address his or her case management needs. Start by reviewing the overall purpose of the service request form. Review with the client his or her responses to specific items. As a check on the accuracy of the information, ask the client whether this feedback fits with his or her own views about his or her case management needs. This will help determine whether the client is committed to following through on the case management plans. With clients who seem reluctant to carry out their plans, it can help to explore how the referral sources (e.g., obtaining housing assistance) might lead to improvements in the substance use problems. To illustrate:

> CASE MANAGER: You seem uncertain about seeking housing assistance even though you mention it as a high priority in the report.
>
> DAVID: Yeah, I'm not sure that I want to live in a new neighborhood since all my friends are here.
>
> CASE MANAGER: So, one of the things you like about your current neighborhood is that you don't feel isolated. Is there a downside?
>
> DAVID: It's been hard for me to stay away from drugs while living in my old neighborhood. The place is infested with dealers and all my friends are users.
>
> CASE MANAGER: How might the move help?
>
> DAVID: I won't have the same temptations or pressures and might even make new friends who do not use.

In the feedback session, the case management helps David weigh the advantages and disadvantages of obtaining housing assistance with the goal of shifting the balance in favor of locating new housing.

Formulating Goals

Begin by summarizing what you have learned thus far from the assessment process. Summaries should include a statement on (1) how the requested service is connected to the drinking or drug use problems, (2) how the requested service could help to achieve overarching treatment goals, and (3) how certain issues (e.g., marital conflict stress) might become obstacles that could interfere with fulfilling these goals. You can conclude by reminding the clients about taking responsibility for addressing the issues, affirming them for their willingness to do so, and expressing optimism for change. An example is provided below:

> CASE MANAGER: David, you checked the item on finding employment as the highest priority. Tell me a bit more about that. How would changing your employment help you to stay sober?
>
> DAVID: I've always worked as a bartender. In fact, our apartment was right over the bar. I just had to go downstairs to get to work. It's hard to resist the urges, even though I wanted to cut down. I was surrounded by booze. I couldn't stop, especially when I wasn't feeling so good.
>
> CASE MANAGER: It's a real problem to stay sober when you tend bar all day. I'm impressed that you're ready to give up something that has provided you with regular income. But clearly this is something you want, so perhaps we can talk about how you might go about making this change.

Before ending the discussion on goals, consider asking the scaling question. "On a scale of 1–10, how important is it to _____ to resolve drinking and drug use problems?" This helps to establish priorities with respect to case management goals and moves you to the next issue, namely, determining the necessary steps or tasks to achieve those goals.

Negotiating Tasks

Once a goal has been agreed upon, you need to consider steps that need to be taken to achieve the goal. Think about whether the proposed tasks are compatible with the individual's preferences, capacities, and education/training to attain the goal. If not, consider turning to another task, one that is more acceptable to the client. Also, you need to consider whether there are resources available in the community to fulfill the clients' needs.

The excerpt below illustrates how the case manager interacts with David about pursuing appropriate tasks:

> DAVID: I really don't want to find work again as a bartender. I always end up drinking again. But I don't know what else to do. This has been the only job I have had in the past 15 years. I guess I should start looking for another job but I have no idea what I really want to do.
>
> CASE MANAGER: Perhaps we can explore this further. Let's look at the options. You could continue with your present job, but based upon what you have already said, it has not worked out. Another

possibility is to meet with a job counselor. Is this something you might consider?

DAVID: I don't know. Haven't thought much about it. What does that mean?

CASE MANAGER: The job counselor will explore your interests, discuss the practicalities involved, and refer you to a particular position if you were interested. There is no guarantee that you would find employment immediately but it could be a beginning step. That is the positive aspect. Is there a downside for you?

DAVID: I would have to depend on my wife's income until I find a job. But she'd probably be okay with that if it helped me to stop drinking.

CASE MANAGER: So maybe you want to think more about this before making a decision. If you do decide to pursue job counseling, then I could provide you with a resource and you could call the person yourself for an appointment. Or you could make an appointment with the counselor right now in my office. However, I can't decide for you. You should decide what will work for you.

Once you have arrived at a consensus about tasks, make sure to talk about indicators of success, such as actually attending an appointment with a job counselor. It may help to quantify these steps by assigning a specific number to a particular activity—for example, calling at least five potential employers per week. These incremental accomplishments will help to build clients' self-esteem and confidence.

Addressing Barriers

Not all clients can readily pursue case management objectives. Some may be too overwhelmed with everyday hardships related to financial, employment, and family matters to undertake relevant tasks. Others may be immobilized by their emotional or mental health conditions. Some clients may not have adequate social support. Rather than view these individuals merely as "resistant" clients, you need to obtain a good understanding of the circumstances and conditions that are interfering with developing a case management plan.

As a first step, initiate a simple conversation about practical barriers. Ask clients directly about various factors that are interfering with their proposed plans. You might learn that just providing transportation or arranging for child care might be sufficient to enable the individual to undertake relevant tasks, whereas other people may need help in managing psychiatric symptoms before pursuing some tasks.

Another task is to determine whether there are interactional or communication difficulties between you and the client that is interfering with carrying out the proposed plans. Clients might not be willing/ready to state openly that they disagree with the plans if they feel insecure in their relationship with you. They may be reluctant to discuss their differences if they feel you would be disappointed in them. They may "act out" these feelings by canceling or not showing up for appointments.

In such cases, it helps to take a nonjudgmental stance. Here it is important to communicate that you are "ready/willing" to hear the client express his or her disagreement with you. This is accomplished by offering a reflective statement about these differences, normalizing the disparities, and providing a summary of the issues that are interfering with the case management process.

The scenario below shows how discrepancies between the case manager and the client can be resolved:

CASE MANAGER: You checked off a number of areas in which you requested help. One of the areas you marked is "parenting issues." In the column on tasks, you indicated that you would be calling the child guidance clinic last week. We both agreed that contacting the agency was a good idea. Yet the task has not been completed. Can you tell me more about it?

CLIENT: I was too busy with other matters.

CASE MANAGER: Aside from your involvement with your everyday activities, has anything happened that caused you to think otherwise?

CLIENT: I guess I decided that going to the clinic would not help. My kids are not that bad. Besides I don't like talking about my problems with another stranger. It is enough that I talk to you.

CASE MANAGER: So, you are not thinking the same way as the last time we talked. Right now, contacting the child guidance clinic is not really what you would like to do about the "parenting issues." That's okay. People have second thoughts or change their mind outside the sessions. Can you tell me what happened to change your mind?

CLIENT: My husband freaked out when I told him. He said that it is enough that I see you. Doesn't want me to talk to other strangers about our family problems. He thinks you are making matters worse by digging up other problems.

CASE MANAGER: It sounds like you had a change of heart after your husband found out about it.

CLIENT: Yeah, I guess that's true. If it causes more friction at home, I would rather not pursue it.

CASE MANAGER: You seem to have a dilemma here. You don't want to make matters worse at home and at the same time, you want to get help with the children since the stress with the children is making you want to drink again. What are your options here?

CLIENT: Well, it would help if he realized that if he wants me to stay sober, he needs to let me get help with the children. His arguing with me about it just makes it worse. I tried telling him this but he wouldn't listen. Perhaps, my husband would listen if <u>you</u> told him.

CASE MANAGER: Would you be willing to invite him to one of our sessions?

CLIENT: I could try but I'm not sure how he would respond.

CASE MANAGER: If you are clear about wanting me to talk with both of you, we can talk further about how you might approach your husband to enable him to attend the sessions.

In this session, the case manager provides the client with an opportunity for problem solving by asking about what prevented her from completing the task, eliciting potential solutions, and examining issues that might result in pursuing a certain plan. Personal choice is emphasized throughout the session.

Clients may not be ready to take certain actions if it might cause other problems. For instance, leaving a stressful job might create or exacerbate financial and marital difficulties, even though it might initially benefit the drinking or drug use problems. It might place the client in the difficult situation of having to apply for financial assistance to support the family. In such cases, it might be useful to help the client create a "decisional balance" form (Miller & Rollnick, 2002). Ask the client to write down the pros and cons of seeking a specific service. Have the client weigh the "good things" and the "not so good things" about carrying out a particular task such as finding a new job. This is a useful approach in ascertaining whether the individual's case management plan is consistent with his or her interests and expectations. In carrying out this activity, the person may decide that keeping the old job is not worth it if it leads to a recurrence of drug use and related problems.

Clients who feel overwhelmed by a task (as described below) sometimes benefit from developing small, incremental steps with a predefined timeline. In this context, the task is presented as a pilot study or interim approach. In this way, the proposed plan is less threatening and more manageable and success is more immediate. At the same time, you are communicating an understanding and acceptance of the client's tentativeness or ambivalence concerning the proposed plan, which in turn helps facilitate a working alliance. The vignette below highlights this process.

> CLIENT: I just can't get the energy to go to the AA meetings you talked about. I have so many other things going on. I need to meet with my probation officer, apply for food stamps, and take care of the kids while my wife is working. I know that you said attending self-helps group might be helpful, but since I returned home from jail, I just can't find the time.
>
> CASE MANAGER: You're dealing with a lot of things. It's been difficult to tackle all these things at once. It might be that you're feeling the need to postpone that task at this time. How can I help?
>
> CLIENT: I need some advice about what to do.
>
> CASE MANAGER: Well, there might be something that you could do to alleviate some of the demands in order to attend AA meetings—although I am not sure you are ready to do it. You could find out where and when AA meetings are being held. You could also talk with your parole officer about rearranging your appointments so that you could attend AA. You could ask family members if they could help by babysitting for you while you attend AA meetings. But again, you're the one who has to make the choice. Of all the things I just mentioned, which ones seem to be most doable for you?
>
> CLIENT: All of them. At the very least, I could check the days and times of AA meetings and see if my parole office would be willing to rearrange our meeting days and times. I think I need to get to AA if I want to stay sober.
>
> CASE MANAGER: Sounds like you have a plan. Remember this is something that you need to decide for yourself.

If the client continues to resist case management plans, it may be worthwhile to shift to another goal that is more amenable to the client. The choice of the goal should balance the needs of the client with what he or she feels capable of doing at the present time. You can ask the client what other goals on the list he or she might be willing to pursue. Another approach is to postpone the discussion of goals and tasks altogether. You could mention that at this juncture, case management planning might be counterproductive. In this context, it may be worthwhile to use the time primarily for rapport building such as asking open-ended questions, affirming, listening reflectively, expressing empathy, and eliciting change talk (see Miller &

Rollnick, 2002, for a full discussion of these rapport-building strategies). Such an approach is regularly employed in MI when a client is "not ready" to carry out an agenda and there is need to build commitment for change (Miller & Rollnick, 2002). Frequently, delaying aversive decision making is met with a sigh of relief on the part of the client, which eventually leads to an improved optimism about change.

Conducting Follow-Up

A final aspect of case management is routine follow-up. This may include monitoring and evaluating progress, modifying plans if the goals are no longer viable, and affirming the client for any progress. Follow-up helps to maintain and extend the benefits derived from the earlier course of treatment.

How Is Case Management Structured in Addiction Treatment Settings?

As mentioned earlier, individuals with substance use disorders often require a range of interventions to deal with concomitant matters. The chances of improvement are greater if different aspects of the problems can be addressed at the same time. Thus, clients may need to be involved in different kinds of settings to fulfill their resource needs. However, it can be difficult to coordinate care between these different settings, particularly if providers differ in their thinking on how best to serve individuals with addiction problems.

Addictions treatment providers hold a remarkable range of views about the etiology and resolution of substance abuse. For instance, some providers view addiction from a public health perspective where substance use problems are seen as a chronic, cyclical, and variable phenomenon often requiring clients to undergo a series of "ups and downs" before intervention can have a lasting effect. Other providers may view addiction from a more traditional perspective where clients are expected to achieve and sustain abstinence following an acute course of addiction treatment. In this model, any deviation from abstinence is seen as a treatment failure. Within this understanding, the main way to improve motivation is to allow clients to experience the negative consequences of substance use (i.e., "hitting bottom"). Any interference with this process is considered to be "enabling" clients. Programs that adhere to this conventional model might remove clients from stable living situations, take away custody of their children, or eliminate financial benefits after finding out that a "slip" has occurred. In such settings, a client may withdraw from a program precipitously after a single drinking or drug use episode rather than reveal that he or she has been drinking or seeking additional help.

The case manager can play a pivotal role in the aforementioned situations by educating providers on the natural course of relapse and recovery in addictive behaviors. He or she can inform providers that having slips or setbacks is natural and can be expected over the course of the recovery period. For most people in recovery, relapse is the rule rather than the exception. The case manager can reframe such events as learning opportunities to help improve clients' coping skills to prevent similar episodes from occurring in the future.

In contacts with these programs, the case manager provides a status report on the client's progress to ensure that staff concerns are being addressed. Efforts are coordinated between the settings by openly discussing relapse precipitants. This allows clients an opportunity to turn to providers in the different settings for assistance and support if setbacks do occur, which in turn may prevent such occurrences from becoming a full-blown relapse event.

Incorporating Case Management in an Integrated Model of Care

To increase the effectiveness of case management, we need to consider how case management can be incorporated into an integrated model of care. This model recognizes that substance use disorders are chronic problems that often require different aspects of the problem to be addressed concurrently over an extended period of time (Saitz, Larson, LaBelle, Richardson, & Samet, 2008; McKay, 2005). Integrated models have been effective in identifying early warning signs associated with relapse, improving access to relevant resources, supporting involvement and retention in treatment, and consequently can become a salient factor in the recovery process (Miller et al., 2011). To develop an integrated model, it is essential to link together various services that address different aspects of the substance use problem.

The case manager is essential in this process, because he or she functions as a liaison between the settings. He or she is involved in exchanging relevant information and resolving misunderstandings among different providers. The case manager ensures continuity of services by monitoring the care of clients from detoxification through intensive outpatient services. He or she is responsible for conducting a comprehensive assessment, facilitating client participation and retention in treatment, and enabling various providers to work collaboratively to resolve problems when they arise.

Embedding the Case Manager in an Interdisciplinary Team

Another challenge in an integrated care system is whether or not to incorporate case management within a treatment facility as part of a multidisciplinary team or employ case management as a "carve-out" program to link clients with external resources (Vanderplasschen et al., 2004). The major difficulty with the carve-out model is that professionals are located in different places, which places greater demands on the case manager for coordination (and communication), often leading to fragmented or disjointed services. For example, providing medications to treat psychiatric symptoms and alcohol problems can become problematic if the prescribing physicians are located in different settings. Administrating certain psychiatric medications in one setting may exclude a person from receiving an effective alcohol medication from a physician in another setting.

Professionals have argued that a single multidisciplinary team is more beneficial than developing a separate entity. In the interdisciplinary approach, the practitioner can have a dual role of treating clinician and case manager. He or she ensures a continuity of care by monitoring the client from detoxification to aftercare. He or she is responsible for conducting a comprehensive assessment, facilitating client participation and retention in treatment, and resolving differences between staff so that they can work more effectively to stabilize the client's situation when problems arise during the course of treatment.

Costs of Integrated Care

A major obstacle to integration is the cost. Reimbursement codes do not provide payment for the coordination of services upon discharge from specialty facilities. Under managed care, funding is most often limited to "threshold visits" for medical or behavioral interventions (Rose, Zweben, Ockert, & Baier, 2011). In addition, the employment of additional staff for the planning of services may be too costly if reimbursement is not available. On a positive note, one state (New York) is seeking to eliminate so-called threshold visits for outpatient services by providing reimbursement for each service offered during client visits. This fosters the use of case management services for planning and integration of services during treatment, which in turn helps clients to adjust to the high-risk period that follows treatment discharge (Rose et al., 2011).

Education and Training of Case Managers

Evidence suggests that the use of core case management functions such as assessment, goal formation and planning, education about community resources, proactive monitoring, and referral compliance are optimal for producing change (Alexander et al., 2007; Morgenstern et al., 2008; Noel, 2006; Vanderplasschen et al., 2004). With respect to the referral adherence, MI can again be helpful in assisting clients with gaining access and becoming involved in such services. MI is effective in increasing awareness of the seriousness of problems, enhancing confidence about changing problems, and establishing a working alliance. All of these factors increase the probability of a positive outcome (Miller et al., 2011).

In addition, medication has been increasingly viewed as an important adjunct to treatment (Weiss, 2004). Consequently, it is important for case managers to have a working knowledge of genetic and biological elements of addictions (see Chung, Ross, Wakhlu, Chapter 11, and Carroll & Kiluk, Chapter 12, this volume). Such knowledge can be used to educate clients and their families about the importance of medications in the treatment of addictive behaviors. For example, helping alcohol-dependent clients find appropriate pharmacotherapies requires extra effort since the majority of specialty programs do not routinely employ alcohol medications (Abraham, 2010).

Case managers would also benefit from understanding how to match individuals to suitable treatments. Of interest here is determining what kinds of clients would benefit most from conventional 12-step programs, cognitive-behavioral treatment, medication, motivational enhancement therapy, or a combination of these treatments. This requires being familiar with standard assessment tools and effective behavioral therapies and pharmacotherapies to learn how to "match" treatments to clients' capabilities and treatment needs.

What Needs to Be Known to Improve Case Management?

Given the chronic nature of many addiction problems, case management is a useful service for changing addictive behaviors. Yet there are many questions about case management services that remain and, if adequately addressed, could help to improve the delivery of such services. A number of important questions are listed below.

1. Of interest is the identification of active ingredients of the case management approach. What are the components of case management that are most important for the success of the process? Which of the features of case management are most salient for improving outcomes—goal setting, feedback, proactive monitoring, advocacy, service coordination, and referral compliance techniques (e.g., rapport building, strengthening self-efficacy, evoking change talk, and other MI strategies)?

2. How do you apply case management elements across different client populations, such as clients with co-occurring disorders, individuals just released from prison, and those with special needs such as women seeking help in public assistance programs?

3. How do you modify the case management approach for use in different kinds of settings, including specialty and nonspecialty settings, primary care clinics, and social service contexts?
4. Should case management services be incorporated into the roles/functions of addiction counselors or should it be assigned to special providers? What are the benefits and costs of combining the roles of case manager and addiction counselor?
5. What kind of training is needed to improve the effectiveness of case managers in different kinds of settings?

Answers to the above questions would help to tailor case management to the circumstances of client populations seen in diverse settings, and thereby improve the overall delivery of substance use services.

Conclusion

Case management is one way of linking substance abuse clients to supplementary services in order to support and maintain the benefits of addiction treatment. Effective implementation of the core components and, in particular, referral enhancement techniques can improve the effectiveness of the referral process. Case managers require training and education to adequately prepare them to deliver the effective components of case management. Much work still remains on improving the case management process so that different groups can benefit from the approach. Future investigations should focus on better integrating case management into an integrated care model of services in order to provide high-quality care for people with addiction problems.

References

Abraham, A. (2010). *Implementation of alcohol pharmacotherapies in specialty AUD treatment settings. How are programs using medication in routine treatment practice?* Paper presented at the 33rd Annual Scientific Meeting of the Research Society on Alcoholism, San Antonio, TX.

Alexander, J. A., Pollack, H., Nahra, T., Wells, R., & Lemak, C. H. (2007). Case management and client access to health and social services in outpatient substance abuse treatment. *Journal of Behavioral Health Services Research, 34,* 221–236.

Conrad, K. J., Hultman, C. I., Pope, A. R., Lyons, J. S., Baxter, W. C., Daghestani, A., et al. (1998). Case managed residential care for homeless addicted veterans: Results of true experiment. *Medical Care, 36*(1), 40–53.

Cox, G. B., Walker, D., Freng, S. A., Short, B. A., Meijer, L., & Gilchrist, L.

(1998). Outcome of a controlled trial of the effectiveness of intensive case management for chronic public inebriates. *Journal of Studies on Alcohol, 59*, 523–532.

Kirby, M. W., Braucht, G. N., Brown, E., Krane, S., McCann, M., & VanDeMark, N. (1999). Dyadic case management as a strategy for prevention of homelessness among chronically debilitated men and women with alcohol and drug dependence. *Alcoholism Treatment Quarterly, 17*(1–2), 53–72.

McKay, J. R. (2005). Is there a case for extended interventions for alcohol problem and drug use disorders? *Addiction, 100*, 1594–1610.

McLellan, A. T., Hagan, T. A., Levine, M., Meyers, K., Gould, F., Bencivengo, M., et al. (1999). Does clinical case management improve outpatient addiction treatment? *Drug and Alcohol Dependence, 55*, 91–103.

Miller, W. R. (Ed.). (2004). *Combined behavioral intervention manual: A clinical research guide for therapists treating people with alcohol abuse and dependence* (Vol. 1). Bethesda, MD: National Institute on Alcohol Abuse and Alcoholism.

Miller, W. R., & Rollnick, S. (2002). *Motivational interviewing: Preparing people for change* (2nd ed.). New York: Guilford Press.

Miller, W. R., Forcehimes, A., & Zweben, A. (2011). *Treating addiction: A guide for professionals.* New York: Guilford Press

Morgenstern, J., Blanchard, K. A., Kahler, C., Barbosa, K. M., McCrady, B. S., & McVeigh, K. H. (2008). Testing mechanisms of action for intensive case management. *Addiction, 103*(3), 469–477.

Najavits, L. M., Weiss, R. D., Shaw, S. R., & Muenz, L. (1998). Seeking safety: Outcome of a new cognitive-behavioral psychotherapy for women with posttraumatic stress disorder and substance dependence. *Journal of Traumatic Stress, 11*, 437–456.

Noel, P. E. (2006). The impact of therapeutic case management on participation in adolescent substance abuse treatment. *American Journal of Drug and Alcohol Abuse, 32*(3), 311–327.

Rapp, R. C. (2002). Strengths-based case management: Enhancing treatment for persons with substance abuse problems. In D. Saleebey (Ed.), *The strengths perspective in social work practice* (3rd ed., pp. 124–142). New York: Allyn & Bacon.

Rose, S., Zweben, A., Ockert, D., & Baier, A. (2011). Interface between substance abuse treatment and other health and social systems. Manuscript in preparation.

Rothman, J. (2003). An overview of case management. In A. R. Roberts & G. J. Greene (Eds.), *Social worker's desk reference* (pp. 467–480). Washington, DC: National Association of Social Workers.

Saitz, R., Larson, M. J., LaBelle, R. N., Richardson, J., & Samet, J. H. (2008). The case for chronic disease management for addiction. *Journal of Addiction Medicine, 2*(2), 55–65.

Siegal, H. A., Li, L., & Rapp, R. C. (2002). Case management as a therapeutic enhancement impact on post-treatment criminality. *Journal of Addictive Diseases, 21*, 37–46.

Siegal, H. A., Rapp, R. C., Kelliher, C. W., Fisher, J. H., Wagner, J. H., & Cole, P. A. (1995). The strengths perspective of case management: A promising inpatient substance abuse treatment enhancement. *Journal of Psychoactive Drugs, 27,* 67–72.

Siegal, H. A., Rapp, R. C., Li, L., Saha, P., & Kirk, K. D. (1997). The role of case management in retaining clients in substance abuse treatment: An exploratory analysis. *Journal of Drug Issues, 27,* 821–831.

Substance Abuse and Mental Health Services Administration. (1998). *Comprehensive case management for substance abuse treatment* (Center for Substance Abuse Treatment: Treatment Improvement Protocol [TIP] Series, Vol. 27). Rockville, MD: U.S. Department of Health and Human Services.

Sullivan, W. P. (2003). Case management with substance-abusing clients. In A. R. Roberts & G. J. Greene (Eds.), *Social worker's desk reference* (pp. 492–496). Washington, DC: National Association of Social Workers.

Test, M. A. (2003). Guidelines for assertive community treatment teams. In A. R. Roberts & G. J. Greene (Eds.), *Social worker's desk reference* (pp. 511–513). Washington, DC: National Association of Social Workers.

Vanderplasschen, H. M., Rapp, R., Broekaert, E., & Fridell, M. (2009). Case management for persons with substance use disorders (Review). *The Cochrane Collaboration, 4,* 1–37.

Vanderplasschen, W., Rapp, R. C., Wolf, J. R., & Broekaert, E. (2004). The development and implementation of case management for substance use disorders in North America and Europe. *Psychiatric Services, 55*(8), 913–922.

Walsh, J. (2003). Clinical case management. In A. R. Roberts & G. J. Greene (Eds.), *Social worker's desk reference* (pp. 472–476). Washington, DC: National Association of Social Workers.

Weiss, R. D. (2004). Adherence to pharmacology in patients with alcohol and opioid dependence. *Addiction, 99,* 1382–1392.

Zweben, A., Pettinati, H., Weiss, R., Youngblood, M., Cox, C., Mattson, M., et al. (2008). Relationship between patient adherence and treatment outcomes: The COMBINE study. *Alcoholism: Clinical and Experimental Research, 32,* 1661–1669.

Zweben, A., Rose, S. J., Stout, R. L., & Zywiak, W. H. (2003). Case monitoring and motivational style brief interventions. In R. K. Hester & W. R. Miller (Eds.), *Handbook of alcoholism treatment approaches: Effective alternatives* (3rd ed., pp. 113–130). Boston: Allyn & Bacon.

Zweben, A., & Zuckoff, A. (2002). Motivational interviewing and treatment adherence. In W. R. Miller & S. Rollnick, *Motivational interviewing: Preparing people for change* (2nd ed., pp. 299–319). New York: Guilford Press.

Index

Page numbers followed by f or t indicate figures or tables.

422